For over thirty years I have recommended the Gerson Therapy to persons fighting cancer, and have never once had cause to regret it. This new Gerson manual is the best ever written on the subject: comprehensive, up to date, exhaustively referenced, and very readable. It explains the therapy as it instructs on exactly how to do it yourself. Most importantly, *Healing the Gerson Way* is about healing chronic diseases other than cancer, including many that are supposedly "hopeless." Don't let anyone tell you otherwise: There is much more than hope for "terminal" patients: there is Gerson. This is a compendium of knowledge, based on decades of success, that you will want to share with everyone you know.

—*Andrew W. Saul, Assistant Editor,*
Journal of Orthomolecular Medicine

In *Healing the Gerson Way,* the chapter describing toxicity and deficiency accurately describes our collective state of health—and the rest of the book gives tools to effectively overcome such problems. Important additions to the Gerson Therapy are found in "The Therapy Moves On" and include grapefruit seed extract, Tahebo herbal extract, selenium, glucose-potassium-insulin treatment, and chromium picolinate. These additions address the worsening chronic diseases of our time including cancer, Candidiasis, viral infection, and diabetes.

—*Carolyn Dean, MD*
author of The Magnesium Miracle

Healing the
Gerson Way

*Defeating Cancer
and Other Chronic Diseases*

Healing the Gerson Way

Defeating Cancer and Other Chronic Diseases

Charlotte Gerson
with Beata Bishop

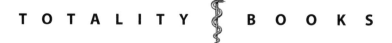

TOTALITY BOOKS

Totality Books
316 Mid Valley Center #230
Carmel, California 93923

ISBN: 0-9760186-0-8
ISBN-13: 978-0-9760186-0-5

Printed in the United States of America.

The marks Gerson, Gerson Therapy and Gerson Institute are trademarks and/or service marks owned and proprietary to the Gerson Institute, San Diego, California, and are covered by appropriate domestic and/or foreign registration and/or protective laws. All other trademarks and/or service marks referred to herein are owned by and/or proprietary to their respective owners.

Front cover image of Charlotte Gerson provided by Bob Stone, Carmel, California.

Additional cover photographs provided by Thomas A. Ekkens, Pacifica, California (www.backspaceink.com/taegallery).

Cover and interior design, editing and production by Joanne Shwed, Backspace Ink, Pacifica, California (www.backspaceink.com).

Contents

List of Tables

Acknowledgements

This book is first of all a tribute to my father, Dr. Max Gerson. He was not just a doctor but a true healer. He deeply understood the basic organization of the incredibly complex and wonderful organism that is the human body, and through his genius he learned how to restore and heal those who were failing. He was not only a healer, but he hoped to bring healing to all the world, to end disease and suffering.

Built on his vast knowledge and experience, we have often been able to bring complete healing, a return of life and health, to those who were once pronounced "incurable" and who faced death or long years of suffering. In this volume, we aim to bring the details of his approach to those who will use it to return to happy and productive lives.

In the past 30 years, the world has changed, conditions have worsened and the healing knowledge has had to be adapted to these changes. It has taken many people of knowledge, experience and vision to achieve these adaptations. It took many more people to help us to record the infinite details of the Gerson treatment.

It is virtually impossible to thank by name all who were involved in the production of this book. They are the Gerson-trained physicians, the nurses and the helpers who produce the hourly juices—and of vital importance, the dedicated caregivers who carry out the daily routine needed for healing. The patients, too, are our heroes, disciplined and steady in their adherence to the therapy. It took those friends, acquaintances and family members who encouraged patients to stay on course and not to give up just because their original doctor gave them a death warrant.

It took my son, Howard Straus, to contribute to this book with uncounted hours of research for references, ideas and suggestions, to put the information on the World Wide Web and to lecture in the U.S., Canada and Asia; it took my daughter, Margaret Straus, whose lectures, seminars and articles introduced the Gerson Therapy into England and Italy, and whose help and encouragement of patients inspired one of our most famous successes, my dear friend, Beata Bishop. First as a dedicated patient, rewarded with a dramatic recovery, Beata gave unending time and energy toward writing and editing this book and carrying on the Gerson work in the United Kingdom where, together with Janet Pottinger, she founded the British Gerson Support Group. We are also very grateful to this group for allowing us to use most of the recipes from their publication, *Gerson Gourmet*. Other contributors to the recipe chapter include Yvonne Nienstadt, Susan DeSimone and several recovered Gerson patients. It took many, many more people, too numerous to name individually, to help, encourage and support us, psychologically and often financially, to bring this project to fruition. To all of those dedicated supporters continuing Dr. Gerson's healing work—I devote this book with the deepest gratitude.

—Charlotte Gerson
Bonita, California
May 2007

An Important Message
to the Reader

The book you are holding in your hand can be the most precious tool to maintain and improve your health if you are fit and well or to regain it if you are ill. You will find all the guidance you need for either purpose, but there are a few points that need emphasizing should you choose the Gerson Therapy for healing yourself. In your own interest, please take them to heart and bear them in mind.

The Gerson Therapy is a finely tuned precision instrument, whose every component plays an important role and affects all other parts. It must be practiced in its entirety without omitting a single detail. To do otherwise not only undermines the healing power of the therapy but can also cause further health problems.

Do not embark on the Gerson Therapy on an experimental basis, thinking that you can always drop it if you find the program too demanding. The program *is* demanding, intensive and extended—a far cry from the pill-popping instant ways of conventional medicine. Instead of suppressing symptoms, it can truly heal and offer a healthy future. *The choice is yours.* Study this book and find out exactly what it means to undertake the therapy. Please, in your own best interest, only embark on it if you are committed to staying on it until you are fully and truly healed. All over the world, there are people who did just that, and who returned from life-threatening diseases to radiant health and a life more abundant. You are more than welcome to join them.

As you read this book, you will find many references to Dr. Max Gerson's epoch-making work, *A Cancer Therapy—Results of Fifty Cases,*[1] which first appeared in 1958, one year before the author's death. It is now in its sixth edition and has been translated into four languages. In the years since its inception, medical technology and research have made enormous progress, offering possibilities that in Dr. Gerson's day would have been hard to imagine. For that reason, today's reader may find parts of *A Cancer Therapy* dated or no longer relevant. However, what has remained topical and more relevant than ever is Dr. Gerson's startlingly original approach to the causation, treatment and healing of cancer, which is totally different from current oncological practice. The organism's breakdown of law and order on the cellular level, resulting in cancer, is the same today as it has ever been, and the Gerson Therapy's ability to deal with that breakdown also remains unchanged.

It should also be remembered that, besides being a practicing physician, Dr. Gerson was also an eminent scientist, closely involved in the debate in the U.S. Congress on policies for cancer treatment, and was acknowledged for his brilliance by Nobel Laureate Dr. Albert Schweitzer. His papers met all the traditional requirements for evidence-based medicine; today's modern scientific approaches have begun to shed some light onto why and how his therapy worked.

REFERENCE

1. Gerson, M. *A Cancer Therapy: Results of Fifty Cases and The Cure of Advanced Cancer by Diet Therapy: A Summary of Thirty Years of Clinical Experimentation,* 6th ed. San Diego, CA: Gerson Institute, 1999.

Introduction

We live in critical times, experiencing an unprecedented attack on health: our own and that of the planet. The two are linked and cannot be separated. This is a crisis that we aren't able to blame on outside forces—we have brought it upon ourselves.

It is stating the obvious to say that over many centuries we have been mistreating the Earth, our only habitat, brutally exploiting it, as if it were a lifeless lump of valuable raw materials for us to utilize. Today, rather late in the day, we have come to realize that in fact our planet is a complex living organism of huge but finite self-regulating power—and that it can hit back in dramatic ways if human activities push it too far. Today it takes extraordinary blindness not to notice that this process has already begun.

All this affects us directly. By not respecting nature, we have become alienated from it, both globally and in our individual lives. Hi-tech brilliance, electronic marvels, space travel, unlimited computing power and all the comforts of the consumer society have made us forget the basics of human existence, namely that:

- All life on Earth depends on some 10 inches of fertile topsoil able to support plant life, which in turn sustains animal and human life. This precious substance is rapidly being lost worldwide through floods, erosion, intensive farming methods, deforestation and other destructive practices. If this destruction continues, no amount of high technology will be able to feed us.

- We are parts of nature, having evolved over millennia alongside other forms of life, so that our organisms can only thrive on natural nurture, clean air, pure water and a toxin-free environment.

Unfortunately, that is not how we live in the developed world. Despite high standards of living, good hygiene, the marvels of modern medicine and growing prosperity, the general health of the population is poor and is getting worse. Granted, people live longer, but extended lifespans are worthless if the old spend their extra years plagued by diseases ranging from crippling arthritis to Alzheimer's, poor mobility, poor digestion and worse, subsisting on masses of medication. At the other end of the age range, children are succumbing at ever-earlier ages to chronic degenerative diseases, which not so long ago only affected the middle-aged and elderly. Obesity, with its dire health consequences, is a worsening epidemic among all age groups. Considering the astronomical sums spent on medical research and health care, the general picture is dismal.

Ironically, in developing countries where the traditional way of life, including farming methods, has largely survived, and despite varying levels of poverty, people are generally healthier. They have not become divorced from their roots in nature—and only begin to sicken when they switch to our misguidedly envied Western lifestyle.

Clearly, we need to change our ways. "Let us return to Nature!" suggested the 18th century French philosopher Rousseau, and that is exactly what we need to do. We must find our way back to an unadulterated natural lifestyle and learn how to restore our health by dealing with the causes, not just the symptoms, of our problems.

The Gerson way of healing, which is the subject of this book, enables us to do that—whether we need to heal one of countless chronic degenerative diseases or to move from a state of nonspecific subhealth, with its many minor symptoms, to energetic fitness and well-being.

The basic principle of this program is totality (also known as holism). It means taking into account the entire organism and dealing with *all* its problems and weaknesses, not homing in on just one symptom or organ, as if it were independent from the rest of the body. It also means considering the setting and physical conditions of the individual's daily life, his or her occupation and lifestyle. This approach is very different from that of conventional allopathic medicine, which is characterized by increasing specialization, concentrating on the symptom, seeking a single cause for it and trying to suppress it with drugs.

It is often said that modern allopathic medicine is the only major science stuck in the pre-Einstein era. Indeed, it still operates in the spirit of Louis Pasteur, the 19th century French scientist and so-called "father of the germ theory." Pasteur maintained all his life that diseases were caused by germs (which he was the first to identify) and that cure was achieved by destroying the germs (bacteria). Unlike his contemporary and opponent, Antoine Béchamp, who claimed that what mattered was not the germ but the condition of the organism which it attacked, Pasteur stuck to his dogma until the very end. Only on his deathbed did he admit that "the germ is nothing, the terrain is everything."[1] Unfortunately, this late change of mind has remained largely unknown, leaving modern medicine in the trap of the germ theory, the neglect of the "terrain" and relentless specialization.

The Gerson program goes the opposite way. Its healing method is nonspecific, which explains why it is able to deal with a wide range of conditions: It aims to restore the "terrain" (i.e., the total organism), which then becomes able to heal itself. The body's amazing self-healing ability, fully utilized in this program, is sadly neglected and even ignored in allopathic medicine. Of course, nonselectivity (the opposite of specialization) is anathema to conventionally trained doctors. This was true for the young Dr. Max Gerson when he discovered that he could get rid of his frequent debilitating migraine attacks by adopting a low-fat, low-salt vegetarian diet. This began a process, which eventually made Dr. Gerson realize that his diet was curing the total organism, not a specific complaint, and that hence there was practically no limit to its healing power. The amazing nearly 80-year-long track record of the therapy proves that he was right.

Today, when the world is infinitely more toxic, and the Western diet vastly more harmful than in Dr. Gerson's lifetime, his therapy is still achieving extraordinary results, although the work of healing is harder and takes a longer time. However, it must be emphasized that *the Gerson way of healing is neither a universal panacea nor a miracle cure and may fail for a variety of reasons* (e.g., if the patient comes to it too late, after the full range of conventional treatments has failed to produce a remission; doesn't observe the rules; or has had an essential organ removed). Such cases aside, the Gerson program's success rate with advanced cancer and many other serious degenerative diseases far outstrips that of conventional treatments. The following chapters will explain in detail why and how it works.

REFERENCE

1. "The germ is nothing, terrain is everything," Claude Bernard (1817-1878). While Pasteur preserved his stance until the end of his life, he conceded on his deathbed that Claude Bernard had been correct. "Claude Bernard was right," conceded Pasteur. "The microbe is nothing, the terrain is everything." Louis Pasteur (1822-1895). Expounded by Louis Pasteur Valery-Radot, sentence pronounced on his deathbed (www.originalquinton.com/history.php).

PART I

Health and Healing in a Sick World

Knowledge is power. It helps us to find our way through unfamiliar territory, such as the Gerson path to healing and health. The first section of this book provides you with all you need to know about the background and strictly scientific theory of this method. "Theory" may sound dry; in this case, it is the opposite. It presents the dismal health problems of modern civilization from a startlingly original revolutionary angle. We must know what is wrong with our lives before we can put it right.

Please read the following chapters carefully. They are your key to the door that leads to the invigorating, healing practice based on the theory. All in all, what you learn will enable you to take responsibility for your health and well-being—and safeguard them rather than engage in damage control and repair work.

CHAPTER 1

The Story Begins

Great spirits have always encountered violent
opposition from mediocre minds.

— *Albert Einstein*

Some of the greatest scientific discoveries resulted from a sudden
insight or inspiration that came unexpectedly, like a bolt from the
blue. Others were made after long years of patient, painstaking effort.
The most fascinating achievements are the ones that grew out of a series
of apparent coincidences, leading to an astonishing outcome. The Gerson Therapy belongs to this last category. It came into being because
one exceptional man, the German-born physician Dr. Max Gerson, pos-
sessed the ability to ask the right questions at the right time and seek the
answers with the utmost scientific rigor. His story helps us to understand how the life-saving therapy that bears his name came into being.

As a small boy, Max Gerson showed some scientific curiosity. He
liked to play in the garden of his grandmother, who grew flowers as well
as fruits and vegetables for her table. On one occasion, when she
decided to try out some new artificial fertilizer, which was supposed to
produce bigger and better crops, Max watched with consternation that
the earthworms were leaving the beds treated with the new chemicals
and migrating to the beds treated with the old, time-honored natural
substances. Young Max concluded that there must have been something
harmful and disturbing in the new chemicals, which the earthworms

couldn't stand and which made them flee to the natural environment. He never forgot this early experience.

Upon graduating from high school, Max decided to become a physician and went on to study at the universities of Breslau, Wuerzburg, Berlin and Freiburg. Throughout his studies and for the rest of his life, he remained eternally curious, always playing with possibilities, wondering "What would happen if …?" As a young doctor, working as assistant to Professor Ottfried Foerster in Breslau, he ordered the finest rose bushes from Holland, planted them and changed their fertilizer, their food and—by installing light filters—even the amount of sunshine they received. With these methods, he succeeded in changing the colors of the roses.

This taught him that nutrients and light could change the metabolism of a living plant, but he had no idea how to apply this discovery to human beings, let alone to healing them. It took his own serious health problem—his recurring severe cluster migraines—to show him the way ahead.

The migraines were so devastating and recurred so frequently that he was desperate to do something about them. His teachers and professors, whom he had consulted, had been unable to suggest a treatment. They had said that he'd feel better when he got to be in his mid-50s, but the young doctor couldn't envisage life for the next 30 years with those migraines. They sometimes kept him in bed, in a darkened room, with violent pain and nausea, for two or three days a week! There had to be a better answer and he was determined to find it.

To start his search, he read everything apparently relevant that he could find. Nothing positive turned up. He visited a number of professors as a patient and found no help. By accident (if we believe in accidents), one day he came across a paper describing how a woman, suffering from migraines, was helped when she changed her diet. *Diet!* Nobody had taught him anything about diet nor had his teachers ever mentioned the possibility that any chronic disease was connected with diet. As always, he was willing to experiment, even using himself as a guinea pig. He abandoned his normal choice of food and tried out several different diets. It took him a while and a number of failures before he established that a salt-free vegetarian diet kept him free from the pain and nausea of migraines.

Then he started to use dietary treatment in his practice. When patients came to his Bielefeld office suffering from migraine, he told them frankly that, according to all the medical texts, there was no cure for this problem. He also told them that he had been suffering from migraine until a change of diet had brought him relief and suggested that the patients try the same method. When these patients returned to see him some three or four weeks later, they regularly reported that they were free from migraines—as long as they adhered to the strict dietary rules and didn't cheat.

This experience made Dr. Gerson refer to his method as the "Migraine Diet," the single treatment for a single complaint, as specified in conventional medicine, until something happened to change his view. One day, a migraine sufferer consulted Dr. Gerson and was urged to adopt the "Migraine Diet," which he did. When he returned a month or so later, he had something extraordinary to report. His migraines were gone, and the skin tuberculosis (TB) (lupus vulgaris) from which he had been suffering was also healing. Dr. Gerson was skeptical. "No, you couldn't have had lupus. It must have been something else. Lupus is incurable," he declared. The patient produced the results of laboratory tests, which proved that indeed there had been tubercle bacilli in the tissues of his lesions. Dr. Gerson was stunned. He couldn't see a connection between migraine and lupus, so why did both conditions heal?

This was another decisive moment in his life when he had to ask a question and find an answer. To start, he asked his patient whether he knew other lupus sufferers and, if so, would he send them to him for treatment, free of charge. Some came and were cured. Dr. Gerson had to accept that his "Migraine Diet" could also heal the reputedly incurable skin TB.

His remarkable results reached the ears of the famous lung TB specialist, Ferdinand Sauerbruch, of Munich, Germany. He put 450 of his "incurable" lupus patients on Dr. Gerson's diet, saying that if Gerson could stop the progress of the disease in a single patient, he would believe everything the young doctor claimed. The Gerson diet not only arrested the disease process, it actually cured 446 of those seriously ill patients. Sauerbruch's response was to publish "his" results in numerous scientific papers.[1]

Dr. Gerson was not satisfied. He reasoned that if skin TB responded positively to diet, wouldn't other forms of TB do so? What about the killer disease lung TB? What about kidney, bone, encephalitic and other forms of the disease? He started to treat such patients, too, with his diet—among them the wife of Dr. Albert Schweitzer—and found that they also recovered. More importantly, many of those patients had other problems along with their TB: high or low blood pressure, allergies, asthma, kidney disease and more. These diseases also disappeared with the "Migraine Diet"!

At this point, it became very clear to Gerson that he was no longer healing a disease with dietary changes; the patients' metabolism and immune system were responding, which meant that he was healing the whole body. This opened the door to curing all "incurable" chronic diseases. From that moment, his path led him in a totally different direction from that of orthodox medicine. His patients were now healed, not drugged.

The first big step toward healing cancer came in 1928 when a lady called him to her bedside. In Dr. Gerson's own words, "I asked her what was wrong, but she didn't want to tell me on the phone."[2] When he arrived at her home, the patient told him that she had an operation for cancer of the bile duct; now she was jaundiced, ran a high fever and needed help. Dr. Gerson told her that he didn't know how to treat cancer, but she insisted, quoting his success with TB cases. Then she asked him to look at the big book on her table, open at the chapter called "The Healing of Cancer." In this book on folk medicine, Dr. Gerson recalls, "There was something about Hippocrates who lived 425 years before Christ. … He had the idea that the patient has to be detoxified with a special soup and with some enemas."[3]

He told the patient once again that he was unable to treat her but, at her insistence, he agreed to try. He wrote down a treatment plan for her—essentially the same as his treatment for TB. As he records it, "I tried—and about six months later the patient was cured! She was up and about in the best condition. She sent me two other cancer cases. One had metastasized glands around the stomach—also cured! The third case was also cured! Three cases were tried and all three were cured!"[4]

Later, in Vienna, he tried again, treating six cases, but all six failed. He was shocked and discouraged, but "… once it was in my head and my hands and my heart, I could no longer separate myself from that problem."[5]

Some years later, Gerson settled in the U.S. In order to obtain his license to practice, he first had to pass a medical exam; then he was unable to find a hospital where he could treat patients. "I couldn't get the first three cases out of my mind. I kept thinking, 'It must be possible. It would be a crime not to do it.'"[6]

He studied all the medical literature and research material he could find, and discovered that there was a difference between chronically ill patients and those suffering from cancer. He later described this difference by specifying that "the chronic disease patient has a weak, damaged liver; the cancer patient has a toxic liver."[7] Gerson also found that the cancer patient could not completely digest and assimilate fats and oils. These undigested residues were picked up by the tumor tissue, which grew and thrived on them. After years of trial and error, amassing direct experience at the sickbed, he developed a remarkably effective treatment that worked—even for terminally ill patients.

Gerson's startlingly original ideas and new methods did not fit into the allopathic medical system. He wrote a number of articles on his work and on patient outcomes, and submitted them to several medical journals; all were refused with various excuses. Subsequently, patients who inquired about Gerson at the American Medical Association were told that his method was "secret," as "he refused to publish."[8]

The Board of Censors of the New York Medical Association wrote to Dr. Gerson five times, asking him to submit records proving his work.[9]

Five times he patiently assembled more of his records and, on occasion, even presented some of his recovered patients. His only request was that the board publish their findings; they never did.

Wanting to ensure the continuation of his work, Dr. Gerson was anxious to train other doctors and/or assistants in the practice of his therapy. On several occasions, young medical doctors, not yet established in their practice, would approach Gerson and ask to be accepted as assistants to learn the treatment. Always ready to pass on his experience to a keen young colleague, he accepted such offers.

The "assistanceship" never lasted more than four or five days. After that time, the young doctor would, in embarrassment, explain to Dr. Gerson that he had received serious threats should he continue to work with him, that he would be banned from hospital associations, that no other doctors would send him patients and that he would be unable to practice. Having a great deal of debt on his shoulders from his medical schooling, the young doctor could not afford to be forced into such a situation and, sadly, had to give up working with Dr. Gerson. (Similar situations occur these days, too, when a not-yet sufficiently established doctor wishes to visit the Gerson clinic in Mexico to study the therapy, and his superiors explain to him that such a move would jeopardize his career development. This explains why there are so few doctors trained in the Gerson protocol.)

Undeterred by all the obstacles, Dr. Gerson carried on with his work, perfecting his treatment as he went along. Since, despite all his efforts, he was prevented from publishing his work in medical journals, he eventually gathered his material and wrote it up in his last book, which is also his lasting medical testament.

A few years ago, we received some amazing information from a well-known health writer and publicist in New York. He was collecting material for his work and wanted to publish Dr. Gerson's testimony, given in 1946 before a congressional committee,[10] under the sponsorship of Senator Claude Pepper. The researcher traveled to Washington, D.C., to look for the report of the testimony in the Congressional Record, which, as an official U.S. government document, is not supposed to be altered or tampered with. He knew that the testimony took up several pages, including Dr. Gerson's answers to a number of questions about his work, and his presentation of five of his recovered patients, who had originally been sent home to die of terminal cancer. The researcher inspected the Congressional Record and found only an empty space under the date where the testimony should have appeared. Against all the rules, it had been removed without explanation.

Orthodox "scientific" medicine routinely rejects studies based on a small number (less than 250) of subjects, irrespective of their merits. Here is a relevant quote, not unconnected with Dr. Gerson's story:

"The small number of subjects used exposed the study to the ridicule that medical science has been using for over a hundred years to flay experiments that do not fit its bias. 'What were the controls?' 'Where are the statistics?' 'How do you know the patients didn't get better because of something else?' 'Statistically the mathematics don't hold up.' 'Did they really control all the variables?' 'How do you know that drugs aren't just as good?' 'Pacemakers work just as well.' 'What we have already is good enough if used right.'"[11]

REFERENCES

1. Ferdinand Sauerbruch, *A Surgeon's Life* (London: Andre Deutsch, 1953); *see also* Howard Straus, *Dr. Max Gerson: Healing the Hopeless* (Carmel, CA: Totality Books, 2002).
2. M. Gerson, *A Cancer Therapy: Results of Fifty Cases and The Cure of Advanced Cancer by Diet Therapy: A Summary of Thirty Years of Clinical Experimentation,* 6th ed. (San Diego, CA: Gerson Institute, 1999), Appendix II.
3. Ibid.
4. Ibid.
5. Ibid., pp. 403-405.
6. Margaret Gerson, *Dr. Max Gerson: A Life Without Fear* (New York: unpublished manuscript, 1968-1969).
7. Note 2 (Gerson), supra..
8. Patricia Spain Ward, "History of the Gerson Therapy," under contract to the U.S. Congressional Office of Technology Assessment: "Compared to

Miley's testimony, Gerson's was innocent, concentrating on the histories of the patients he brought with him and on the likely mechanisms whereby his diet caused tumor regression and healing. Only under pressure from Senator Pepper did Gerson state that about 30% of those he treated showed a favorable response (U.S. Congress, 1946, 115). Nonetheless, *JAMA* devoted two pages to undermining Gerson's integrity (*JAMA*, 1946). Showing no restraint where Gerson was concerned, Fishbein, contrary to fact, alleged that successes with the Gerson-Sauerbruch-Hermannsdorfer diet 'were apparently not susceptible of duplication by most other observers.' He also falsely claimed that Gerson had several times refused to supply the AMA with details of the diet. (Fishbein said he could provide them in this editorial only because 'there has come to hand through a prospective patient' of Gerson a diet schedule for his treatment.) Fishbein emphasized, without comment, Gerson's caution about the use of other medications, especially anesthetics, because they produced dangerously strong reactions in the heightened allergic state of his most responsive patients." The statement was in Morris Fishbein's editorial, cited by Ward above. "Gerson's Cancer Treatment," editorial, *Journal of American Medical Association* 132 (Nov. 16, 1946): 645-646.

9. S. J. Haught, *Censured for Curing Cancer: The American Experience of Dr. Max Gerson* (San Diego: Gerson Institute, 1991).

10. Ibid. *See also* the transcript of Dr. Gerson's testimony before the Pepper-Neeley Subcommittee. "Cancer Research, Hearings before a Subcommittee of the Committee on Foreign Relations, United States Senate, Seventy-Ninth Congress, Second Session on S. 1875, A Bill to Authorize and Request the President to Undertake to Mobilize at Some Convenient Place in the United States an Adequate Number of the World's Outstanding Experts, and Coordinate and Utilize Their Services in a Supreme Endeavor to Discover Means of Curing and Preventing Cancer. July 1, 2 and 3, 1946" (Washington, DC: United States Printing Office, 1946).

11. R. J. Glasser, *The Body Is the Hero* (New York: Random House, 1976), p. 242.

CHAPTER 2

The Therapy Moves On

Newcomers to the Gerson way of healing sometimes express the view that a therapy developed some 60 years ago and left unchanged ever since must surely be obsolete. After all, medicine has made huge progress since Dr. Gerson's death in 1959. This criticism is wrong on all counts.

Human physiology and the nature of chronic disease have not changed, and therefore the Gerson approach to healing has not become obsolete. On the contrary, recent worldwide research has come up with results that confirm and justify Dr. Gerson's choice of methods and materials.[1] Over the years, far from remaining stagnant and unchanged, the therapy itself has been enriched with carefully chosen additions, in the spirit of Dr. Gerson, who was never satisfied with the results he obtained no matter how excellent or dramatic they were. He felt that they could always be improved.

Since his death, the work of healing has become increasingly difficult. Air, soil and water are globally polluted; food grown on impoverished soil has lost a major part of its nutritional value as well as being heavily processed and adulterated with chemical additives. Worse still, the use of drugs, both prescribed and over-the-counter, has vastly increased. Certain self-destructive habits (e.g., smoking, alcohol abuse and so-called recreational drugs) have become part of the modern lifestyle. As a result, people are more severely toxic and their bodies are more damaged.

Accordingly, at the Gerson clinic in Mexico, we noted early on that the results obtained with Dr. Gerson's strict therapy were not as good and dramatic as the ones he had recorded. Moreover, some of the original medications had been altered while others were no longer available or usable. For example, Dr. Gerson used crude liver extract (Lilly) to boost his patients' liver function. Today's liver extract is much more refined and presumably not as effective. He also used freshly prepared raw calves' liver juice to help repair the damage caused by pesticides to the patient's liver. This can no longer be done because it was found that even the young livers from the best available sources were infected with campylobacter—a bacterium that can cause diarrhea, abdominal pain, fever, nausea and vomiting.

To make up for the resulting deficiencies, several new items and procedures have been added to the Gerson protocol. One of them is Coenzyme Q10, which replaces some of the contents of the raw liver juice, boosts the immune system and enables the body to resist certain infections and types of cancer. Another is defatted colostrum, the first fluid that is secreted into a mother's breast (or into the equivalent gland of all vertebrate animals) to feed the new baby. This valuable material helps to set up and organize the new infant's immune system, and it does the same to strengthen the flagging defense system of immune-deficient patients.

Pancreatic enzymes have been an essential medication from the very beginning. Dr. Gerson used them to attack, break down and digest tumor tissue. To help today's more severely damaged patients, the therapy has been reinforced with increased amounts of pancreatin at higher concentrations. Also, Wobe-Mugos tablets, containing a range of immune-supportive and antitumor substances, prove to be helpful. One of the functions of this medication is to destroy the external coating of cancer cells so that they can be recognized and destroyed by the precisely targeted elements of the therapy.

Gerson doctors also use artificial fever treatment (hyperthermia) to generate improved immune function and to speed up healing reactions. This treatment involves the use of laetrile (also known as vitamin B_{17}), derived from apricot pits. Developed by Ernst Krebs, Sr., MD, with his son, Ernst Krebs, Jr., laetrile contains a cyanide fraction which is able to attack and destroy cancer cells without harming healthy cells. It has also been found that an intravenous injection of laetrile raises the temperature of tumor tissue by as much as one full degree—a great bonus, since tumor tissue cannot survive in elevated temperatures that normal body tissue easily tolerates. To enhance this effect, the patient is immersed in a hot bath (hyperthermia), which further raises the total body temperature, causing the patient to develop a "fever." In its totality, this treatment promotes tumor destruction, pain reduction and improved well-being. (Of course, an entire tumor is not immediately destroyed by one treatment!)

Please note: While laetrile can be helpful in reducing tumor masses as well as pain—particularly bone pain—it does *not* restore body systems and organs nor does it help to carry off toxins. It is a useful addition to the therapy, but it is *not* a cure.

Another helpful addition to the Gerson protocol is ozone (used via rectal insufflation) or as peroxide (applied as a skin rub). Accordingly, it is available in two forms: hydrogen peroxide or ozone gas. In either case, it kills germs and viruses, destroys cancerous tissue, oxygenates the blood supply—and thereby all the organ systems—and converts harmful free radicals into excretable compounds. Hydrogen peroxide, in liquid form at 3% or lower concentration, as sold in drug stores, is rubbed all over the patient's body once or twice a day, to be absorbed into the system through the pores. If hydrogen peroxide is only available in higher concentration, it *must* be diluted to 3% or below. It must never be used internally.

Room ozone generators are routinely used in Gerson clinics and are recommended to patients living at high altitudes (above 3,000 feet) and/or in areas where toxic sprays have been used, or where there is a great deal of industrial air pollution. Inhaling ozonated air is refreshing and energizing and has even improved patients' moods.

An innovation in the field of diet affects certain patients who are lactose-intolerant (i.e., they are unable to tolerate the defatted and predigested milk proteins, such as yogurt and cottage cheese, that are normally added to the protocol after six to 10 weeks). In these cases, vegetarian, protein-rich materials, such as spirulina, are used.

GRAPEFRUIT SEED EXTRACT

Since patients' immune competence is generally low, great care is taken to protect them from catching colds or, worse still, flu. Grapefruit seed extract, which has antiviral and antibacterial properties, was recently added to the program and has been useful. Taken orally and used as a gargle, it can ward off a cold if taken at the very first suspicion of trouble. Another excellent preparation is the homeopathic flu solution by Dolisos America, Inc. (www.dolisosamerica.com).

TAHEBO, PAU D'ARCO OR LAPACHO

Tahebo or Pau d'Arco is the inner bark of the Andean pine tree, traditionally used for healing purposes by many tribes in the South American Andes. Made into tea, it has been used, in addition to the Gerson treatment, on a number of patients who found it a valuable extra, increasing their well-being and even helping to reduce tumors. Tahebo consists of thin woody splinters, which have to be steeped for five to 10 minutes in simmering water and strained before serving. As this remedy is being used by a number of tribes, it is known as Tahebo, Pau d'Arco or Lapacho.

SELENIUM

This chemical element has been found by several researchers—including Professor Gerhard N. Schrauzer of the University of California at La Jolla[2] and Professor Harold D. Foster of Victoria, B.C., Canada[3]—to be an important stimulant for the immune system. For that reason, it is included in the Gerson treatment of many patients.

GLUCOSE-POTASSIUM-INSULIN TREATMENT

The intravenous glucose-potassium-insulin drip was developed by famous heart specialist Demetrio Sodi-Pallares, MD. The glucose and insulin provide the energy needed to transport the potassium across the cell membrane into the tissues. Since the Gerson protocol is high in both glucose and potassium from the juices and the potassium salts, only a small amount of insulin (3-5 mg) is used, administered subcutaneously (i.e., injected under the skin).

CHROMIUM PICOLINATE

It has been found that chromium, in the form of picolinate, stimulates the production of insulin by the pancreas. Capsules or tablets of 200 mg of this substance have been added to the protocol, particularly for diabetics, to help alleviate their deficiency.

TO SUM UP

These are just some of the items added in recent times to the basic Gerson program in order to increase its effectiveness. Obviously, they must be proven to be "nontoxic." By testing promising innovations and possible additions with extreme caution, it can be ensured that the Gerson Therapy does its work well under today's increasingly difficult circumstances.

REFERENCES

1. Carmen Wheatley, in Michael Gearin-Tosh, *Living Proof: A Medical Mutiny* (London: Simon & Schuster, 2002), Appendix.
2. L. Olmsted, Gerhard N. Schrauzer, M. Flores-Arce and J. Dowd, "Selenium supplementation of symptomatic human immunodeficiency virus infected patients," 1: *Biol Trace Elem Res.* (April/May 1989); 20 (1-2): 59-65. Department of Family Medicine, School of Medicine, University of California, San Diego, La Jolla. "The mean whole blood selenium levels in

male San Diego, CA patients with acquired immune deficiency syndrome (AIDS) are 0.123 +/- 0.030 micrograms/mL (n = 24), and 0.126 +/- 0.038 micrograms/mL (n = 26) in patients with AIDS-related complex (ARC), compared to 0.195 +/- 0.020 micrograms/mL (n = 28) in San Diego healthy controls (males). To establish whether intestinal absorption of dietary selenium is impaired in AIDS or ARC, a supplementation trial was conducted in which 19 symptomatic HIV-antibody positive male patients with AIDS or ARC were taking 400 micrograms of selenium/d in form of selenium yeast for up to 70 d. The mean whole blood Se levels increased to 0.28 +/- 0.08 micrograms/mL after 70 d of supplementation, the selenium supplements were well tolerated. A rationale for adjuvant selenium supplementation of symptomatic and asymptomatic HIV carriers is proposed." PMID: 2484402 [PubMed - indexed for MEDLINE].

3. Harold D. Foster, *What really causes AIDS* (Victoria, BC: Trafford Publishing, 2002).

CHAPTER 3

Knowing the Enemy

T he Gerson approach to health and sickness is so different from the usual medical procedures that it is important to thoroughly understand its basic principles. Once that happens, the therapy's theory and practice become totally clear and display their profound logic. In fact, many recovered patients admit that they chose the Gerson program in the depths of a life-threatening health crisis because it made sense and held the credible promise to cure them.

The therapy's aim is to deal with the cause of disease, not with its symptoms. Its focus is on what it sees as the two major enemies of health: toxicity and deficiency. Both are the result of today's denatured, artificial lifestyle; both are, to some extent, connected to the modern Western diet and to our polluted environment. Let us take a close look at them.

TOXICITY

The air we breathe—the absolute necessity of life—is contaminated with the exhaust fumes of road traffic, the invisibly tiny particles that fly off tires and nestle in our lungs, the residues of aircraft fuel descending from the sky and the poisonous fumes of countless industrial procedures belching out of factory chimneys or from the neighborhood dry-cleaning establishment. Water—another basic essential of life—is just as bad, contaminated with chlorine and fluoride and with the residues of a wide variety of drugs, which resist all existing purification techniques (except distillation). Industrial and agricultural run-off contaminates rivers and lakes.

The latest addition to environmental pollution is electrosmog, the invisible but constantly thickening electromagnetic fields surrounding us everywhere. Indoors, they are produced by television sets, refrigerators, computers, microwave ovens and cellular phones. By interfering with the natural electromagnetic fields of the human body, they have a harmful impact on health.[1] Outdoors, radio masts serving cellular phones are causing serious concern: clusters of diseases, mainly cancer, have been found in the vicinity of newly erected masts.[2] (See Chapter 5, "Breakdown of the Body's Defenses," p. 29.)

Toxicity starts in the soil and in the plants that grow in it. Highly poisonous pesticides, fungicides, herbicides and other chemicals used in commercial agriculture, often until the day of harvesting, leave residues on the plants that become our food. Many of these poisons are systemic (i.e., they permeate the produce and cannot be removed by washing). Unless we eat only organically grown foods, our daily intake is richly laced with a cocktail of agrochemicals whose cumulative effect has never been tested.

In the course of food processing, vast numbers of chemical additives are introduced, many of which are unsafe.[3] Their purpose is to extend shelf life almost indefinitely, to make the product look more attractive and to substitute artificial flavors for the missing natural ones. "Food cosmetics," as they are ironically called, solely serve the profit-centered interests of the manufacturers and have nothing to do with healthy nutrition.

However, the dangers of food additives should not blind us to the fact that the first major culprit of the average modern diet is salt (sodium)— the very substance that is hardest to avoid. Despite official warnings against its overuse,[4] salt consumption in the Western world is alarmingly high, causing the body to retain water in the cells, leading to edema. Salt also puts an unreasonable burden on the kidneys, raises blood pressure, deadens the taste buds so that more and more is needed to produce an effect and interferes with the digestive process. Salt, as we shall see later, also plays a dangerous role in the cellular process leading to cancer.

Since meat is a valued staple item of the modern diet, it may sound surprising that excess animal proteins behave as toxins in the body. The fact is that the human organism, with its long intestinal tract, is not designed to cope with a diet high in animal proteins. (By contrast, the intestinal tract of carnivores, such as lions and other big cats, is short— hence the waste products of the digested meat are quickly eliminated.) The ideal diet for humans should be predominantly plant based, with a minimum of animal protein; today, the opposite applies.

As we go through life, we become less able to digest animal proteins. These poorly digested, incompletely broken down parts linger in the body as toxins. The animal fats contained in almost all meat, poultry and dairy produce are also inadequately digested as the body ages and its enzymes no longer function efficiently. Food animals are raised on unhealthy food treated with hormones, antibiotics and synthetic growth promoters. Whatever they are forced to consume remains in the meat, eggs and milk products that finally land on our tables, adding to the already heavy toxic load we are unwittingly carrying.

The body attempts to get rid of all these harmful substances to protect itself. Unfortunately, in addition to the massive burden of toxins with which it needs to deal, it also confronts the problem of deficiency.

DEFICIENCY

Just like toxicity, this enemy of good health also starts in the soil. For well over 150 years, artificial fertilizers have been increasingly used in commercial agriculture, providing the soil with three major minerals: nitrogen, phosphorus and potassium. They do not provide the 50 or so minerals and trace elements which are essential to keeping the soil healthy, fertile and rich in enzymes and micro-organisms that characterize naturally fertilized, humus-rich land. As a result, the impoverished soil can only produce deficient, nutrient-poor plants, which become our equally deficient daily food.

This is further depleted by processing. All canned, jarred, boxed, smoked, pickled, bottled and otherwise preserved items are drained of their few remaining nutrients and damaged by high heat and preservatives. They lack vitamins and enzymes. The latter, vitally important for good digestion, are destroyed at a temperature of over 140° F (60° C) and can only be supplied to the body by fresh raw fruits and salads. However, few people eat enough of these to get adequate enzymes needed for a healthy system.

By now, it should be clear that the two main enemies of good health— toxicity and deficiency, which the Gerson program attempts to tackle as a first priority—add up to a single vicious circle. If our food were truly nutritious, our bodies would be better able to deal with toxicity, but it is not. As a result, sooner or later the degenerative process sets in, opening the door to serious chronic disease. Obviously, both enemies of health have to be dealt with in order to initiate healing and to restore the body's natural defenses. This is the subject of the following chapters.

REFERENCES

1. Robert O. Becker, MD, as quoted in *Icon* magazine in Eileen O'Connor, Trustee of the EM Radiation Trust, "Mobile Phone Mast Radiation and Breast Cancer: Eileen O'Connor's Personal Story," The Interdisciplinary Centre for Obesity, Nutrition and Health (ICON-Health), University of Leeds (UK), No. 34 (Winter 2006); *Gerson Healing Newsletter* (San Diego: Gerson Institute, March/April 2007); Joseph Mercola, MD, "Are EMFs Hazardous to Our Health?" (www.mercola.com/article/emf/emf_dangers.htm).

2. Note 1 (Becker), supra; *see also* Ronni Wolf and Danny Wolf, "Increased Incidence of Cancer near a Cell-Phone Transmitter Station," *International Journal of Cancer Prevention* 1 (2) (April 2004).

3. Sally Fallon, "Dirty Secrets of the Food Processing Industry," presentation given at the annual conference of Consumer Health of Canada (March 2002) (www.westonaprice.org/modernfood/dirty-secrets.html).

4. "Excessive Sodium is One of the Greatest Health Threats in Foods," World Health Organization (WHO) report from October 2006 meeting in Paris, part of the implementation of the WHO's Global Strategy on Diet, Physical Activity and Health.

CHAPTER 4

The Body's Defenses

The human body is a wonderful living precision instrument whose every part is closely connected to every other part. Each of its trillion cells has its own intelligence, function and place in the total system. It is no exaggeration to say that the body is a living miracle whose potential is far from being fully understood. Despite the rapid development of high-technology research, scientists are only just beginning to unravel the enormous complexities of life on the cellular level.

The body, left to its own devices and given the right conditions, functions in order to survive and remain in the state of homeostasis (i.e., a state of dynamic equilibrium). In this state, the human organism maintains stability while adjusting to changing conditions. As soon as this stability becomes endangered, several built-in defense systems spring into action. Let us explore these sophisticated systems in depth.

THE IMMUNE SYSTEM

All through nature, millions of living organisms prey on others. This also applies to the human body, as it is daily exposed to attacks by germs, viruses and parasites that carry disease. Its main protector is the immune system, which has in recent times gained some recognition among the general public, mainly through advertisements offering preparations "to strengthen the immune system." Irrespective of whether or not these work, people buy them without knowing anything about the immune system—what it consists of or where it is located—yet the subject deserves attention.

The immune system is not a single organ or a single gland; its parts are located all over the body. Several organs (e.g., the liver, the brain and the pancreas) are so important that they have their own immune mechanism—the reticuloendothelial system—which gives them extra protection.

There is also the lymphatic system, which transports excess fluid from body tissues into the bloodstream. The lymph itself is a straw-colored liquid containing cells which fight infection. The system consists of some 700 nodes in a normal person, distributed all over the body. Unlike the bloodstream, circulated through the pumping action of the heart, the lymph is moved around the body by muscular action.

However, the main basic component of the system is located in the bone marrow, where the white blood corpuscles are formed. When they are released, they are not complete. Some wander to the thymus gland, where they are completed, and released as T lymphocytes; others drift to the spleen and lymphoid tissue and mature into B lymphocytes. All of them ingest germs, viruses, malignant cells or toxic substances, killing or otherwise neutralizing them.

As all other parts of the organism, the immune system is made up of cells that need to be nourished. They require a full complement of minerals, enzymes and vitamins in their natural form which is easily assimilated. Pills and drugs cannot cover that need; sometimes they are not absorbed at all. Here, as in the rest of the body, the need is for fresh, living, organic substances to nourish and maintain this essential life-preserving system.

THE ENZYME SYSTEM

Enzymes are often poorly understood by the lay person. According to one authoritative definition, they are "complex proteins that are capable of inducing chemical changes in other substances without being changed themselves."[1] Everything that happens in the body—from taking a breath in order to supply oxygen to the blood, to digesting food and then to combining digested foods with oxygen in order to produce energy—hundreds of such processes require enzyme activity.

The body must build its own enzymes since it cannot utilize the ones found in raw foods or animal products. In order to produce the hundreds needed, the organ systems require specific minerals as catalysts. (Catalysts are substances that speed up a reaction without themselves being altered.)

Researchers Dixon and Webb[2] performed a detailed study into how the body builds enzymes. They found that, in most of the enzymes they studied, the body needed potassium as a catalyst, while sodium acted as an enzyme inhibitor (i.e., a blocking substance). Since enzymes are destroyed at temperatures above 140° F (60° C), the body receives no enzymes from cooked or processed foods. If it doesn't receive fresh living nutrients, such as the Gerson Therapy supplies, serious difficulties will arise. This is particularly true for patients already facing major health problems such as poor digestion, poor appetite, constipation, diarrhea and painful gas. The pancreatic enzymes are not doing their job of attacking tumor tissue and the oxidizing enzymes are not producing adequate energy, to name just a few deficiencies.

The reason why enzymes, especially pancreatic ones, are able to attack and destroy tumor tissue while digesting foods is because they recognize tumor cells as "foreign," needing to be eliminated. However, the basic function of these same enzymes is to digest proteins. Since the average diet is high in animal proteins, most of the pancreatic enzymes are used for digestion and little—if any—is available to destroy tumor tissue, allowing the latter to grow and spread.

Clearly, inadequate enzyme activity is one of the major problems with which sick people, especially cancer patients, must contend. The answer lies in providing them with toxin-free, fresh organic food and speeding up their intensive detoxification by means of coffee enemas. Moreover, supplying extra doses of digestive and pancreatic enzymes is an integral part of the Gerson protocol, alongside fresh juices with their high oxygen content.

THE HORMONE SYSTEM

Hormones are substances produced in certain glands that release them directly into the bloodstream and are therefore called endocrine (i.e., ductless) glands. Most people associate hormones specifically with sexual function, yet there are many others playing significant roles in the body (e.g., insulin, thyroxin and adrenaline). Hormones, especially thyroxin and adrenaline, regulate the entire metabolism.

The thyroid deserves special attention as it is an important part of the immune system. Among its many other functions, it regulates body temperature, including fever. If and when the organism is invaded by germs or viruses, the immune system responds by producing excess heat, namely fever. We must remember that most germs and viruses, and even tumor tissue, do not tolerate elevated temperatures, which healthy cells can easily bear. Hence, the well-functioning thyroid helps to restore health if it is supplied with iodine, which it needs in order to manufacture its vitally important hormone—thyroxin.

These days, iodine is unfortunately in short supply. Chlorine in the water supply is able to remove it from the thyroid. Fluoride, a dangerous toxin,[3] is even more powerful in blocking this important hormone. In addition, as a consequence of commercial farming methods, the soil contains too little iodine, thus producing iodine-deficient plant foods. In recognition of this, the governments of many countries have made it compulsory to add iodine to ordinary table salt on the grounds that, as the public already used a great deal of salt, everybody was likely to consume some iodine with it. High salt consumption, on the other hand, is now known to be unhealthy and is, in fact, officially discouraged,[4] resulting in a serious shortfall of iodine even in people on a good diet.

Other enzyme inhibitors include food additives such as preservatives, emulsifiers, coloring agents, artificial flavors and many other so-called food cosmetics, plus pesticides and other agricultural poisons in our food supply. Some pesticide residues have even been found to inhibit the production of male sperm.[5] The hormone system, an important part of the body's defenses, is itself under severe attack.

THE ESSENTIAL ORGANS

Certain organs (e.g., the liver, the pancreas, the lungs, the kidneys, the heart and the brain) are called "essential." While they certainly deserve that name, one should not assume that, for instance, the colon is not essential! The same applies to the small intestine, the bone marrow, the spleen—even the appendix, which is part of the immune system. In fact, there is nothing nonessential in the body.

In the course of healing, it is therefore extremely important to deal with all the body systems. Since the liver plays a major part in healing the body, the Gerson Therapy pays particular attention to restoring its functioning as quickly and as thoroughly as possible. The liver is an amazing organ. It is the only one in the body that is able to regenerate and regrow if parts of it are removed. It is involved in most bodily processes; all physiological activities begin and end in it. Often described as an organ of detoxification, which it certainly is, the liver has many more functions—dozens, if not hundreds—which even the high-technology facilities of modern medicine have not been able to define.

According to Dr. Gerson, each new generation of liver cells takes about five weeks to come into being. He assumed that it would take 12 to 15 generations of new cells to form a totally new, healthy liver. He specified a period of 18 months in order to fully heal and restore the liver of even advanced cancer patients and, with it, the whole organism. Unfortunately, that is no longer a valid model.

In the past 50 years or so, owing to deterioration of the environment and of the food supply, people have become much more seriously damaged than those whom Dr. Gerson had treated. Even more seriously, a percentage of cancer patients choosing the Gerson Therapy have been pretreated with chemotherapy, which means more damage to their systems. Nowadays, it takes two years—not 18 months—to recover fully; those pretreated with chemotherapy may take even longer to detoxify and heal.

THE MINERAL BALANCE

In order to function well and keep its defenses strong, the body needs a large number—some 52 or so—minerals. On the Gerson Therapy, this requirement is amply fulfilled by the generous supply of fresh organic juices made from produce grown on rich soil. However, Dr. Gerson also recognized that two minerals, sodium and potassium, were mainly involved in creating mineral imbalance in the body.

Over millennia, the human body has become a "potassium animal," needing some 90% potassium versus 10% sodium in its diet—the approximate percentage found in natural, fresh, organic vegetarian foods. Yet, these days, the average modern diet is far removed from these proportions; instead, it is overloaded with sodium, which the body must excrete. Excess sodium is an enzyme inhibitor, as described by Dixon and Webb.[6] It has also been shown to stimulate tumor growth and produce edema,[7] as the body ties it up with water to reduce its toxicity.

To remedy this situation, Dr. Gerson introduced large amounts of potassium to the patient's diet—up to 40 teaspoons a day of a 10% solution for the first two to three weeks, in addition to the naturally potassium-rich diet. This resulted in an immediate reduction of edema, ascites and pain. He also noticed that adding any other minerals, such as magnesium, calcium or iron, disturbed the patient's mineral balance and caused damage. His main warning was against adding calcium to the diet. He discovered—with his close friend, top biochemist Rudolf Keller[8]—that calcium belonged to the sodium group of minerals and stimulated tumor growth. Even in cases of severe bone destruction by tumor tissue, or in osteoporosis, the Gerson treatment—with its high level of well-balanced minerals—is capable of achieving bone restoration. In light of all this, it is easy to see why mineral balance is an important component of the body's defenses.

REFERENCES

1. *Taber's Cyclopedic Medical Dictionary* (Philadelphia: F. A. Davis Company, 1993).
2. Malcolm Dixon and Edwin C. Webb, *Enzymes* (New York: Academic Press, Inc., 1964).
3. John Yiamouyiannis, *Fluoride: The Aging Factor* (Delaware, OH: Health Action Press, 1986).
4. "Excessive Sodium is One of the Greatest Health Threats in Foods," World Health Organization (WHO) report from October 2006 meeting in Paris, part of the implementation of the WHO's Global Strategy on Diet, Physical Activity and Health.
5. D. Whorton, R. M. Krauss, S. Marshall and T. H. Milby, "Infertility in Male Pesticide Workers," *The Lancet* 2 (8051) (1977): 1259-1261.
6. Note 2 (Dixon/Webb), supra.
7. M. Gerson, *A Cancer Therapy: Results of Fifty Cases and The Cure of Advanced Cancer by Diet Therapy: A Summary of Thirty Years of Clinical Experimentation,* 6th ed. (San Diego, CA: Gerson Institute, 1999), p. 210.
8. Rudolf Keller, as quoted in Note 8 (Gerson), supra, p. 64.

CHAPTER 5

Breakdown of the Body's Defenses

In the previous chapter, we explored the body's multiple defenses which, under ideal circumstances, enable it to maintain its dynamic equilibrium known as homeostasis. However, if we consider today's high level of ill health in the developed world, it becomes clear that those sophisticated defense systems are unable to do their work and homeostasis can no longer be taken for granted. To understand why this has happened, we need to consider the problem from a wide perspective.

As mentioned before, the human organism evolved over millions of years as part of nature, alongside plants and animals. It was only exposed to natural substances; environment, food and shelter contained nothing artificial or alien. Our remotest ancestors' lives were undoubtedly hard and short, but their slow evolution was totally natural and well adapted to the world in which they lived.

Changes set in with civilization, but they only became drastic and rapid after the arrival of the Industrial Revolution in the late 18th century. A second wave of even more drastic innovations followed in the developed world after World War II, changing people's daily lives, working routine, living conditions and, above all, their diet—the most important factor affecting us all. The huge development of commercial agriculture and the apparently limitless expansion of the food industry changed our "daily bread" almost beyond recognition.

However—and this is the main point—the infinitely complex human organism hasn't had time to adapt and adjust to these fundamental changes and therefore its defenses can't cope with the multiple challenges facing them. They fight to keep functioning normally but, undermined by polluted air, water and wrong food, they break down sooner or later. Unfortunately for each new generation, the breakdown now comes sooner.

In this chapter, we shall examine the causes of the breakdown in more detail.

CHEMICAL AGRICULTURE

Artificial fertilizers have been in increasing use for well over 150 years, damaging and impoverishing the soil and the microorganisms on which the health of the soil and of all plant life depends. Plants, in turn, are the food of animals and humans, and their reduced nutritional value has far-reaching effects. Dr. Gerson was one of the few visionary scientists who realized early on that there was a definite link between dietary deficiencies and diseases—and between diseases and a sick, depleted soil. He wrote, "There is an external and an internal metabolism upon which all life depends; both are closely and inextricably connected with each other; furthermore, the reserves of both are not inexhaustible."[1]

Once the reserves of the soil were exhausted, the plants also began to sicken. Having become deficient, they lost much of their defenses against pests, rust, fungi and a multitude of other invaders. Hence, fungicides, pesticides and other toxic chemicals were developed to overcome the attackers. Of course, it was assumed that these agrochemicals were harmless if applied "as directed"; unfortunately, this was not the case.

The heavy pesticides—specifically DDT (dichloro-diphenyl-trichloroethane)—were first distributed halfway through World War II, around 1943. As Dr. Gerson reports in his book,[2] this and other toxic materials were found in meat, butter, milk and even mother's milk within 18 months!

Subsequently, it became clear that the toxic agrochemicals were also penetrating into the soil and the water table. These results can be seen today in several areas of California, heavily treated with huge amounts of pesticides every year, where the water and the soil are so toxic that an epidemic of primary liver cancer has hit children who played outdoors.[3]

The situation has gone from bad to worse. After DDT had been used for some time, the insect pests became resistant to it, so that heavier, even more toxic materials, such as dieldrin, had to be produced. At the same time, it transpired that the human body was *not* able to develop a resistance to those poisons. Their effect on adults is bad enough; tragically, embryos, tiny babies and small children with their delicate constitutions suffer more serious damage to their developing bodies. It is a sobering thought that cancer, formerly a degenerative disease of the elderly, is now afflicting children. Obviously, the cancer incidence among the general public is increasing at a much faster rate.

To illustrate the extent and speed of the increase, it is worth recalling that, in 1937, when the Gerson family had just settled in the U.S., posters at street corners proclaimed that one person in 14 died of cancer. In 1971, President Nixon declared the "War on Cancer," and assured the public that if enough money were spent on research, a cancer cure would be found.[4] In that year, some 215,000 people died of cancer[5]; 25 years later, in 1996, *U.S. News & World Report* published the result of the research: after $29 billion was spent, that year 555,000 people were expected to die of cancer.[6] The research had been done on chemicals, more and more toxic chemotherapy drugs—*not* nutrition. As a matter of interest, more than two in five people today are expected to develop cancer[7] and, according to Canadian estimates,[8] that proportion is moving towards one in two.

Over the years, the harmful effects of agrochemicals in food have become better understood. A Swedish study[9] produced evidence to show that non-Hodgkin's lymphoma (NHL) is linked to pesticides. (An earlier study in 1981 specified phenoxy herbicides as the culprits.[10]) Another herbicide implicated in the increased incidence of NHL is glyphosate, marketed by Monsanto under the trade name of Roundup®. Rather alarmingly, resistance to this poison is now incorporated in the genetically altered seed produced by Monsanto, allowing more pesticide to be used without killing the plant.[11] An earlier study by the same Swedish group has implicated Roundup in causing hairy cell leukemia,[12] while animal studies have shown that Roundup can cause gene mutation and chromosomal aberrations.[13]

The pesticide DDE (dichlorodiphenyldichloroethylene), a breakdown by-product of DDT, is known to interfere with male sexual development by deactivating the male sex hormone testosterone.[14] Throughout Europe, male fertility—measured by sperm count—is in decline.[15] (The highest sperm count was found among Danish organic farmers who have no contact with toxic agrochemicals.[16]) Equally alarming is the spread of breast cancer among women of all age groups. Every week in the United Kingdom, about 250 women die of the disease,[17] and at least 850 are newly diagnosed with it.[18] Although other factors also contribute to this trend, the effects of agrochemicals cannot be discounted.

As if dealing with the existing problems caused by agrochemicals were not enough, human health is facing the further threat posed by genetically modified (GM) food. This is an area where the conflict between powerful commercial interests and public health has come out into the open, despite GM-producer Monsanto's best efforts to suppress data casting serious doubts on the safety of GM foods for human consumption.[19] This is in keeping with the normal routine of agrochemical manufacturers who invariably set out to prove the safety of one or another of their products. However, anyone on an average modern diet is bound to consume the residues of several toxic substances contained in fruits and vegetables, yet no one has ever researched the cumulative effect of this kind of toxic cocktail.

The picture is gloomy, yet all is not lost. From small beginnings, the organic production of fruits and vegetables has grown exponentially in recent years, allowing the enlightened consumer to live on poison-free produce. Organic food, grown on traditionally fertilized soil, has the further advantage of containing all the minerals, trace elements, enzymes and vitamins needed for good health. This is why, in order to achieve healing, Gerson patients must use nothing but organic produce.

Enough has been said to show the vicious circle in which people on an average modern diet are caught. In due course, people who live on toxin-rich but nutrient-poor food—especially "fast food"—begin to suffer from headaches, arthritis, insomnia, depression, frequent colds, infections, digestive problems and more. They use more over-the-counter drugs, and doctors prescribe more painkillers, sleeping pills, antidepressants and other symptom-relieving drugs, which don't deal with the underlying problems. As all drugs are toxic in the long run,[20] the body's defenses are weakened and eventually break down. The link between the sick soil and the sick human being is painfully obvious.

DRUGS

One of the first duties of the physician is to educate the masses not to take medicine.

—*Sir William Osler, 1849-1919, medical historian, called "the most influential physician of his age"*

Half of the modern drugs could well be thrown out of the window, except that the birds might eat them.

—*Dr. M. H. Fischer, MD*

"A pill for every ill" sums up the extreme reliance on drugs that has become an integral part of today's lifestyle. One only has to turn on the television or radio to hear an endless recitation of the latest drugs being promoted to overcome every kind of human ill. Invariably, there is also a rapidly recited and deemphasized list of the many harmful side effects of each one. This denial of risks is not always successful: witness the scandal that broke in late 2004 around the drug giant Merck & Co., Inc., in connection with their arthritis drug VIOXX®.[21] At first, Merck publicly admitted that some 16,000 people had died worldwide from the drug's side effects in the two or three preceding years and withdrew VIOXX from the market. Remarkably enough, Merck had for some years published the life-threatening side effects and warnings concerning this drug in the Physicians' Desk Reference (PDR).[22] As the inquiries widened, Merck eventually had to admit that some 55,000 people had died of the side effects of a drug they had taken to ease the pain of arthritis. The truly scandalous fact is that the U.S. Food and Drug Administration (FDA) invited Merck to put the killer drug back on the market, claiming that its benefits exceeded its risks.[23]

Another overused drug increasingly in the public eye is Ritalin®, routinely prescribed to children suffering from so-called attention deficit hyperactive disorder. The PDR, which lists and describes all drugs on the market for use by physicians, specifies that it should not be used by children under the age of six years, and lists the following side effects: suppression of growth, loss of appetite, abdominal pain, weight loss, insomnia and visual disturbances.[24] (It does not mention the many documented cases[25] of suicide and unprovoked killings by youngsters on Ritalin.)

Despite the warning, children as young as two and four years old are known to have been put on the drug, which is also highly addictive, causing severe withdrawal symptoms. Peter R. Breggin, MD, Director of the International Center for the Study of Psychiatry and Psychology, published a book entitled *Talking Back to Ritalin*, in which he lists the many scientific studies that have been ignored by the advocates of Ritalin. He writes: "Ritalin does not correct biochemical imbalances—it causes them. There is some evidence that it can cause permanent damage to the child's brain and its function."[26] It is not hard to imagine what it does to its entire developing organism and still immature natural defenses. At the time of this writing, over five million American children are on Ritalin.[27] What will their state of health be like in, say, 15 years' time? (See "Hyperactivity" in Chapter 6, "Diseases of Modern Civilization," p. 89.)

Looking at the overuse of drugs in general, the real trouble is that they only suppress symptoms and allow people to carry on with their daily routines, at least for a while. However, they never heal nor clear the underlying cause of the pain or malfunction. The problem continues and gets worse; being masked by the drug, it becomes harder to diagnose. Since the body is an indivisible whole, the drug's toxicity affects not just the liver—the heart, the lungs, the kidneys and the digestive system also suffer—and the body's defenses weaken accordingly.

Because virtually all medical drugs are toxic,[28] Gerson patients are advised to keep clear of them. However, antibiotics are an exception. While their overuse in general medical practice has weakened people's immune system and strengthened bacteria by making them resistant, occasionally they need to be used by Gerson patients. We must remember that a cancer patient has a seriously weakened immune system, otherwise he or she wouldn't have cancer!

Since the immune system cannot be restored to normal in a few weeks or even months (it may take nine to 12 months), in case of an acute infection, antibiotics are required. For dental work, the dentist's recommendation should be followed. Antibiotics are also used to help fight colds and cases of flu. Of course antibiotics don't kill viruses; however, they help to control infections—the opportunistic infectious agents that set in due to the body's weakened condition. The least toxic antibiotics are used when dealing with colds, namely penicillin, unless the patient is allergic to it. Otherwise, the appropriate antibiotic has to be used for a particular infection. In all cases, the effectiveness of the antibiotic can be vastly strengthened, without increasing the dosage, by taking it together with one aspirin, one 500 mg tablet of vitamin C and 50 mg of niacin.

Once we understand the severe, all-over damage caused by the overuse of drugs, it becomes clear why the so-called recreational drugs are such a menace. Used by young—and not so young—people as casually as if they were candy, these drugs can eventually lead to addiction that destroys lives. On top of all the other harmful components of the modern lifestyle, these drugs, taken for fun, can be the last straw that breaks the body's defenses.

FOOD ADDITIVES

One way of healthy eating goes under the name of the "Stone Age Diet," which says: "Eat only foods from which nothing has been removed, to which nothing has been added, and which would go bad if you didn't eat it immediately."[29] You would have a hard time if you tried to find such foods in any supermarket on Earth. What those temples of the food industry sell—unless they have a range of organic produce—is the exact opposite of the above rule.

The ubiquitous use of food additives, whose number is at present about 4,000,[30] serves the sole purpose of making industrially produced foods look better, taste good despite the fact that they contain inferior raw materials, have a longer shelf life and thus be more profitable. Food chemistry is so highly developed that it can mimic almost any natural flavor or scent. What it cannot do is fool the human organism into responding to these fakes as if they were the genuine article, and only delivers chemicals of varying toxicity instead of essential nutrients.

The most widely used additives include sodium nitrite, saccharin, caffeine, olestra (a fat substitute), artificial colorings and flavorings, antioxidants, emulsifiers, flavor enhancers, thickening agents, aspartame, transfats and monosodium glutamate—plus unhealthy amounts of sugar, salt and fat. They can cause a multitude of allergic reactions, such as fatigue, behavioral problems, mood swings and, after long-term use, may even lead to heart disease and cancer.

Aspartame

Aspartame—sold as NutraSweet®, Spoonful®, neotame and Canderel®—deserves special scrutiny because it is present in over 5,000 food items[31] including fizzy drinks, jam, breakfast cereals, vitamins, and diet and diabetic food. It contains no calories and is therefore attractive to weight-conscious people with a sweet tooth. After its discovery in the U.S., originally developed as an ulcer medication, the FDA refused to license it for eight years, considering it unsafe for human consumption.[32] However, after years of lobbying by the manufacturers, in the early 1980s, despite the misgivings of scientists,[33] aspartame was officially sanctioned as a food additive.

Aspartame contains some six chemical substances, including methanol (wood alcohol), a cumulative poison, which converts into formaldehyde, a known carcinogen[34]; DKP (diketopiperazine), which in animal experiments has produced brain tumors[35]; and phenylalanine, which can produce severe neurological problems.[36] As for its claim to help people control their weight, the epidemic of overweight and obese people all over the U.S., the U.K. and elsewhere contradicts that claim.

More alarmingly, reactions among large-scale consumers of aspartame in, for instance, diet soda, can mimic conditions such as multiple sclerosis, depression, diabetes, lymphoma, arthritis, Alzheimer's disease, panic attacks, epilepsy/seizures, Parkinson's disease and hypothyroidism. Diabetes specialist, H. J. Roberts, MD, of The Palm Beach Institute for Medical Research, has coined the phrase "aspartame disease"[37] to cover the many pathological conditions among his patients. Nearly two-thirds of his patients improved as soon as they excluded aspartame from their diet.

Monosodium Glutamate

The flavor enhancer MSG (monosodium glutamate), which is tasteless by itself, was developed by a Japanese food chemist in 1907. In its original form, it was a salt derivative of a natural amino acid called glutamate, a common substance found in every plant and animal species. Eventually, turned into MSG, it found its way into almost every kind of convenience food—from soups, canned gravy, salad dressings, frozen-ready meals to potato chips, and into the meals served in the worldwide chains of fast-food restaurants. (On food labels, it often hides behind the name "hydrolyzed vegetable protein.")

The reason for this lavish use of MSG was discovered by John E. Erb, a research assistant at the University of Waterloo, Ontario, Canada, when he found out that laboratory mice and rats, used for studies on obese animals, had to be injected with MSG soon after birth to make them fat.[38] Under natural circumstances, no rodents become obese. They only do so when the injected MSG triples the amount of insulin their pancreas produces. Once fat, they are known as "MSG-treated rats."

Away from the research laboratory, MSG is added to human food for its addictive effect. As long ago as 1978, it was scientifically proven to be an addictive substance.[39] Since the food manufacturers' lobby openly states that the purpose of MSG is to make people eat more,[40] this additive clearly plays a major role in the current obesity epidemic. Huge numbers of people suffer from the serious side effects of MSG, which include headaches, palpitation, vomiting, nausea, numbness, chest pain, drowsiness, facial pressure and weakness. Some of these side effects are also referred to as "Chinese restaurant syndrome."

John E. Erb summed up his findings in *The Slow Poisoning of America*,[41] his book on the harmful activities of the food additive industry. Although the dangers of MSG have been widely known for decades, the FDA has set no limits on how much of it may be added to foods.

ALTERED FOODS

Transfats

Described variously as the world's unhealthiest food and/or as "heart attack in a box," these ubiquitous food components are produced by hydrogenating vegetable oil to turn a liquid into a solid substance. Transfats or hydrogenated vegetable oils (HVOs) are known to increase the levels of LDL (low-density lipoprotein) or "bad cholesterol," while reducing those of HDL (high-density lipoprotein), the "good" variety. They leave fatty deposits in the arteries, cause digestive disorders and reduce the absorption rate of essential vitamins and minerals.

Transfats are created by heating vegetable oil to a very high temperature, turning it solid so it can be used in margarine, pastry, pies, ice cream, confectionery and countless convenience foods. (Uninformed shoppers often fall for advertisements which claim that margarine, made from sunflower oil, is healthier for the heart than, say, butter; they don't stop to wonder just how the golden liquid oil had become snow white and solid.)

Hydrogenated fat is cheap, has no flavor and secures any product a long shelf life, hence its popularity in the food industry. However, recent evidence has indicated that instead of protecting the heart, transfats actually damage it, are essentially toxic, cause obesity and have even been linked to some forms of cancer. A long-term study carried out at the Harvard School of Public Health on 18,555 healthy women trying to get pregnant found that, for every 2% increase in the amount of calories a woman got from transfats, her risk of infertility increased by 73%.[42]

The British transfat expert, Alex Richardson, MD, commented, "Transfats shouldn't be in our diet. They are toxic and have no known health benefits and many known health risks."[43] In 2003, the World Health Organization (WHO) recommended that trans fat intake be limited to less than 1% of overall energy intake[44] and, in Britain, all the leading supermarket chains have pledged to ban hydrogenated oils from their own brand foods and drinks as fast as possible.[45]

The Harvard School of Public Health has estimated that at least 30,000 people—probably 100,000—die every year in the U.S. from cardiovascular disease, caused by eating HVOs found in most convenience foods.[46] The American nutritionist, Mary Enig, has stated that transfats disrupt the cellular function of the body, weakening its power to expel wastes and toxins.[47] This opens the door to heart disease, diabetes, cancer, poor immunity and obesity.

The good news is that, since January 2006, under U.S. government regulations, food manufacturers must state the amount of transfats contained in their products.[48] Some have already started to remove transfats from their output. The British Soil Association, flagship of the organic movement in the U.K., has recently declared that all additives, including transfats, MSG and aspartame, are absolutely banned from all organic products.[49]

The only way to exclude these and countless other harmful additives from one's diet is to avoid all manufactured foods; take the more labor-intensive but health-restoring path of eating only fresh, organic natural foods; and limit restaurant meals to rare occasions.

Additive-filled junk food not only harms the body, but is also a powerful trigger for antisocial behavior. Researchers both in California and in England have run experiments in prisons housing young male criminals, giving them supplements containing vitamins, minerals and essential fatty acids over several months, and monitoring their behavior. In both countries, minor offenses dropped by 33%; serious ones, including violence, dropped by 37% to 38%.[50] Take those findings out of the prison setting and it becomes obvious that much antisocial behavior in society can be ascribed directly to harmful toxic food additives—yet another powerful argument for avoiding junk food of all kinds.

FLUORIDE

Among the factors undermining the body's defenses, fluoride deserves special attention. While exorbitant dental health claims are made for it by commercial interests, it is in fact a dangerous poison, an industrial waste containing small amounts of lead, mercury, beryllium and arsenic.[51] The official reason why the U.S. government promotes the compulsory addition of fluoride to drinking water is to improve children's dental health, which, as common sense recognizes, is not undermined by a shortage of fluoride but by an unhealthy diet, insufficient dental hygiene and too many sweets. According to some experts,[52] fluoride only protects the teeth of children up to the age of five. Since that age group comprises only a small percentage of the population, it seems indefensible to force this highly controversial chemical onto everybody, irrespective of their age and dental condition.

Moreover, there is evidence[53] to show that fluoridation does not lastingly improve children's dental health. On the other hand, it causes fluorosis in one of every eight children, resulting in mottled, discolored teeth.[54] In the U.S., according to figures released in 2003, despite fluoridation, more than half of children aged six to eight years and two-thirds of all 15-year-olds suffer from dental decay.[55] It is also claimed that the prolonged intake of fluoride can be linked to increased risk of cancers, hip fractures, osteoporosis, kidney trouble and even birth defects.[56]

The late Dean Burk, MD, who had worked for more than 30 years as chief chemist at the U.S. National Cancer Institute (NCI), declared, "Fluoride causes more human cancer deaths, and causes it faster, than any other chemical."[57] Following a 17-year study, the NCI found that, as fluoridation increased, so did oral cancer and osteosarcoma, a rare form of bone cancer, in young men.[58] An increase in both oral cancer and osteosarcoma noted in the past decade is consistent with the finding of statistically significant relationships between fluoridation of the water supply and toothpaste and carcinogenicity of sodium fluoride in these two cancers.[59]

Despite the NCI study's conclusions, the profluoride camp is doing its utmost to hide and deny the harmful effects of the chemical. One such attempt led to an uproar among scientists in 2006, when it transpired that Professor Chester Douglass of the Harvard Dental School had kept secret the findings of his graduate student Elise B. Bassin for four years. In her 2001 thesis, Bassin discussed the association between fluoride and cancer, particularly osteosarcoma—bone cancer—in young males. When her findings were finally published in May 2006, and the truth came out to general consternation among researchers, Harvard exonerated Professor Douglass from any wrongdoing and conflict of interest, although he is widely known to be a paid consultant for the toothpaste industry, which is a major user of fluoride.[60] Up to 500 letters of protest have been sent to Harvard's President Bok, among them a blistering one from Professor Samuel Epstein, Chairman of the Cancer Prevention Coalition, demanding "a full and watertight explanation of this extraordinary action."[61] At the time of this writing, the issue has not been resolved.

This story is just one of many examples showing how assiduously vested interests fight to protect their profitable products, even at the risk of endangering public health. To guess the truth about the claimed harmlessness of fluoride, we only have to read the warning on any tube of commercial toothpaste: "Keep out of the reach of children less than six years of age. If more than used for brushing is accidentally swallowed, get medical help or contact a Poison Control Center right away. Children two to six years: use only a pea-sized amount and supervise child's brushing and rinsing to minimize swallowing."

Many brands of toothpaste, infant formulas and commercially prepared beverages use fluoridated water. Great care must be taken to avoid them all.

NICOTINE AND ALCOHOL

The health ravages caused by smoking have been widely known for a long time, yet the habit persists. Smokers use cigarettes either as a stimulant or as an aid to relaxation. In either case, the desired effect wears off quickly and has to be renewed, hence the self-destructive routine of chain smoking.

The main active ingredient of tobacco is nicotine, authoritatively described as "one of the most toxic and addictive of all poisons that acts as swiftly as cyanide,"[62] yet nicotine is not the only toxic product of smoking. The tars produced by the burning process line the lungs and eventually cause emphysema and cancer.[63] Smokers tend to assume that they are only damaging their lungs.

However, the poisons contained in cigarettes pervade the entire organism, damaging all organs. Bladder cancer, for instance, occurs more frequently among smokers than abstainers.[64] There is also the detrimental effect of the well-documented "second-hand smoke" on the smoker's family and workmates.[65] What may appear to many—even today—as an acceptable social habit is in fact a serious attack on our natural defenses.

The same applies to alcohol, which ideally should only be consumed occasionally and in small amounts. If consumed in excess, alcohol can lead to chronic alcoholism. It is poisonous to the brain and even more so to the liver, and can cause gastritis, pancreatitis, seizures and delirium. In extreme cases, it leads to cirrhosis of the liver and death.[66] Since the liver is a key organ, it is easy to see how its destruction by uncontrolled drinking undermines the entire organism.

COSMETICS

Compared to heavily toxic substances, such as nicotine and alcohol, cosmetics may seem somewhat out of place on our black list. After all, they have been used to enhance beauty and glamour for thousands of years; archeologists have found many remains of precious ointments, lotions and other cosmetics in ancient royal sites and temples.

However, today's cosmetics are vastly different from the natural substances used in ancient Babylon and Egypt. They contain an astounding number of ingredients, many of which (e.g., the wide range of parabens) are toxic. Sodium lauryl sulphate (used to clean garage floors and degrease engines), dioxins (suspected of being carcinogenic) and formaldehyde (a highly irritant toxic substance) are also used. Since all toxins help to break down the body's defenses, it stands to reason that all sources of toxicity must be eliminated from our daily lives, which includes toxin-rich cosmetics.

The fact is that up to 60% of all substances sprayed or rubbed into the skin are promptly absorbed and travel straight into the bloodstream. Orthodox medicine makes use of this with the application of various patches, which deliver substances, mostly painkillers, into the bloodstream. By the same token, powders, creams, ointments, sprays and perfumes also enter the organism at speed. Some estimates suggest that women absorb around 2 kg of chemicals through toiletries and cosmetics every year.[67] Worse still, whatever is absorbed through the skin bypasses the body's normal metabolic system and doesn't get broken down or neutralized, including carcinogenic substances. (We always say to our women patients, "If you wouldn't eat or drink it, don't put it on your skin or lips!" However, we make one tiny concession: eyebrow pencils are permitted.)

One of the riskiest "grooming" substances is the underarm deodorant. Almost all brands contain aluminum, which is seriously harmful,[68] especially when we remember that there are many lymph glands in the underarm area, which pass on absorbed toxins to the lymphatic system. Even those creams and sticks that are genuinely free from toxic

43

materials and claim to be organic have to be avoided because they interfere with the body's attempt to eliminate poisons by the simple act of perspiration!

Patients on the intensive therapy often experience night sweats, representing the body's effort to detoxify when at rest. Brainwashed into thinking that perspiration is not "nice," they may reach for the deodorant cream, spray or stick; healthy people perspiring on a hot day or during physical exertion may want to do the same. In either case, this would be a serious mistake. When the body attempts to detoxify through the sweat glands, the process must not be stopped or hampered.

Blocking the underarm passages with a deodorant will force the toxins back into the lymphatic system around the chest and shoulders and increase the risk of breast cancer, even in men.[69] Since male grooming aids have become widely used, the incidence of male breast cancer has been increasing. We may assume that much of this development is due to men's routine use of underarm deodorants.

So how should we deal with the problem of perspiration? The first rule is to avoid toxic (i.e., nonorganic) foods and drinks so that the body doesn't need to work hard to get rid of the residues. Soap and water are the best cleansers. Healthy perspiration is odorless and requires no chemical weapon to eliminate it.

Talcum powder should also be banned. Besides blocking the pores, it has been shown to cause lung cancer in babies when it is inhaled[70] and ovarian cancer in women who apply it to the genital area.[71]

Another highly toxic item used by both men and women is the wide range of hair dyes. The scalp is thoroughly "vasculated" (i.e., rich in blood vessels close to the surface) so whatever is put on it gets quickly absorbed into the bloodstream. Most hair dyes are highly toxic.[72] Even the more recent types, containing mainly nontoxic vegetable materials, introduce an alien substance into the organism. This is why Gerson patients are not allowed to use hair dyes of any kind and may only use the mildest shampoos. They are also advised to avoid perfumes, which contain synthetic aromatics, but may use diluted pure glycerin (without rosewater) to moisturize dry skin. Men patients in turn have to do without after-shave lotions and aerosol shaving creams.

There are some gentle, nontoxic cosmetics and grooming aids on the market, which are made from natural raw materials, that can be used by recovered patients and those not on the therapy. You may have to search diligently and read the tiny print on the containers before buying them but, when it comes to safeguarding your health, no trouble can be too much.

IMMUNIZATION—VACCINATION

Vaccines can be lifesavers; they can also be lethal. Their story goes back to the work of British physician Edward Jenner, MD (1749-1823). He observed that milkmaids, who contracted cowpox, only suffered a mild form of the disease and were subsequently immune to smallpox. From this he concluded that a mild form of the disease produced immunity to a more deadly form.[73] The assumption was correct but, in later attempts to obtain the same results, it was not taken into consideration that the milkmaids were young and presumably healthy; thus, their immune systems were able to respond. Since then, many generations of children have been vaccinated against smallpox; by the 1980s, the medical authorities declared that smallpox had been wiped out.[74]

For years, however, American children have been receiving the DPT (diphtheria-pertussis-tetanus) vaccination at an ever-younger age. The late Robert S. Mendelsohn, MD (1926-1988), one-time head of the American Pediatric Society and of the Chicago Pediatric Hospital, never stopped warning against the immunization of babies, reporting on the many children who were permanently injured, including cases of extensive brain damage. He noted that Dr. William Torch of the University of Nevada School of Medicine at Reno reported two-thirds of 103 children who died of Sudden Infant Death Syndrome (SIDS) had been immunized with the DPT vaccine in the three weeks before their deaths, many dying within a day after getting the shot.[75] A 1994 study found that children diagnosed with asthma (a respiratory ailment not unlike SIDS) were five times more likely than not to have received pertussis vaccine. Another study found that babies die at a rate eight times greater than normal within three days after getting a DPT shot.[76] When Japan banned immunization of infants under two years old, their SIDS problem virtually disappeared.[77] In due course, the U.S. government had to guarantee the safety of the DPT injections, since the pharmaceutical companies producing them were faced with so many lawsuits for damage and death caused by the shots.[78]

The DPT shots are still being used in the U.S. Their use is actually unscientific, since a small baby does not yet have its own immune system and is therefore unable to respond. A baby is born with about six months' worth of its mother's immunity, yet pediatricians continue to start immunization against DPT with babies at two to three months of age. Clearly, this interferes with the natural development of the child's immune system at a later stage.

In Britain, controversy has been raging over the safety of the measles-mumps-rubella vaccine, routinely given to babies, and claimed by some doctors to have the potential of causing autism and bowel disease[79]— claims vigorously rejected by medical authorities.[80] In the U.S., the presence of thimerosal (ethyl mercury) in vaccines administered to babies and small children has caused much heated debate, linking the toxic mercury to many cases of autism, speech delays and tics in youngsters, and contributing to mental and immune disorders in a significant proportion of the population.[81] By now, all routinely administered pediatric vaccines are being manufactured either in thimerosal-free or thimerosal-reduced forms. All in all, many questions concerning routine immunization remain unanswered.

All too often, what seems like a valuable medical innovation turns out to have considerable drawbacks. Generally speaking, powerful chemical interventions—whether by food additives, drugs or environmental toxins—weaken the body's natural defenses and thus open the way to serious disease, hence the need to restore them the Gerson Way, as we shall set out in the following chapters.

ELECTROMAGNETIC FIELDS

Every living thing is surrounded by its own electromagnetic field—an invisible but measurable layer of radiating energy. For millions of years, these fields existed undisturbed. In the late 19th century, the first incandescent filament light bulb was invented in Britain and then later in America. With that invention, electricity became a vital part of everyday life and its use has grown exponentially.

Today, all populations on Earth are exposed to varying degrees of electromagnetic fields. Lamps, television sets, radios, refrigerators, regular and microwave ovens, computers and latterly cellular phones all emit invisible electromagnetic frequencies. If we add natural geopathic radiation to our household implements, it is no exaggeration to say that we exist in an electronic soup or to see that this is bound to have a harmful impact on human health and well-being.

As the use of cellular phones increases worldwide, more and more radio masts are erected to service them. So far, official bodies have claimed that these masts presented no health risks to people living near them,[82] but concerned individuals tell a different story, reporting on clusters of diseases, mainly cancer, erupting in the vicinity of a recently erected mast.[83] Sleep disturbances, headaches, skin rashes, heart palpitations and vertigo have also set in within the same period.[84]

Some scientists agree with the concerns of the lay public. For example, Robert O. Becker, MD, twice nominated for the Nobel Prize, called the proliferation of electromagnetic fields "the greatest polluting element in the earth's environment."[85] Both the WHO and the European Parliament have held discussions on the environmental impact of electromagnetic fields.[86]

Applying the precautionary principle, "If in doubt, don't," everything possible must be done to limit the risks of the all-pervasive electronic smog. Cellular phone use must be cut to a minimum, switched off immediately after use and not carried on the body even when switched off. If possible, hands-free devices should be used to keep phones away from the head and body.

Phones aside, it is wise not to keep any electronic devices near beds where the sleepers would be exposed to radiation throughout the night. All electronic equipment should be switched off when not in use, not left on stand-by. Some common houseplants (e.g., a Peace Lily) are said to absorb harmful radiation[87] and should be kept in the home in large numbers.

STRESS: THE ENEMY WITHIN

Beside the harmful influences that attack the body's defenses from the outside, there is another self-made internal one, namely stress, that must be considered. Stress is very much taken for granted as part of today's rushed and restless lifestyle, yet it wasn't even identified, let alone explored, until the first half of the 20th century.

It was then that the eminent Hungarian-born endocrinologist, Hans Selye, MD (1907-1982), first began to wonder why so many people were suffering from what he called a state of sub-health, being neither ill nor well and lacking in vitality. He eventually identified the cause as stress, which he defined in the following words: "Stress is the nonspecific response of the body to any demand, whether it is caused by, or results in, pleasant or unpleasant conditions. How you take it determines whether you can adapt successfully to change."[88] In other words, stress in itself isn't bad. On the contrary, to quote Selye again, "It is generally believed that biological organisms require a certain amount of stress in order to maintain their well-being. However, … excess stress that the system cannot handle, produces pathological changes."[89]

The problem is that modern human beings respond to real or imaginary danger with the same instantaneous biological changes as our most remote ancestors did when confronted with an attacking mammoth or the flint axe of an enemy: the "fight or flight" response clicks in, giving the organism a burst of energy to fight the attacker or flee with above-average speed. The alarm reaction causes the pituitary-adrenocortical system to respond by producing the hormones essential to either fighting or fleeing. The heart rate increases, the blood sugar level rises, the pupils dilate to see better and the digestion slows down to divert energy to the limbs. Adrenaline and cortisol rush into the system. All these changes disappear when the situation is resolved, either by fighting the enemy or fleeing to safety.

These days, the threats are mainly nonviolent, and the challenges tend to cause frustration, simmering rage or repressed tension, which find no outlet. After all, we can't wrestle with a hypercritical boss or escape from a maddening traffic jam, so the organism stays in an unnaturally aroused state. Just like our cave-dwelling ancestors, modern people also go through the three phases of alarm, resistance and, finally, exhaustion. In due course, the stress-induced hormonal changes can lead to a wide range of diseases, including hypertension, coronary thrombosis,[90] brain hemorrhage, gastric or duodenal ulcers,[91] arteriosclerosis,[92] arthritis, kidney disease and allergic reactions.[93] Above all, the immune system is weakened and we know how dangerous that is.

Hardly anyone gets through life without experiencing periods of great stress. Business failure, financial problems, serious debt, divorce, sickness in the family or loss of a job—the list is long. People often respond by putting in extra hours of work, living on junk food and unhealthy snacks, taking sleeping drugs to fight insomnia and "wake-up drugs" to cope with the new day, drinking more coffee and alcohol and smoking more cigarettes—all of which speed up the descent into ill health. However, it is their reaction to stress—not the stress itself—that causes the trouble. Stress and its consequences may act as the proverbial last straw that breaks the camel's back, especially if we are dealing with one of Selye's "sub-healthy" individuals whose liver is already in a sorry state, with the rest of the organism toxic and malnourished.

Stress must be included among the factors that undermine the body's defenses and we need to deal with it sensibly. Relaxation techniques, yoga, breathing exercises and counseling help to reprogram one's spontaneous, deeply damaging reactions to life's inevitable turmoil. (See Chapter 25, "Overcoming Stress and Tension," p. 263.) Combined with optimum nutrition, this may result in the ideal set out by Dr. Selye when he recommended, "Stress without distress."[94]

REFERENCES

1. M. Gerson, *A Cancer Therapy: Results of Fifty Cases and The Cure of Advanced Cancer by Diet Therapy: A Summary of Thirty Years of Clinical Experimentation,* 6th ed. (San Diego, CA: Gerson Institute, 1999).
2. Ibid., pp. 145-173.
3. B. P. Baker, Charles M. Benbrook, E. Groth III and K. Lutz Benbrook, "Pesticide residues in conventional, integrated pest management (IPM)-grown and organic foods: insights from three US data sets," Taylor and Francis Ltd., *Food Additives and Contaminants* 19 (5) (May 2002): 427-446(20).
4. State of the Union address by Richard M. Nixon (1970), which led to the National Cancer Act of 1971.
5. Dispatches from the "War on Cancer, Special Report," *U.S. News & World Report* (Feb. 5, 1995).
6. Ibid.
7. "Probability of Developing Invasive Cancers Over Selected Age Intervals by Sex, US, 2001 to 2003," American Cancer Society, Surveillance Research (2007) (www.cancer.org/downloads/stt/CFF2007ProbDevelInvCancer.pdf).
8. "Chasing the cancer answer," Canadian Broadcasting Corporation broadcast (Mar. 5, 2006).
9. L. Hardell and M. Eriksson, "A case-control study of non-Hodgkin lymphoma and exposure to pesticides," *Cancer* 85 (6) (1999): 1353-1360.
10. L. Hardell, "Relation of soft-tissue sarcoma, malignant lymphoma and colon cancer to phenoxy acids, chlorophenols and other agents," *Scandinavian Journal of Work, Environment, and Health* 7 (2) (1981): 119-130.
11. Charles M. Benbrook, MD, "Evidence of the Magnitude and Consequences of the Roundup Ready Soybean Yield Drag from University-Based Varietal Trials in 1998," Ag BioTech InfoNet Technical Paper, No. 1 (Jul. 13, 1999).
12. "Occupational exposures, animal exposure, and smoking as risk factors for hairy cell leukaemia evaluated in a case-control study," *British Journal of Cancer* 77 (1998): 2048-2052.
13. Caroline Fox, "Glyphosate Factsheet," *Journal of Pesticide Reform* 108 (3) (Fall 1998).
14. Gina M. Solomon, MD, "Breast Cancer and the Environment," School of Medicine, University of California, San Francisco, and the Natural

Resources Defense Council (revised April 2003)
(www.healthandenvironment.org/breast_cancer/peer_reviewed).

15. Elizabeth Carlsen, et al., "Evidence for decreasing quality of semen during the past 50 years," *British Medical Journal* 305 (1992): 609-613.

16. Annette Abell, et al., "High sperm density among members of organic farmers' association," *The Lancet* 343 (June 11, 1994): 1498.

17. "UK Breast Cancer statistics," Cancer Research UK, (http://info.cancerresearchuk.org/cancerstats/types/breast/).

18. Ibid.

19. G. Lean, "Revealed: health fears over secret study into GM food," *The Independent on Sunday* (London) (May 22, 2005).

20. Carolyn Dean, MD, *Death by Modern Medicine* (Belleville, Ontario: Matrix Vérité, Inc., 2005); Carolyn Dean, MD, and Gary Null, "Death by Medicine" (www.healthe-livingnews.com/articles/ death_by_medicine_part_1.html). For their statistics on the number and cost of annual U.S. adverse drug reaction deaths, *see also* J. Lazarou, B. Pomeranz and P. Corey, "Incidence of adverse drug reactions in hospitalized patients," *Journal of the American Medical Association* 279 (1998):1200-1205; D. C. Suh, B. S. Woodall, S. K. Shin and E. R. Hermes-De Santis, "Clinical and economic impact of adverse drug reactions in hospitalized patients," *Annals of Pharmacotherapy* 34 (12) (December 2000): 1373-9; Abram Hoffer, MD, "Over the counter drugs," *Journal of Orthomolecular Medicine* (Ontario, Canada) (May 2003). It is reprinted in *Death by Modern Medicine* (supra), Appendix C, pp. 349-58.

21. "News Release: Merck Announces Voluntary Worldwide Withdrawal of VIOXX®" (Whitehouse Station, NJ: Merck & Co., Inc., Sept. 30, 2004).

22. Note 20 (Dean), supra, p. 182. ("The FDA covered itself by telling Merck to amend their package insert for Vioxx to include precautions about cardiovascular disease, but on the other hand it still let the drug be mass marketed on the media.")

23. Mike Adams, "Health freedom action alert: FDA attempting to regulate supplements, herbs and juices as 'drugs,'" NewsTarget/Truth Publishing (Tuscon) (Apr. 11, 2007).

24. PDR Drug information for RITALIN® HYDROCHLORIDE (Novartis) (methylphenidate hydrochloride) tablets USP RITALIN-SR® (methylphenidate hydrochloride) USP sustained-release tablets (www.ritalindeath.com/Ritalin-PDR.htm).

25. "Learning and Learning Disabilities: Ritalin Side Effects," Audiblox (www.audiblox2000.com/learning_disabilities/ritalin.htm).

26. Peter R. Breggin, *Talking Back to Ritalin* (Monroe, ME: Common Courage Press, 1998).

27. "Ritalin: Keeping Kids Cool and in School" ("There are currently an estimated 5 million school-age children on the drug. Another 2 million children are thought to be on other psychiatric drugs, such as Adderall and Dexedrine. Production of these drugs has grown 2000%, according to the Drug Enforcement Agency.") (http://social.jrank.org/pages/1011/Special-Needs-Gifts-Issues-Ritalin-Keeping-Kids-Cool-in-School.html).

28. Note 20 (Dean/Null), supra. For their statistics on the number and cost of annual U.S. adverse drug reaction deaths, *see also* J. Lazarou, B. Pomeranz, and P. Corey, "Incidence of adverse drug reactions in hospitalized patients," *Journal of the American Medical Association* 279 (1998): 1200-1205; D. C. Suh, B. S. Woodall, S. K. Shin, and E. R. Hermes-De Santis, "Clinical and economic impact of adverse drug reactions in hospitalized patients," *Annals of Pharmacotherapy* 34 (12) (December 2000): 1373-9.

29. Richard Mackarness, *Eat Fat and Grow Slim* (London: Harvill Press, 1958; London: Fontana/Collins, revised and extended edition, 1975).

30. Tuula E. Tuormaa, "The Adverse Effects of Food Additives on Health," *Journal of Orthomolecular Medicine* 9 (4) (1994): 225-243.

31. The Nutrasweet Co. (www.nutrasweet.com).

32. "Aspartame, Decision of the Public Board of Inquiry" (Sept. 30, 1980), Department of Health and Human Services, Food and Drug Administration [Docket number 75F-0355] (www.sweetpoison.com/articles/pdfs/fdapetition.pdf).

33. Ibid. Note 20 (Dean), supra.

34. Betty Martini, MD, "Aspartame: No Hoax, Crime of the Century (Front Groups in Violation of Title 18, Section 1001 When They Lie About the Aspartame Issue and Stumble Others)" (Duluth, GA), Mission Possible International (Jul. 18, 2004) (www.wnho.net/aspartame_no_hoax.htm).

35. Luis Elsas testifies before Congress. Animals developed brain tumors; *see also* Note 34 (Martini), supra.

36. Ibid.

37. H. J. Roberts, MD, *Defense against Alzheimer's Disease* (West Palm Beach, FL: Sunshine Sentinel Press, January 1995); *see also* Note 20 Dean), supra.

38. John E. and T. M. Erb, *The Slow Poisoning of America* (available on-line at https://www.spofamerica.com).
39. Ibid.
40. Note 34 (Martini), supra.
41. Note 38 (Erb), supra.
42. J. E. Chavarro, J. W. Rick-Edwards, B. A. Rosner and W. C. Willett, "Dietary fatty acid intake and the risk of ovulatory infertility," *American Journal of Clinical Nutrition* 85 (1) (January 2007): 231-237.
43. Alex Richardson, MD, "Brain food: Why the Government wants your child to take Omega-3, the fish oil supplement," *Food and Behaviour Research* (Jun. 11, 2006) (www.fabresearch.org/view_item.aspx?item_id=956).
44. "Diet, Nutrition and the Prevention of Chronic Diseases," World Health Organization, report of a Joint WHO/FAO Expert Consultation, WHO Technical Report Series 916 (2003).
45. Jeremy Laurence, Health Editor, "Should trans fats be banned?," *The Independent* (Nov. 17, 2006).
46. D. Mozaffarian, et al., "Trans Fatty Acids and Cardiovascular Disease," *New England Journal of Medicine* 15 (354) (Apr. 13, 2006): 1601-1613; *see also* "Trans Fatty Acids and Coronary Heart Disease" ("In an updated analysis of the trans fat-heart disease link, HSPH researchers have found that removing trans fats from the industrial food supply could prevent tens of thousands of heart attacks and cardiac deaths each year in the U.S.(1) The findings are published in the April 13, 2006 issue of the New England Journal of Medicine. . . . Trans fats have also been associated with an increased risk of coronary heart disease in epidemiologic studies.[4] . . . Based on the available metabolic studies, we estimated in a 1994 report that approximately 30,000 premature coronary heart disease deaths annually could be attributable to consumption of trans fatty acids.[4]" Note 4: W. C. Willett, A. Ascherio, "Trans fatty acids: Are the effects only marginal?," *Am J Public Health* 1994; 84: 722-724.) (www.hsph.harvard.edu/reviews/transfats.html)
47. Interview with Richard A. Passwater, "Health Risks from Processed Foods and the Dangers of Trans Fats."
48. "Food Labeling: Trans Fatty Acids in Nutrition Labeling . . ." U.S. Department of Health and Human Services, FDA 21 CFR Part 101, Federal Register (Jul. 11, 2003), p. 41434.
49. "What we can say—the quality and benefits of organic food," British Soil Association information sheet, Version 4 (Nov. 24, 2005).

50. B. Gesch, London press conference, Royal College of Psychiatrists (Jun. 25, 2002); S. Schoenthaler, *Anti-Ageing Medical Publications*, Vol. III. (Marina del Rey, CA: Health Quest Publications, 1999).

51. Emma Young, "Trace arsenic in water raises cancer risk," *New Scientist* (Sept. 14, 2001).

52. J. A. Brunette and J. P. Carlos, "Recent Trends in Dental Caries in U.S. Children and the Effect of Water Fluoridation," *Journal of Dental Research* 69 (Spec. Issue February 1990): 723-727.

53. Ibid.

54. M. A. Awad, J. A. Hargreaves, and G. W. Thompson, "Dental Caries and Fluorosis in 7-9 and 11-14 Year Old Children Who Received Fluoride Supplements from Birth," *Journal of the Canadian Dental Association* 60 (4) (1991): 318-322.

55. C. H. Shiboski, et al., "The association of early childhood caries and race/ethnicity among California preschool children," *Journal of Public Health Dentistry* 63 (1) (2003): 38-46.

56. Elise B. Bassin, D. Wypij, R. B. Davis and M. A. Mittleman, "Age-specific fluoride exposure in drinking water and osteosarcoma (United States)," *Cancer Causes and Control* 17 (2006): 421-428.

57. Dean Burk, MD, Congressional Record (Jul. 21, 1976).

58. Perry D. Cohn, "A Brief Report on the Association of Drinking Water Fluoridation and the Incidence of Osteosarcoma Among Young Males," Environmental Health Service, New Jersey Department of Health (Nov. 8, 1992). In 1992, the New Jersey State Department of Health released the results of a study which found six times more bone cancer among males under the age of 20 living in communities with fluoridated water.

59. K. H. Gelberg, E. F. Fitzgerald, S. Hwang and R. Dubrow, "Fluoride exposure and childhood osteosarcoma a case control study, *American Journal of Public Health* 85 (1995): 1678-1683; *see also* J. K. Maurer, M. C. Cheng, B. G. Boysen and R. I. Anderson, "Two-year carcinogenicity study of sodium fluoride in rats," *Journal, National Cancer Institute* 82 (1990): 1118-1126.

60. Juliet Eilperin, "Professor at Harvard Is Being Investigated, Fluoride-Cancer Link May Have Been Hidden," *The Washington Post* (Jul. 13, 2005), p. A03.

61. Letter from Professor Samuel Epstein to Harvard University President Derek C. Bok (Aug. 31, 2006).

62. *Taber's Cyclopedic Medical Dictionary* (Philadelphia: F. A. Davis Company, 1993).
63. "Questions About Smoking, Tobacco, and Health," American Cancer Society (www.cancer.org/docroot/PED/content/ PED_10_2x_Questions_About_Smoking_Tobacco_and_Health.asp).
64. "Detailed Guide: Bladder Cancer, What Are the Risk Factors for Bladder Cancer,?" American Cancer Society (www.cancer.org/docroot/cri/content/ cri_2_4_2x_what_are_the_risk_factors_for_bladder_cancer_44.asp).
65. "Secondhand Smoke—It Takes Your Breath Away: Secondhand Smoke is unhealthy ..." New York State Department of Health (www.health.state.ny.us/prevention/tobacco_control/second/second.htm).
66. Howard J. Worman, MD, "Alcoholic Liver Disease," Columbia University Department of Medicine (http://cpmcnet.columbia.edu/dept/gi/ alcohol.html).
67. "Is make-up making you sick? The hidden dangers on your bathroom shelf," *The Telegraph* (UK) (Mar. 18, 2005).
68. M. S. Petrik, M. C. Wong, R. C. Tabata, R. F. Garry and C. A. Shaw, "Aluminum adjuvant linked to gulf war illness induces motor neuron death in mice," *Neuromolecular Medicine* 9 (1) (2007): 83-100.
69. P. D. Darbre, et al., "Chemical Used in Deodorant Found in Breast Cancer Tissue," *Journal of Applied Toxicology* 24 (1) (2004).
70. M. A. Hollinger, "Pulmonary toxicity of inhaled and intravenous talc," *Toxicology Letters* 52 (1990): 121-127.
71. B. L. Harlow, D. W. Cramer, D. A. Bell and W. R. Welch, "Perineal exposure to talc and ovarian cancer risk," *Obstetrics & Gynecology* 80 (1992): 19-26.
72. F. N. Marzulli, S. Green and H. K. Haibach, "Hair dye toxicity—a review," *Journal of Environmental Pathology, Toxicology and Oncology* 1 (4) (March-April 1978): 509-30.
73. John Baron and H. Colburn, "The life of Edward Jenner," with illustrations of his doctrines, and selections from his correspondence (London, 1838).
74. "What You Should Know About a Smallpox Outbreak," Department of Health and Human Services, Centers for Disease Control and Prevention (www.bt.cdc.gov/agent/smallpox/basics/outbreak.asp).
75. Robert S. Mendelsohn, MD, "The Medical Time Bomb Of Immunization Against Disease," *East West Journal* (November 1984) (www.whale.to/ vaccines/mendelsohn.html).

76. Shirley's Wellness Cafe (www.shirleys-wellness-cafe.com/vaccine_sids.htm)

77. Personal communication to Charlotte Gerson from Professor Takaho Watayo, MD, Subdirector of the Ohtsuka Hospital in Tokyo (September 2006).

78. National Vaccine Injury Compensation Program (Oct. 1, 1988).

79. Bill Parish, "MMR Vaccine and Subsequent Cases of Autism Suspected," *Sightings,* Parish s& Company (May 23, 2000), FreeRepublic.com (www.freerepublic.com/forum/a3931156b1dee.htm).

80. "Frequently asked questions about Measles Vaccine and Inflammatory Bowel Disease (IBD)," Department of Health and Human Services, Centers for Disease Control and Prevention (www.cdc.gov/nip/vacsafe/concerns/autism/ibd.htm).

81. James F. and Phyllis A. Balch, *Prescription For Dietary Wellness: Using Foods to Heal,* 2d ed. (New York: Avery (Penguin Group), May 26, 2003).

82. "Cell Phone Facts: Consumer Information on Wireless Phones," U.S. Food and Drug Administration (www.fda.gov/cellphones/qa.html#4).

83. "Cancer clusters at phone masts," *The London Sunday Times* (Apr. 22, 2007).

84. Eileen O'Connor, "EMF Discussion Group at the Health Protection Agency for Radiation Protection (HPA-RPD) on 2nd March 2006" (October 2006), Mobile Phone/Mast Radiation (www.mast-victims.org/index.php?content=journal&action=view&type=journal&id=111).

"Six other short-term mobile phone mast studies have also found significant health effects such as headaches, dizziness, depression, fatigue, sleep disorder, difficulty in concentration and cardiovascular problems:

"1) H-P Hutter, H Moshammer, P Wallner and M Kundi (http://oem.bmjjournals.com/cgi/content/abstract/63/5/307) Subjective symptoms, sleeping problems, and cognitive performance in subjects living near mobile phone base stations: Conclusion: Despite very low exposure to HF-EMF, effects on wellbeing and performance cannot be ruled out, as shown by recently obtained experimental results; however, mechanisms of action at these low levels are unknown. . . .

"2) Santini et al (Paris) [Pathologie Biologie (Paris)] 2002 (http://www.emrnetwork.org/position/santini_hearing_march6_02.pdf)

"3) Netherlands Ministries of Economic Affairs, Housing, Spatial Planning and Environment and Health Welfare and Sport. (TNO) 2003 (http://www.unizh.ch/phar/sleep/handy/tnoabstractE.htm)

"4) The Microwave Syndrome – Further Aspect of a Spanish Study – Oberfeld Gerd. Press International Conference in Kos (Greece), 2004 (http://www.mindfully.org/Technology/2004/Microwave-Syndrome-Oberfeld1may04.htm)

"5) Austrian scientists Dr Gerd Oberfeld send out a press release 1 May 2005 with this report: 'A study in Austria examined radiation from a mobile phone mast at a distance of 80 metres; EEG tests of 12 electro-sensitive people proved significant changes in the electrical currents of the brains. Volunteers for the test reported symptoms like buzzing in the head, palpitations of the heart, un-wellness, light headedness, anxiety, breathlessness, respiratory problems, nervousness, agitation, headache, tinnitus, heat sensation and depression.

"6) Bamberg, Germany 26-April, 2005 Dr C Waldmann-Selsam, Dr U. Säeger, Bamberg, Oberfranken evaluated the medical complaints of 356 people who have had long-term [radiation] exposure in their homes from pulsed high frequency magnetic fields (from mobile phone base stations, from cord-less DECT telephones, amongst others)."

See also Warren Brodey, MD, "Radiation and Health," Oslo, Norway (Sept. 13, 2006), p. 14 (www.computer-clear.com/radiation_and_health.pdf).

85. Linda Moulton Howe, "British Cell Phone Safety Alert and An Interview with Robert O. Becker, MD," Council on Wireless Technology Impacts (www.energyfields.org/science/becker.html).

86. "Minutes of the Seventh International Advisory Committee Meeting," The International EMF Project (Geneva), World Health Organization (Jun. 6-7, 2002) (www.who.int/peh-emf/publications/IAC_minutes_2002MR_update.pdf).

87. Mary Lambert, *Clearing the Clutter for Good Feng Shui* (New York: Michael Friedman Publishing Group, Jan. 1, 2001). Lambert suggests that the following plants are especially good for absorbing electromagnetic emissions from computers and other electronics: Peace Lily, Peperomias, Cirrus peruvianus (a cactus) and Dwarf Banana Plants. Studies conducted by the National Aeronautics and Space Administration have shown it to be particularly effective in absorbing formaldehyde, xylene, benzene and carbon monoxide from the air in homes or offices.

88. Hans Selye, MD, *The Stress of Life* (New York: McGraw-Hill, 1956).

89. Hans Selye, MD, "The stress concept and some of its implications," in Vernon Hamilton and David M. Warburton, *Human Stress and Cognition: An Information Processing Approach* (New York: John Wiley and Sons Ltd., 1979).

90. Vijay Sood and R. N. Chakravarti, "Systemic stress in the production of cardiac thrombosis in hypercholesterolaemic rats," *Research in Experimental Medicine* 167 (1) (February 1976): 31-45.

91. "Digestive Disorders: Stomach and Duodenal Ulcers (Peptic Ulcers)," University of Maryland Medical Center (www.umm.edu/digest/ulcers.htm).

92. E. C. Lattime and H. R. Strausser, "Arteriosclerosis: is stress-induced immune suppression a risk factor?," *Science* 198 (4314) (Oct. 21, 1977): 302-303.

93. M. Lekander, "The immune system is affected by psychological factors. High stress levels can change susceptibility to infection and allergy," *Lakartidningen* 96 (44) (Nov. 3, 1999): 4807-11.

94. Hans Selye, MD, *Stress Without Distress* (Philadelphia, PA: Lippincott, 1974).

CHAPTER 6

Diseases of
Modern Civilization

I t is an astonishing fact of the 21st century that, instead of enjoying good health and fitness, so many people in the developed world suffer from a multitude of complaints and diseases, which a few generations ago were much less widespread. Worse still, these conditions are no longer limited to the middle-aged and elderly but instead attack ever-younger generations. Because of their comparative novelty, they are often called "diseases of modern civilization."

This sounds like a kind of justification, as if they were the price we have to pay for our unprecedented degree of technological development, comfort and consumer choice; in other words, they are a direct consequence of today's denatured, overcivilized lifestyle. Whether or not that is so, orthodox medicine deems these diseases incurable. All it can offer is symptomatic treatment, which only works up to a point and for a limited time, and has serious side effects.

What exactly is it in modern civilization that can be blamed for the deterioration of public health? The accepted culprits are widespread pollution of air, water and soil; the consequences of climate change; vastly increased levels of noise, violence and general insecurity; social tensions; stress; and the breakdown of law and order in many areas of life. All of this is true and valid. Oddly enough, the one overwhelming factor that affects every living person is not included in the list of harmful influences, namely the huge dietary changes that have taken place in the developed world over the past century or so. (See Chapter 3, "Knowing the Enemy," p. 17.)

This is amazing if we consider that the quality of the food and drink we consume every day of our lives is bound to have a powerful effect on our state of health. It becomes less surprising if we remember that the science of nutrition is conspicuously absent from the training of doctors. The resulting ignorance deprives them of a powerful yet gentle method of healing that is able to turn officially incurable conditions into curable ones. One can only hope that, at some time in the future, this method will enter mainstream medicine.

Meanwhile, with its nutritional program, the Gerson Therapy has been successfully curing most "diseases of modern civilization" over several decades. In this chapter, we list some of them and explain how and why the irreducible basis of the therapy, namely the rebuilding of the immune system and restoring all body defenses, is able to reverse and heal them.

DEFEATING THE KILLERS

Cancer

Of all the diseases under review, cancer is undoubtedly the one that strikes the greatest fear into most hearts and minds. Its incidence is rising, its effects are devastating—the same as the side effects of the available orthodox treatments—and its mortality rate is high. Above all, it remains apparently incurable. Taking all this together, it is not hard to understand that most people's reaction to the very mention of cancer is one of dread.

Let us take a closer look at this scourge, which the medical dictionary describes as "an uncontrolled growth of cells derived from normal tissues,"[1] adding that the disease comprises more than 200 different kinds. This raises some questions: Why is the growth uncontrolled? What are the normal controls and why do they fail? Why is cancer a killer? There can be "uncontrolled" growth in so-called benign tumors.

Those are noninvasive (i.e., they don't spread), can be removed fairly easily and generally do not recur. How do they turn into malignant killers?

While benign tumors are not cancers, they are growths that do not belong in the body and represent an early breakdown of the body's defenses. They do not necessarily recur but tend to turn malignant in time as the body's defenses continue to weaken. Tumors are identified as malignant when they invade adjacent tissues and also release tumor cells into the bloodstream. These cells circulate and are able to set up new colonies, known as metastases, which grow into other tissues. In due course, they invade and destroy essential organs, leading to death.

The body has a system of defenses that maintain homeostasis, the state of dynamic equilibrium of the internal environment. (See Chapter 4, "The Body's Defenses," p. 21.) It is the disturbance of this equilibrium that starts the process of cell deterioration, and the disturbance itself can be caused by various chemicals, specifically carcinogens, viruses, radiation, ultra-violet light and tobacco. Interestingly enough, it can also be caused by cytotoxic chemicals used to treat cancer[2] and, of course, by a faulty diet.

Cancer cannot occur in a normally functioning body because its defenses recognize and destroy any malignant cell that may develop or do not allow it to come into being at all. The immune system plays the leading role in the group of defenses. It recognizes a malignant cell as a foreign invader and attacks and destroys it, as it would any intruding germ or virus. However, the immune system, along with the other defenses (e.g., the enzyme and hormone systems and the proper mineral balances), consists of organs and glands that need proper nutrients, which can function only if they are not blocked by toxins. When those conditions don't apply, the defenses are unable to fulfill their task, and there is nothing to stop the malignant cell from surviving and multiplying.

The reason that cancer is credited with having more than 200 different types is that the cells of each variety look different under the microscope, depending on the kind of tissue where they originate. Still, in all cases, cancer essentially represents the uncontrolled proliferation of cells. This definition even includes leukemias and myelomas, which do not belong to the group of solid tumors, since they affect the bone marrow where, however, their malignant cells proliferate without control just the same.

Instead of causing solid tumors, some cancers break down the tissues they invade and cause severe open lesions. Their margins usually consist of swellings filled with malignant tissue that invades and breaks down any healthy tissue it touches. This type also proliferates.

Cancer is further broken down into two major and several minor categories, depending on the tissue where they originate. Cancers derived from epithelial tissues, which line all organs and blood vessels and the body's mucous membranes, are called carcinomas. They represent the largest number of malignancies. Those that originate in connective tissue, bones, blood vessels and the lymphatic system are called sarcomas. Their treatment with the Gerson Therapy is equally effective for both and requires little adjustment.

The most aggressive cancers (e.g., melanomas, aggressive lymphomas and small-cell lung cancers) respond most rapidly to the Gerson treatment. It could be that they are the most thoroughly altered from normal cells and therefore the newly recovering immune system is able to recognize them easily. Likewise, excellent results are obtained with ovarian cancers, even after some treatments with chemotherapy. That does not imply that other malignancies do not respond. However, as Dr. Gerson pointed out, some of the glandular cancers, including breast and prostate cancers, are located in glands whose entrance and exit are plugged with tumor cells. This can make it awkward for the newly oxygenated blood, enriched with enzymes and immune substances, to reach the malignant cells and kill them. In time, that problem is resolved and those tumors are also destroyed. However, this may explain why breast and prostate tumors take a little longer to reduce.

Patients must understand that, even when their tumor is gone, they are not healed yet. Where Dr. Gerson most clearly diverged from orthodox oncology was in his realization that, in cancer, the tumor is *not* the disease, only the symptom of the underlying breakdown of the body's systems; in other words, cancer is not a thing (i.e., the tumor) but a process involving the entire organism.

Therefore, most importantly, the disappearance of the tumor only means that the responses have been restored to the point of removing the threat to the patient's life, but that does not equal healing. True, total healing can only occur when all the patient's organs have been restored, literally rebuilt, with the best organic foods and continued detoxification. Healing is only complete when the damaged toxic liver is cleansed and rebuilt to as near normal as possible. The difficulty is that no tests exist to show how well the liver is restored and functioning. The liver enzyme tests are helpful but incomplete. A patient can have "normal" test results even if malignancies are still present. The blood chemistry, blood count and urinalysis only show that the basic organs are again functioning to the extent that the body has become able to heal.

The recovering patient may feel disturbed or disappointed when all this is explained to her or him, yet the need to achieve *complete* healing must override all other considerations. Without fully understanding the reason for this, there is a risk. When all tests come back "normal," the tumors are no longer evident. The local doctor, unfamiliar with the Gerson principles, then tells the patient that, "to all practical purposes," they are healed. They break off the therapy, relapse and die. Unfortunately, this has happened more than once, wasting much effort, hope and precious lives.

Case Histories

Because of the Gerson Therapy's long, successful record of healing cancer, enough case studies to fill this volume could be included. Indeed, separate booklets recording the healing of a wide variety of cancers are available (see Additional Reference Material on p. 403). Here, we describe two cases to illustrate how the body has to be damaged more and more before a malignancy can appear. In both cases, the patients were too young (ages 32 and 42) to suffer from an age-related cancer.

D. L. had pneumonia at age three. A year later, her appendix was removed. During her teens, she suffered some minor problems and, in her early 20s, developed a series of bladder infections, which were treated with antibiotics. These overcame the infections but candida set in. Drugs eliminated the problem but the bladder infections recurred, to be again cleared with antibiotics, setting up a cycle lasting for several years. D. L. became depressed and was treated with antidepressants. After the continual drug treatments, she developed an unusually aggressive lymphoma, which, she was told, would not respond to conventional treatments. Instead, she was offered a bone marrow transplant. She refused this and instead embarked on the intensive Gerson Therapy, which she followed faithfully for some three years. At the end of that period, she was free from all her problems—lymphoma, bladder infection, candida and depression—and has remained well ever since.

D. W. suffered from depression and panic attacks as a young girl and was kept on antidepressants throughout her 20s and 30s. Despite constant drug treatments, her panic attacks worsened until she was unable to be alone in a room, go out in the street or meet people. In her late 30s, she developed diabetes. In 1995, aged 42, suffering from severe pain, she presented at the San Antonio Community Hospital in Upland, California. The diagnosis was carcinoma of the left ovary, with metastases to the uterus and right ovary.

D. W. underwent a hysterectomy, with repairs to the wall of the rectum. At the same time, multiple nodules were found on the bowel and abdominal wall, but many small nodules, as well as seedlings on the vaginal wall, were left in place. In addition, an MRI (magnetic resonance imaging) scan disclosed a cyst on the patient's left kidney. Doctors urged D. W. to start chemotherapy at once and she made an appointment accordingly. However, the day before, after extensive research, she found information on the Gerson Therapy, cancelled the chemo and went instead to the Gerson clinic in Mexico. D. W. remained on the Gerson protocol for two years and was healed of all her problems. She didn't need hormones to control her surgery-induced menopause or drugs to control her diabetes. Her panic attacks had ceased and the kidney cyst had disappeared. Subsequently, D. W. was able to get a job, drive and function normally. She states that, at the time of receiving her diagnosis, three of her friends were also diagnosed with ovarian cancer. D. W. has now survived in excellent health for 12 years; sadly, none of her friends receiving orthodox drug treatment survived for more than six months.

Heart and Circulatory Disease

As with other chronic degenerative diseases, the incidence of heart and circulatory disease has vastly increased in the past 50 to 75 years.[3] Dr. Paul Dudley White, the most famous American heart specialist of the 1920s and after, stated that he had witnessed his first-ever heart attack in 1921.[4] The reason why he had not encountered one earlier is that canned, bottled and heavily salted foods had only been on the market for a relatively short time; likewise, the chlorination of municipal water supplies had also begun fairly recently. Therefore, these two factors had not yet been able to cause metabolic disease. Since then, however, they have more than made up for lost time. As it has often been claimed, the first symptom of heart disease in 40% of patients is a fatal heart attack.[5]

Sixty years after Dr. White's first encounter with heart disease, in 1981, at a meeting celebrating the 100th anniversary of Dr. Gerson's birth, one of the speakers was the famous heart specialist Dr. Demetrio Sodi Pallares of Mexico City. Describing the treatment he had developed for his heart disease patients, he declared that cardiac disease was not a local disease (i.e., of the heart) but a metabolic disease caused by the loss of potassium from the body and the penetration of sodium into its cells.[6] This insight was almost identical to Dr. Gerson's fundamental theory and practice. The big difference was that Dr. Sodi used his treatment exclusively for heart and circulatory disease patients while Dr. Gerson had discovered that it was an effective therapy for most chronic diseases.

Dr. Sodi published over a dozen books and hundreds of scientific papers describing his successful method of treatment. One of the techniques he developed, with the French physician Dr. Henri Laborit, was the use of an intravenous glucose-potassium-insulin (GKI) drip. The simple process that the two physicians invented was to use glucose and insulin to provide the energy needed to transport the potassium across the cell membranes into the tissues.

Meanwhile, the physicians using the Gerson Therapy also found the GKI solution very useful to reintroduce potassium into the depleted tissues. However, since the Gerson treatment is already high in glucose (supplied by the large volume of juices) and high in potassium (also provided by the juices and the added potassium salts), only a small amount of insulin needed to be used. As a result, one of the additions to the Gerson treatment is a tiny dose (3-5 mg) of insulin, administered subcutaneously (i.e., under the skin).

What has become of Dr. Sodi's revolutionary treatment for heart disease? One answer comes from a *Bucks County Courier*[7] article:

> "'A long-abandoned heart attack treatment that is so simple and cheap that even Third World hospitals can use it, is showing new promise and could save the lives of up to 75,000 U.S. patients a year,' researchers say. ... A study conducted at 29 hospitals in Latin America found that patients given the intravenous mixture of sugar, insulin and potassium within 24 hours of experiencing a heart attack had half the death rate of those who didn't get the treatment. 'The decrease in the death rate is dramatic—the largest reduction of just about any intervention that's been tried,' said Dr. Carl S. Apstein, professor of medicine at Boston University. 'Newer heart attack treatments, such as clot-dissolving drugs, typically cost hundreds of dollars per patient compared with less than $50 for GKI.'"

While the treatment was supposedly abandoned because of "doubts as to its effectiveness,"[8] the author of the article states his belief that "the doubts were caused by the fact that the treatment was cheap and effective, so that the hugely expensive bypass surgeries, angioplasties, heart transplants, etc., would no longer be needed. It is interesting that the heart specialists now use the excuse that the treatment could be used by people who can't afford more and those who live in the Third World."[9]

The Role of Cholesterol in Heart Disease

In the public mind, cholesterol is vaguely linked to heart attacks and strokes, but not everyone knows how this connection works. Cholesterol, a soft waxy substance found among the lipids (fats) in the bloodstream, is produced naturally in the liver. It is needed for various important body functions, such as the production of hormones, including sex hormones and corticosteroids. Cholesterol is divided into low- and high-density lipoproteins (LDL and HDL, respectively). HDL is considered necessary and beneficial and is able to rid the blood of the harmful LDL. This can have a genetic origin but is more likely to be caused by the average American diet that is far too rich in saturated fats—the obvious source of excess cholesterol.

Some of the food sources highest in cholesterol, according to Dr. W. Virgil Brown,[10] professor at the Mount Sinai School of Medicine in New York, are hamburgers, cheeseburgers, meat loaf, whole milk and cheese, steaks, hot dogs and eggs. Since these foods make up a high proportion of the usual American diet, they clearly introduce far too much LDL cholesterol into the blood. The result is that blood lipids (i.e., fats) are deposited in the walls of arteries and form plaque, which in turn causes atherosclerosis. The plaque reduces arterial blood flow, is rough and easily allows platelets to accumulate, causing clots which then block the artery altogether. If this occurs in the coronary arteries, which surround and supply the heart, it will cause a heart attack; if in the brain, the result will be a stroke.

The Gerson treatment is exceptionally effective in not only reducing harmful cholesterol but also in dissolving plaque and clearing the arteries for normal blood flow. Cases of cholesterol reduction by 100 points in just one week have been seen. The diet free from meats, fats, milk products, eggs, etc., contributes greatly to this success. The use of flaxseed oil is another important factor. Cold pressed from organically grown flaxseeds, as discovered by Johanna Budwig, MD,[11] it is high in the important Omega-3 and low in the Omega-6 fatty acids. This ratio causes the excess cholesterol to be dissolved and carried off via the bloodstream and the liver. (By way of contrast, the high cholesterol diet is high in Omega-6 and seriously deficient in Omega-3 fatty acids.)

As an immediate result of embarking on the Gerson Therapy, patients present a more normal level of cholesterol and are able to stop taking the statin drugs prescribed by their doctors. These drugs represent one of the largest markets for any prescription medication. They are toxic and dangerous,[12] but doctors feel compelled to use them to prevent heart attacks and strokes. By being able to do without statins, patients on the Gerson program avoid yet another source of toxicity. Any remaining cholesterol surplus is easily eliminated by niacin (vitamin B_3), which is an integral part of the Gerson protocol. Of course, smoking—another source of elevated cholesterol—is strictly banned on the therapy.

The Gerson treatment helps to clear arteries of plaque, which medicine claims cannot be done, thus avoiding strokes or more serious second heart attacks. It is a natural method of prevention, even in people who may have a genetic predisposition to heart disease. It has also helped patients who have already suffered a heart attack or stroke to recover and even restore some lost functions.

Case History

The following case history is only one of a large number on record. In December 1993, the 87-year-old father of recovered Gerson patient Margaret W. suffered a heart attack. After the ambulance delivered him to the emergency room, he had a stroke. Subsequently, he spent three weeks in the hospital's intensive care unit, was given a pacemaker and a great deal of drugs, and eventually his wife was told to take him to a nursing home. Margaret, however, persuaded her mother to take him home instead and immediately rushed to join her parents.

She was shocked at the sight of her father, sitting in a wheelchair, head drooping to one side, drooling. She worked with him day and night, cautiously putting him on the Gerson Therapy. At first, she gave him a few juices while he was still taking all the prescribed drugs, and then slowly increased the intensity of the protocol. In three months, the old gentleman was out of his wheelchair. In August 1994, eight months after the heart attack and stroke, he walked into the Department of Motor Vehicles office and applied for—and got—a driver's license. He remained well, celebrated his 90th birthday in August 1996, and passed away a few years later.

Hypertension (High Blood Pressure)

Blood pressure (i.e., the pressure exerted by the blood against the walls of arteries) plays an important role in health or disease. The average normal blood pressure is 120/80. When it rises over 140/90, it is considered abnormal and dangerous, linked to kidney disease and, as a contributory factor, to coronary artery and cerebral vascular disease. The standard medical response is to reduce the pressure with drugs, which, patients are told, they must take for the rest of their lives in order to preserve their kidneys.

The increase in pressure can have many causes. The chief cause is the narrowing of the blood vessels, essentially by cholesterol deposits forming plaque. Other causes include kidney disease, coronary artery disease and hyperthyroidism (i.e., overactivity of the thyroid gland). Stress, nervous tension or excitement can cause a temporary rise of blood pressure.

The standard allopathic medical treatment mainly involves the statin family of drugs. These reduce blood pressure, sometimes by as much as 25-35 mmHg (millimeters on the mercury scale used for measuring). However, they are highly toxic.[13] Moreover, doctors rarely inform their male patients that the statins cause impotence.[14] This is not surprising if we consider that the drug relaxes the pressure exerted on the arteries, including the pressure needed to cause an erection. Many marriages have been destroyed due to the effects of this drug.

Since hypertension is generally believed to respond only to palliative drug treatment while remaining incurable, it may come as a surprise that it is easily overcome with the salt-free, vegetarian basis of the Gerson program. At the start of the treatment, the patient continues to take the prescribed allopathic medication but needs to reduce the dose by 50% after three days on the therapy, which has already started to work. By the sixth day, the drug has to be cut out completely since the patient's blood pressure has become normal, and to lower it further to an abnormally low level might cause him or her to faint.

High blood pressure, together with heart disease, is the #1 disease killer in the U.S.[15] Treated with the Gerson Therapy, to which it responds easily and quickly, it would lose much of its menace, and tens of thousands of lives could be saved every year.

Case History

G. C., at the time aged 54, suffered from a number of serious health problems when he arrived at the Gerson clinic in Mexico, having been given a second death sentence by his doctors a few weeks before. The patient was suffering from liver cirrhosis, acid reflux (i.e., the highly unpleasant return of acid into the esophagus from the stomach), gastric ulcers, sleep apnea (i.e., temporary cessation of breathing), pulmonary lung disease, diabetes, high blood pressure, chronic fatigue and depression. He had undergone triple bypass surgery and had tried Viagra® (and doubled the dose without the hoped-for result).

Seventeen months after starting the Gerson Therapy, all of G. C.'s test results were within the normal range. His last examination was a total metabolic work-up, including tests for his liver, kidneys and all other essential organs. He reports that he is feeling great, has good energy— and no longer needs to even think about Viagra. In addition, the patient's wife had been doing the therapy alongside him. As a result, her monthly migraine headaches, which had landed her in the hospital with dry heaves and even blackouts, have ceased. She stopped smoking, looks younger, has better energy and feels truly well.

Diabetes

Diabetes is the #3 disease killer of Americans, following heart and circulatory disease and cancer.[16] We need to distinguish between two different types of the disease—juvenile or "brittle" diabetes and age-onset diabetes mellitus—and both require a different approach, as set out below. Generally speaking, it's fair to say that "the usual suspect," namely the modern American diet with its excessively high sugar and fat content, is largely to blame for the exponential rise in cases of diabetes mellitus. If you add up all the sugar that an average American adult consumes daily in the form of sweets, cookies, cakes, convenience foods, ice cream and the worst culprits—soft drinks—the sum total is pretty frightening. The human body and its most concerned organ, the pancreas, are unable to deal with this onslaught; after a while, diabetes sets in. However, the causation of juvenile diabetes is a different story.

Juvenile or "brittle" diabetes is described as "insulin dependent,"[17] which is correct, since those suffering from it do not produce enough insulin to satisfy their bodies' needs. Insulin is a hormone, secreted by the Islets of Langerhans in the pancreas. It is essential for the proper metabolism of blood sugar and for the maintenance of proper blood sugar level. Insufficient production of insulin is generally due to severe damage to, or infection of, the pancreas, which leads to the Islets of Langerhans being damaged or partly destroyed. The remaining ones are unable to produce enough insulin.

In many cases, the problem starts in early childhood, hence the name "juvenile." Children tend to catch colds and flu fairly often, and their concerned parents take them to a pediatrician who routinely prescribes antibiotics. These suppress and temporarily clear the symptoms but tend to damage the children's immune system. As a result, more infections develop until at some stage the apparent flu is very severe, persists for some weeks and finally slowly clears. That flu turns out to have been pancreatitis (i.e., inflammation of the pancreas). A short time later, the child is diagnosed with diabetes.

In this case, not enough natural insulin is produced, and the child becomes insulin dependent and must be injected daily with the missing hormone. Sadly, the problem is lifelong and worsens over time. Since the patient is advised to eat a largely protein-based diet, excluding carbohydrates, eventually the kidneys are affected, leading to the need for kidney dialysis. Further difficulties arise, including plaque formation and circulatory problems, and even loss of toes, feet or legs, due to insufficient circulation and resulting gangrene. During adolescence, such children are not able to concentrate or do well in their studies, nor do they grow at the same rate as their peers.

These multiple problems arising at a young age have been relieved by the Gerson Therapy. Obviously, the treatment has to be modified to suit the special needs of the patients: they are given less carrot and apple juice and more green leaf juice. Potatoes are cut out in favor of vegetables and raw foods, and little fruit is given, mainly apples and melons. Insulin is continued as needed. However, most patients are able to cut down considerably on the dosage used.

One 12-year-old boy was able to decrease his insulin requirement by two-thirds of the original dose. He became an "A" student and even caught up with his classmates' growth. In other words, his condition had greatly improved. However, he could not be cured (i.e., totally freed from his need for insulin) for it was impossible to restore the destroyed Islets of Langerhans, which should have produced the necessary natural insulin. This boy's Gerson medication was augmented by chromium picolinate to boost his insulin output, but it did not come back to normal.

Caution: Once a patient has been started on dialysis, the Gerson Therapy cannot be used.

Age-onset diabetes mellitus is curable with the Gerson Therapy. Patients suffering from this condition actually produce an adequate amount of insulin. The problem is that this insulin is unable to reach the relevant receptors within the cells for they are blocked by excess cholesterol.[18]

As far as the majority of diabetes mellitus patients are concerned, they benefit from the Gerson program which, with its exclusion of animal products, is free from cholesterol. More importantly, the restored enzyme activity, together with the high Omega-3 content of the flaxseed oil, is able to clear the cholesterol from the body tissues. In most patients, excess cholesterol gets cleared out within a week or two, even though they no longer take their cholesterol-lowering drugs. It takes only a short time before the available natural insulin reaches its destination in the cells; the excess glucose (sugar) in the bloodstream is reduced to normal so that there is no further need for additional insulin.

These patients are also restricted at the start of the therapy in their intake of carrot and apple juice and sweet fruit, but they can before long embark on a regular Gerson Therapy with the usual juices, potato-rich meals and oatmeal with fruit for breakfast. They, too, are supplemented with chromium picolinate but can drop this provided their blood sugar remains normal.

Case History

Our most severely ill diabetic patient was a 41-year-old man weighing over 300 pounds. His blood sugar ran over 340 (normal is below 120) and was uncontrollable with insulin and/or other medications. He had had a heart attack at age 38 and was left with dangerously high blood pressure—240/110 (normal is 120/80), also uncontrolled by drugs. He suffered from gout as well. If he had omitted his gout medication for a single day, he would have had to endure an excruciatingly painful attack.

On the Gerson Therapy, he was eating mainly vegetables and raw salads with green juices, and his diet was restricted to one potato a day. Instead of oatmeal in the morning, he received a plateful of mixed raw vegetables. He also used the usual enemas and took chromium picolinate along with the other Gerson medication. Insulin had to be continued at the start of the treatment as needed, the requirement being checked by regular blood tests.

The patient lost between one and two pounds a day without ever being hungry. On top of his three regular meals, he was given a plate of vegetables for snacks in his room. (Nondiabetic patients receive a fruit plate to eat as snacks during the night or between meals should they feel hungry.) His vegetable plate contained carrot and celery strips, tomatoes, cauliflower florets and radishes. His gout medication was discontinued immediately after starting the treatment without bringing on an attack.

At the end of 10 weeks, the patient's blood sugar was normal and he was able to discontinue the insulin injections. His weight had come down by almost 100 pounds, and at 6'2" he weighed an almost normal 210 pounds. Finally, his blood pressure had also dropped to a normal level without the need for drugs.

CONFRONTING CHRONIC CONDITIONS

Unfortunately, the diseases described so far are not the only ones inflicted on us by the faulty, health-destroying dietary habits of modern civilization. Nowadays, people truly dig their graves with their teeth, not realizing the harm they are doing to themselves. As various serious diseases have silently crept up on us, becoming part of our way of life, and death, we tend to take them for granted and no longer question their growing prevalence or why they cut short the lives of so many people in their prime.

Now is the moment to ask questions, listen to the answers and change our lives for the better. The good news is that the severe health damage caused by the wrong diet can be undone by the right one. This applies as much to the killer diseases we have reviewed as to the many chronic degenerative conditions that can drag on for many years, causing much pain, discomfort, depression and poor quality of life. Modern medicine can ease the pain with allopathic drugs but is unable to eliminate the basic problem. Indeed, many people believe that their arthritis or osteoporosis is incurable, but they are wrong. Although the Gerson Therapy's best-known achievement is its successful healing of cancer, it also has an extraordinary track record in dealing with so-called incurable chronic conditions.

Chronic Immune-Deficiency Diseases

Chronic Fatigue Syndrome

Chronic fatigue syndrome is also known as myalgic encephalomyelitis. Along with many other diseases caused by inadequate immune competence, it is spreading dramatically. Sometimes referred to as the "Yuppie Syndrome," it used to be known as Epstein-Barr disease. That was a more accurate description since its cause was found to be the body's inability to overcome the Epstein-Barr viral infection. As there are no medical treatments to overcome viruses—antibiotics are useless against them—the disease is considered not only incurable but also untreatable.

In due course, with people suffering from worsening symptoms of weakness, inability to concentrate, aches and muscle pains, it was discovered that the underlying cause was not exclusively the Epstein-Barr virus, namely that this virus had possibly mutated into other forms and that perhaps other viruses were also involved. At this stage, the disease was renamed chronic fatigue syndrome, referring to one of its main symptoms. Unfortunately, the change of name still left it "incurable."

Case History

What we already know about the Gerson Therapy's ability to rebuild a damaged, severely deficient immune system should make it clear why it is so effective against this condition. One patient's dramatic response to the therapy illustrates the process well. It concerns a middle-aged engineer who, after 20 years, was forced to leave his job when the viral infection hit him. He was given the California "Disabled Driver" plaque, although there was some doubt as to whether he was able to drive at all. At times, he was even unable to find his own car, could not balance his checkbook and complained of "the black cheesecloth that falls over me."

On the full Gerson therapy, in his own words, he soon felt "not as well as my colleagues, as I had wished, but much better, with new energy, a brighter outlook and feeling again like 25 at age 55! My coordination, eyesight and hearing are so good—I can do everything today that I couldn't do at 30."

Multiple Sclerosis

Multiple sclerosis (MS) is supposed to be an autoimmune disease. In such diseases, it is claimed that the patient's immune system attacks its own tissues and causes lesions or damage. In MS, it is stated that, "Infiltrating lymphocytes (white blood corpuscles), predominantly T-cells and macrophages, degrade the myelin sheath of nerves."[19] Nerves are conductors of electrical impulses and require insulation in the form of myelin sheaths in order not to short out. When the myelin sheath is damaged, electrical shorts occur, sending false messages along the nerves. These cause the typical symptoms of MS.

MS usually develops in people between 20 and 40 years old and is more common in colder climates than in milder ones. Its symptoms include poor coordination, unsteady gait, nystagmus (i.e., uncontrolled eye movements) and urinary urgency. In the early stage of the disease, it often goes into spontaneous remission, only to recur in a more severe form. Many sufferers eventually have to use a wheelchair; some even become bedfast.

The only difficulty in applying the Gerson Therapy to MS is that, in the early weeks of the treatment, MS patients typically experience a worsening in their condition. This is probably caused by the detoxification process removing the products of the infection from the lesions in the myelin sheaths. The cleansing causes an additional temporary loss of insulation and in consequence a worsening of symptoms. This understandably scares the patients, several of whom have abandoned the therapy, mistakenly assuming that it didn't work and was instead aggravating the disease.

If an MS patient persists, however, the cleared lesions—with the help of the hyperalimentation and detoxification of the Gerson program—allow the sheaths to reform, proving that MS is not incurable. Also, since the therapy actively restores and strengthens the immune system, clearly MS cannot be an autoimmune disease. If it were, an enhanced immune system would make recovery impossible.

Case History

Born in 1960, J. S. was raised on a ranch where he lived all his life, exposed to a wide range of agricultural toxins. He suffered several accidents, the first serious one at the age of six, which left him with an uneven gait. After a severe fall causing injury to his shoulder, he was given powerful painkillers to enable him to function.

The first symptom of an as-yet unknown disease was a fall, caused by his inability to control the movement of his leg. Subsequently, he lost most of his sight in one eye. In March 1995, when he was 35, J. S. was examined by a neurologist at the Benefis Hospital in Great Falls, Montana, and was found to be suffering from MS. Although this disease often brings on partial remissions followed by exacerbation, J. S. enjoyed no periods of ease; his condition went from bad to worse. His doctors told him that there was no hope of a cure.

In February 1996, J. S. embarked on the full intensive Gerson Therapy. His energy increased almost at once, his walk became even and he was able to work on the ranch while staying on the demanding Gerson schedule. By the fall of that year, his eyesight had improved and his other symptoms were gone. By 2002, his only remaining symptom of MS was a somewhat weakened sight in his affected eye. To date, J. S. is able to manage 16-hour days on the ranch and is no longer affected by heat, which used to debilitate him. He stays close to the therapy as does the rest of his family.

Caution: The artificial sweetener, aspartame, sold under the names of NutraSweet and Spoonful, is highly toxic to the nervous system and can mimic many symptoms of MS.[20] It is claimed to have caused the current epidemic of apparent MS,[21] which has nothing to do with the genuine disease. In many cases, the fake condition has been reversed simply by removing aspartame from the patients' diet.[22] (See "Aspartame" in Chapter 5, "Breakdown of the Body's Defenses," p. 36.)

Human Immunodeficiency Virus

Human immunodeficiency virus (HIV), credited with causing AIDS (Acquired Immune Deficiency Syndrome), is spreading rapidly and unchecked. The chemotherapy that has been developed as a treatment is at best yielding only temporary relief. No effective immunization has yet been found. Since the disease is clearly associated with a depressed immune system, it stands to reason that the Gerson Therapy should be able to overcome it. As far as we know, that is happening. However, most of the Gerson work is performed in Mexico, and since the Mexican Health Department does not allow HIV-positive patients to be treated there, we have had very little experience with the condition. In fact, two patients with active HIV infections, who were treated at home with the Gerson Therapy, have recovered and became negative. Still, we feel uneasy to claim that the therapy is successful, with only two recoveries of HIV-positive patients on record.

The only other evidence we have of nutrition, combined with a selenium supplement, being effective in treating HIV comes from the book, *What Really Causes Aids,* by Professor Harold D. Foster.[23] Dr. Foster discovered that, in areas where the soil was rich in selenium, the population had good resistance to HIV. In areas with selenium deficiency in the soil, the opposite applied: people were much less resistant to infections and many diseases, including cancer. He was also able to demonstrate that patients with active HIV disease could be turned around and made negative with the correct diet and adequate selenium supplementation. Surprisingly, he found that the Brazil nut is the natural food highest in selenium—seven times richer in that substance than the next highest selenium-containing food.[24]

Hepatitis B and C

Hepatitis, or inflammation of the liver, should not exist. This vitally important organ has tremendous reserves beside its own immune system. Therefore, under normal circumstances, its powerful resistance to infections protects it from hepatitis. However, the fact that this disease exists and is spreading points once more to the increasingly weakened immune system of the general population.

Essentially, hepatitis B and C are pretty much the same. They are only classified under different names because each is caused by a different virus, known as hepatitis B and hepatitis C virus, respectively. In either case, the disease is contagious and nursing is supposed to pay maximum attention to the cleanliness of linens, dishes, food, etc. The only available orthodox treatment consists of rest and a good diet.

The disease causes liver enzymes to rise. Unfortunately, although these enzymes are often reduced as the patient overcomes the first acute stage of the disease, they do not return to normal. This means that the patient is never wholly clear of the disease. In time, the liver becomes more seriously damaged, the liver enzymes rise again and the viral load increases. This process can eventually lead to hepatoma (primary liver cancer) or other malignancy.

Since the Gerson Therapy is able to strengthen and restore the immune system, we have seen a number of recoveries from hepatitis, including the return to normal of the liver enzymes.

Case History

L. M., aged 54, was sick, had no energy, couldn't walk across the street and was unable to digest her food. Eventually she was diagnosed at the University of Chicago as suffering from chronic active aggressive hepatitis with liver cirrhosis. Her liver enzymes were extremely high—SGOT (serum glutamic oxaloacetic transaminase) 1360 (normal is 0-30)—and her doctors said that she might have two years to live.

She started on the Gerson Therapy in January 1995. Within three weeks, her SGOT dropped dramatically by 200 points but her recovery was slow. It took one and one-half years for her liver tests to become normal; after two years, she was back "to her old self." To quote her recent statement, "I feel better than ever and I have incredible energy."

Collagen Diseases

Collagen is an insoluble fibrous protein found in the connective tissues of the body, including skin, bone, ligaments and cartilage. It represents 30% of the body's total protein content. Collagen diseases are caused by various conditions, such as a weakened liver and digestive system or by the accumulation of inadequately digested animal protein. The following diseases belong to this category.

Systemic Lupus Erythematosus

Systemic lupus erythematosus (SLE) is assumed to be an autoimmune disease. Its "etiology is unknown,"[25] meaning that its cause is not understood. SLE is a serious condition, able to affect every organ. Its symptoms are numerous and severe. One of the early ones is the so-called butterfly rash, resembling the open wings of a butterfly, which appears on either side of the nose. SLE is described as a chronic inflammatory disease of connective tissue in the skin, joints, kidneys, mucous membranes and the nervous system. It is not unusual for the disease to cause the patient's death.

Despite its ominous reputation, SLE is eminently curable with the Gerson Therapy. The time it takes to heal depends on the kind and length of conventional treatment patients have received. In extremely severe cases, treated by prednisone (a steroid hormone used as an anti-inflammatory agent) for a long time, it takes longer to restore the liver, the adrenals and the immune system. Even in such cases, healing is possible.

Case History

A. B. was born in 1951 in Australia. Married at the age of 20, she developed soreness and swelling in her knees and joints. During her second pregnancy, all her symptoms disappeared, only to return after the birth of the baby. For some five years, her doctors were unable to discover what was wrong. In late 1976, a Melbourne specialist diagnosed A. B. as suffering from SLE. His diagnosis was confirmed by the analysis of a specimen in the U.S.

During 1978, A. B. had periods of total incapacitation. In 1979, she was started on cortisone injections. Her knees would swell up to the size of footballs and her doctors would drain them and inject cortisone. In spite of taking painkillers, she spent the nights sobbing. By 1992, the pain was so bad that A. B. required morphine and her doctors admitted that there was nothing else they could do to help her. At some point in 1992, her husband found out about the Gerson Therapy, which seemed to offer some hope, but A. B. objected to the idea of coffee enemas and refused. Some months later, however, she was so ill that she agreed to try the Gerson program.

Shortly after starting on the treatment, A. B. could urinate normally which, her husband reported, she had been unable to do for many months. Her healing reactions were violent but the enemas provided relief. A. B. admitted occasionally straying from the diet, but every such trespass necessitated a trip to the hospital for morphine. By 1994, the patient had improved considerably and, for the first time in 20 months, she enjoyed longer and longer periods without pain. By early 1999, she was drug-free and remains so, able to run their country property—quite an achievement, since a few years earlier she had been unable to lift a plate from the table. She is no longer suffering from the frequent infections which used to plague her.

Rheumatism/Arthritis

There are various forms of rheumatism, mostly referred to as an arthritic condition. In many cases, it manifests simply as a passing inflammation of muscles and joints, which may occasionally recur, but it does not cause a permanent problem. According to medical information,[26] its cause is unknown and there is no specific treatment for it.

Its most widespread form is osteoarthritis, normally a disease of aging, which causes chronic changes, most frequently in the weight-bearing joints (i.e., knees, hips and vertebrae). It is characterized by an overgrowth of bone, forming spurs and a lumpy deformity of the joints. Also, the cartilage (i.e., firm connective tissue ensuring that bones in joints don't touch) becomes thin and wasted so that bone rubs on bone, causing wear and tear and sharp pain.

While conventional medicine can only relieve pain but not halt the progress of the disease, the Gerson Therapy has obtained good responses by relieving pain and dissolving some of the bony deformities. If continued, the therapy can halt the advance of the disease and even reverse it to some extent. However, as in other diseases involving bone lesions, healing is slow, and patients are often unwilling to engage in the long, labor-intensive Gerson treatment. Instead, they are satisfied with as much pain relief as modern drugs can give them.

The etiology of rheumatoid arthritis (RA) is also unknown and the condition is essentially treated with drugs for symptomatic relief. The disease can spread to every joint in the body, causing swelling and deformities and severe pain. It is routinely treated with aspirin, prednisone and more powerful pain-relief drugs. Since RA is also assumed to be an autoimmune disease (i.e., the body's immune system attacks its own tissues), it has even been treated with cancer drugs in order to disable the immune system.

This treatment brought no benefits and instead made the organism more severely ill, so that healing on the Gerson Therapy took longer. Patients not pretreated with such drugs respond extremely well and fast to the Gerson program and its restoration of the immune system. Since RA is aggravated, if not caused, by the excessive consumption of animal protein, the protein-restricted Gerson Therapy produces an immediate reduction of swelling, the easing or total elimination of pain and the start of healing. In time, patients recover completely.

Case History

In 1970, D. P. was a high school athlete of great promise. Her trainer suggested that she drink a lot of milk to strengthen her muscles and supply calcium. Within a year, before her 20th birthday, she developed RA, with swollen and inflamed joints, lumps and calcifications. Orthodox treatment with prednisone and gold proved to be ineffective; by 1976, D. P. was bedfast, suffering constant pain.

All her joints were stiff: fingers, knuckles, wrists, elbows, knees and ankles. In addition, she suffered from heart palpitations and labored breathing. She was pale, anemic and hypoglycemic and could barely walk or sleep. In May 1979, D. P. arrived at the Gerson hospital; in six weeks, she was virtually free from pain, most of the lumps in her joints were dissolving and her wrists started to regain their mobility. By 1981, two years after starting on the Gerson protocol, she was able to water ski, got married and started a family.

Scleroderma

This third member of the group of collagen diseases is also considered an autoimmune disease.[27] Scleroderma causes a chronic hardening and contraction of the skin and connective tissues, which makes movement such as bending, especially of the fingers, difficult if not impossible. The disease can eventually spread to internal organs as well. Despite its apparent hopelessness, this condition also improves rapidly on the Gerson program, which can lead to complete recovery.

Assorted Enemies of Health

In this section, we present a variety of very different conditions and complaints that blight the lives of vast numbers of people in the developed world. They represent only a tiny part of the grand total of hundreds of chronic conditions that are erroneously accepted as inevitable and incurable. Despite their surprisingly varied nature, these enemies of health have one thing in common: they originate in faulty nutrition and therefore respond positively to the Gerson protocol.

Asthma

Asthma, an inflammatory disorder of the airways, is widespread and growing more frequent all the time. An estimated 25 million Americans of all age groups suffer from it.[28] In an asthma attack, the muscles surrounding the airways tighten up; at the same time, the lining of the air passages swell. As a result, less air can pass in and out, causing wheezing, shortness of breath and/or coughing. Attacks can last from a few minutes to a whole day or more. They can become dangerous, cause anxiety and even bring on feelings of panic to the sufferer.

Asthma has many causes. General pollution in the atmosphere, pollen, dust mites and indoor molds are among them; however, food allergies and intolerance and adverse reactions to drugs can be the main culprits. Asthma also has a strong psychosomatic connection, especially in young children in whom it often clears up spontaneously when the emotional roots are eliminated. Here, we are only concerned with the physical-nutritional aspects.

When these aspects are at fault, asthma—especially in the case of children—is easily cured with a relatively minimal change of diet and lifestyle. For any age group, the best-known potential triggers of an attack—namely cheese, chocolate, citrus fruits and wheat—must be eliminated one by one in order to see which one has to be excluded for good. For children, it is essential to omit all milk and milk products. This flies in the face of conventional medical advice as mothers discover when they consult their pediatrician about their child's asthma. They are told to make sure that the child gets adequate milk, which is essential for growth and development; yet, over many months, even years, the prescribed medications are unable to cure the condition. However, it disappears readily if milk is excluded from the child's diet.

In adults, recovery takes a little longer since, as a rule, having been treated with drugs and inhalants for years, they have suffered more severe damage. Therefore, instead of just dropping a few food items, they need to follow the less intensive form of the Gerson Therapy, which excludes animal proteins. Asthma is curable irrespective of age with one warning: If the patient has been treated for a long time with prednisone, healing becomes difficult. In many other diseases, long-term treatment with prednisone produces the same degree of excessive damage and takes longer to overcome.

Case History

D. B.'s story, as recalled by her mother, started when she was six months old and suffered her first asthma attack. By her second birthday, she had an attack every two months, each one lasting seven days. The little girl was tested for 40 different allergens, then given drugs and immune shots every three weeks. This regimen went on for six years. The shots made her sick. Her arms swelled up and her eyes became puffy. Later, her mother discovered that the drugs her daughter was taking caused liver damage. When she asked her doctor about this, he declared that, in view of the severity of D. B.'s asthma, the liver damage caused by the drugs was the lesser evil.

Searching for a better answer, D. B.'s mother accidentally found out that nutrition could have something to do with her daughter's problem. She found out about the Gerson Therapy when D. B. was nine years old and changed the entire family's eating habits. Although D. B. did not take coffee enemas, she adopted the complete Gerson dietary approach and never had another asthma attack. She is now 38 years old, able to have a golden retriever and play with it without any allergic or asthma attacks.

Allergies and Food Intolerance

According to one authoritative definition,[29] allergies are acquired or inherited abnormal immune responses to a substance (allergen) that does not normally cause a reaction. These reactions do not always occur after the first exposure and may need a second or later occasion to be triggered. Allergens can be, for example, foodstuffs, pollen, house dust, detergents, indoor mold or household chemicals. They cause a wide variety of symptoms ranging from skin redness, itching, swelling of the tongue and throat to difficulty in breathing, diarrhea, abdominal cramps and vomiting. The most severe reaction to a food allergen—anaphylactic shock—is sudden, intense and potentially fatal, involving various parts of the organism and needing immediate medical help.

Food intolerance is a much milder reaction to certain edible substances. It does not involve the immune system and its symptoms are limited to gas, bloating and abdominal pain. The obvious answer to this and to stronger food allergies is to monitor the body's reactions and avoid the harmful substances.

Probably due to the increased all-around pollution and the malfunctioning immune system of the general population, allergies of all kinds are more widespread than ever. According to one estimate, one in four Americans are affected by some kind of allergy[30] and more than 50 million Americans are believed to have nasal allergies.[31] Orthodox medicine treats allergies with symptom-suppressing drugs, which may bring relief but invariably have undesirable side effects.

By contrast, Gerson patients generally overcome most of their food allergies on the pure organic foods they consume. The improvement often arrives surprisingly quickly. For instance, one patient's severe allergy to carrots disappeared in one day. Another person's allergy to onions ended within the first week of treatment. On the other hand, hard-to-digest foods, which are actually forbidden for Gerson patients (e.g., seafood, soy, milk, nuts and peanuts) would continue to cause them allergic reactions.

Many patients who suffer from migraines—which they believe are of allergic origin—find almost immediate and lasting relief after starting the therapy. Even intractable allergic reactions to inhaled items, such as pollen or certain smells, are reduced by the therapy; in some cases, they even cease for good. Although Dr. Gerson banned the consumption of berries at the start of the treatment, since they often cause allergic reactions, after 18 to 24 months on the protocol, patients may eat them without suffering adverse reactions.

Addiction

Addictions of all kinds are the plague of our times. They come in many forms and, if they persist, invariably lead to ill health and even death. People become addicted for many reasons. The young start experimenting with street drugs because it's trendy. Others try to soften their psychological/emotional problems by getting drunk or taking hard drugs. Indeed, people can become addicted to almost any substance, such as alcohol, tobacco, sleeping pills, sugar, milk, tranquilizers, painkillers, prescription drugs and, of course, food—the major addiction behind the alarming spread of obesity. Apart from all other factors, most addictions are caused—or at least aggravated—by nutritional deficiency. The body actually craves nutrients, not drugs or drink, and certainly not junk food. The addict does not realize this and keeps consuming the wrong substance, leading to ever-stronger craving.

In the many cases of addiction we have seen, the newly arrived patient, on being given an hourly glass of freshly pressed organic juice, loses the craving almost immediately. However, withdrawal symptoms may appear almost at once, since the body is now able to release the large amount of toxic residues it has stored for a long time. These are carried to the liver via the bloodstream and must be eliminated.

The coffee enema fulfils that task very efficiently, so much so that addiction—even to the heaviest street drugs and the ensuing withdrawal symptoms—has been overcome on the Gerson Therapy in as little as three days. Medical morphine, administered in some cases of severe pain for many months, takes longer to clear.

Case History

Some nine years ago, E. H., a young man aged 34, was admitted to the Gerson clinic in Mexico. He told a sad story: All his friends who had been using street drugs were dead. He was aware of displaying ominous symptoms himself and frankly believed that, if the Gerson treatment could not help him, he would also be dead in about three months' time. E. H. was not only heavily addicted to cocaine, he was also a heavy smoker. The combination of those two poisons caused him severe breathing difficulties and chest pain.

As in most cases of substance addiction, E. H. was terrified of withdrawal symptoms. Indeed, these are sometimes almost unbearable if the patients are unable to get their "fix." Fortunately, tackling drug addiction by the Gerson method makes it possible to more easily deal with withdrawal symptoms. As E. H. was receiving his 13 glasses of freshly prepared organic juices, he immediately noticed that his cravings were almost completely gone. When the withdrawal symptoms quickly set in, he also realized that the coffee enemas dealt with them very well. As a result, he enjoyed very good days, filled with fresh nutrients that overcame all cravings and coffee enemas that cleared withdrawal symptoms.

However, the nights were a different matter. The last juice arrives around 7 p.m. and the last enema is usually taken around 10 p.m., after which the patient goes to sleep, which means that, for some eight hours, his body receives no support. Sure enough, E. H. was wakened by very heavy nightmares some four hours after retiring. The toxins were pouring into his system without anything to control and evacuate them. In such cases, as E. H. was told, a coffee enema has to be taken in the middle of the night. He was provided with some fruit in order to replenish his blood sugar and a little herb tea for fluid, and he took a coffee enema around 3 a.m. This cleared the toxins and E. H. was able to enjoy a dreamless sleep until the morning.

This night-time routine continued for three or four nights, after which the withdrawal symptoms were cleared during the day and the patient's nights were undisturbed. The real problem for recovered addicts like E. H. is their return home. If his regular home life is peopled by friends or relatives who continue to use addictive substances, it's easy for him to relapse and undo all the good work of the Gerson Therapy.

Hyperactivity

Attention deficit hyperactivity disorder (ADHD) is in the news these days. It refers to children who show disturbed, hard-to-manage behavior: constant overactivity, lack of concentration, aggression, impulsiveness and distractibility. In the official view,[32] it could be caused by central nervous system dysfunction—a debatable opinion.

Over 30 years ago, Benjamin Feingold, MD,[33] developed a dietary treatment for this condition, which is in strong sympathy with the Gerson principles. He excluded all artificial flavors and colors, all preservatives, some kinds of sugars, yeast and salicylates, and prescribed instead fresh, preferably organic foods. His method attracted enthusiastic support and sharp criticism, the latter mainly from the food industry.[34]

Since then, many naturopaths and nutritionists have had good results, treating ADHD children by simply changing their diet to wholesome organic food, excluding all additives. Unfortunately, orthodox physicians, who are unfamiliar with dietary principles, prescribe hyperactive youngsters the drug Ritalin, a highly addictive substance closely resembling cocaine. Not surprisingly, the side effects, including permanent brain damage,[35] are dire. The drug is prescribed even for children younger than six years old, sometimes on the say-so of a nurse who considers the child "ill behaved" and wants to keep him or her quiet and obedient—in fact, zombie-like.

It is a terrifying fact that nearly nine million American children are drugged with Ritalin[36] and the number is rising. Mothers are grateful for Ritalin, which eliminates their children's destructiveness and aggression, since they don't understand the true—nutritional—cause of such behavior and therefore don't know how to deal with it sensibly and effectively. Their pediatricians also don't know how to advise them correctly; they are only trained in the use of drugs.

Even the mildest form of the Gerson protocol puts an end to ADHD in no time at all.

Depression

All over the developed world, depression is rapidly becoming a major mental health problem, causing much suffering and incapacity, loss of earnings, plus growing expenditure on treatment, mainly by drugs. According to the WHO,[37] by 2020, clinical depression will become the second leading cause of disability worldwide. Alarmingly enough, already now more and more children and adolescents become depressed; many of them react by developing eating disorders or committing self-harm.

We need to differentiate between two kinds of depression—one caused by psychological factors and the other by physical factors—although they often affect each other. Human life has never been free from problems and difficulties and the resulting depression needs to be alleviated by professional psychological help and support. (Ways to deal with depression caused by a cancer diagnosis are described in Chapter 24, "Psychological Support for the Gerson Patient," p. 251.)

Here we are concerned with the physical basis of depression, turning our spotlight on the brain. Clearly, our thinking, outlook, feeling reactions, handling of daily problems, as well as control of movement, physical coordination and many more vital activities are directly related to the brain. Thus, its function is basic and depends on the health and correct working of the brain cells. Although it is a relatively small organ compared to the total body mass, the brain uses up some two-fifths of the body's intake of oxygen and one-fifth of its blood supply. We may safely assume that it also requires a large amount of nutrients—vitamins, minerals and enzymes—to perform its incredibly complex tasks. Since the so-called normal American diet is chronically short of such nutrients, obviously the brain's needs are not fulfilled. Yet, as part of the central nervous system, the brain's tissues are so specialized that, unlike the tissues of other organs, most of them are unable to regrow (i.e., reproduce themselves).

It follows that, if the brain cells are inadequately nourished, they cannot function properly, their fragile balance is disturbed and certain mental disturbances occur. These include bipolar disorder, schizophrenia, insomnia, chronic anxiety and, above all, depression. Most of these conditions have been alleviated by up to 90% by vitamin (inositol) treatment.[38]

Double Nobel Laureate Linus Pauling[39] has also stated that 60% of schizophrenics treated with megavitamins either improved or had complete relief of symptoms. Abram Hoffer, MD,[40] first discovered that niacin (vitamin B_3) lowered cholesterol, and that excess cholesterol was a contributory factor in schizophrenia. He was able to restore thousands of schizophrenics to normalcy by treating them with megadoses of niacin and ascorbic acid (vitamin C).

Under normal circumstances, the brain is protected from the penetration of toxins (poisons) by the blood-brain barrier (BBB), a membrane that controls the passage of substances from the blood into the brain. The BBB can be damaged and broken down by microwaves, radiation, hypertension (high blood pressure), infection and, most importantly, by severe toxicity of the organism, which stops the barrier from blocking the penetration of poisons into the brain. Hence, the vicious circle of inadequate nutrition and toxicity spins on and depression and other kinds of mental ill health set in.

The recent development of drugs to relieve the condition is almost as bad as the proliferation of clinical depression. These highly toxic drugs are prescribed even for young children, although the well-known side effects include severe worsening of the depression to the point of suicide or homicide.[41] By way of contrast, the standard Gerson treatment is able to alleviate the depression fairly quickly, even in patients who have already undergone drug treatment and are suffering from their side effects. The therapy's detoxifying coffee enemas, and the flooding of all body tissues, including the brain, with the needed nutrients, is the quickest and safest way to relieve depression.

Case History

Some eight years ago, as Charlotte Gerson was traveling all over the U.S., giving lectures to numerous groups, she stayed at a charming little motel. The manager, P. B., was interested in her work and, in the course of their conversation, told her that he was suffering from severe clinical depression, controlling the condition with prescription drugs. He also admitted that he had been in Viet Nam and had been exposed to "Agent Orange."

When Charlotte told him more about the nutritional approach to healing, P. B., aged around 50, purchased the Gerson publications and began to follow the therapy on his own at home the best he could. In December 2006, he reported that he had recovered, was able to discontinue all medical drugs, felt very well since he no longer suffered the side effects of those drugs and led a normal, active life.

Crohn's Disease

The medical term for Crohn's disease is regional ileitis. It is a chronic inflammation of the lower two-thirds of the small intestine (the ileum) and, as a rule, alternates between periods of aggravation and remission. The patient suffers from diarrhea, abdominal pain, weight loss, anemia and, eventually and often after several years, intestinal obstruction. According to *Taber's Cyclopedic Medical Dictionary,* "the cause is unknown."[42] As orthodox medicine has no cure for this condition, the final outcome is usually surgery, removing part of the small intestine or part or the entire large intestine and installing an ileostomy or colostomy bag.

Case History

M. G. was only 15 when she was diagnosed with Crohn's disease. She spent much of that year commuting between her home and General Hospital in Sault Ste. Marie, Ontario, Canada, missing much of her schooling. Several times when visiting the hospital, she was on the verge of developing bowel obstruction; unable to absorb her food, she weighed only 78 pounds. Her physicians suggested surgery but this was refused. Just in time, her family discovered the Gerson Therapy and the young girl started on it at home. Although her bowel was nearly obstructed, the coffee enemas brought immediate relief and she no longer needed to visit the hospital. After three months, the pain was gone and her energy had returned; within one year, she gained 26 pounds and was able to attend school regularly. She remains well and at present is studying medicine.

Migraine

Migraines are described as frequently unilateral (one-sided) paroxysmal (sudden, severe) attacks of headache. The sharp, throbbing pain is normally accompanied by hypersensitivity to light and sounds, nausea and/or vomiting; attacks are recurring and can last from four to 72 hours. Migraines are extremely common: nearly 30 million Americans are regular sufferers[43] Medical treatment is limited to pain-relieving drugs, sometimes as powerful as morphine, with various undesirable side effects. For instance, one of the most commonly prescribed American drugs was recently found to boost the risk of excessive acidity in the blood, leading to the formation of kidney stones.[44]

Migraines can be caused by a number of factors. Some are due to dental problems, such as a poorly aligned bite or muscle imbalance in the jaw. In other cases, the cause is a blockage or a minute dislocation in the spine or neck, which needs to be corrected by expert chiropractic treatment. The overwhelming majority of migraines are caused by allergies or intolerance to certain foods. The most frequently identified "usual suspects" are cheese, chocolate and citrus fruits.

As a young doctor, Max Gerson often suffered from severely debilitating migraines. After experimenting with various diets, he discovered that his problem was caused by toxic foodstuffs, mostly salty and heavily spiced meats. In order to heal, he developed a salt-free, low-fat vegetarian diet that became the basis of his nutritional protocol. After further refinements and improvements, this gave birth to the Gerson Therapy, used worldwide to this day to heal the vast majority of chronic degenerative diseases. Many patients who embark on the Gerson program rapidly recover from their long-standing migraines and remain pain-free unless they revert to the foods that sparked their attacks in the past.

Endometriosis

The endometrium is the mucous membrane lining the uterus. During the fertile years of a woman, this lining is shed every month if the secreted ovum is not fertilized and implanted in the tissue. When the organism or the hormone system is malfunctioning, the endometrium can spread to various sites throughout the pelvic area, including the abdominal wall. As the condition worsens and the menstrual cycle does not become regulated, endometrial tissue may spread throughout the body, becoming a malignancy "resembling metastatic pelvic carcinoma."[45]

Case History

The case of S. T. illustrates this progression perfectly. This patient had gynecological problems at the very start of her menstrual periods. Thirty-five years later, she was diagnosed with endometriosis and had a number of D and C (dilatation and curettage, or scraping of the uterus) procedures to remove endometrial plaque. In the end, she had a partial hysterectomy, yet her problems continued. In 1979, a Pap smear showed cancer of the cervix with "atypical" (irregular, not conforming to the normal) cells in her blood. She also noticed lumps in her breast but these were not further investigated. A hysterectomy was arranged for her, but she declined the operation and changed her diet. Some time before, she had heard a lecture by Charlotte Gerson and had decided at the time that, if any of her family members developed cancer, they would embark on the Gerson Therapy. S. T. stayed on the strict therapy for two years. She was cured and remains fit and well, leading a busy life.

Morbid Obesity

This condition is defined as "obesity of such degree as to interfere with normal activities, including respiration."[46] Weight in excess of 100 pounds above the normal average for the individual's age, sex and build is considered "morbid." Not so long ago, excessively fat people drew curious or critical glances in the street. These days, there are too many of them to receive attention. The rapid worldwide spread of fast-food outlets and the exponentially growing sales of convenience foods have sparked a global epidemic of dangerous obesity in all age groups.

On March 10, 2004, it was repeatedly announced on the radio (KNX-1070 AM in Los Angeles) that the Centers for Disease Control in Atlanta has upgraded obesity in the U.S. as the #1 preventable cause of disease, displacing cigarettes from that position.

The word "morbid" means "of the nature of or indicative of disease" and, indeed, the medical dictionary quotes obesity as a contributing factor to the following diseases: diabetes mellitus (type 2), hypertension and some types of cancer.[47] At the time of the publication of the dictionary (1993), it was estimated that 34 million adults in the U.S. were overweight.[48] A more recent statement (2001) by the Center for Science in the Public Interest[49] declared that almost two-thirds of American adults are overweight. The 1980 figures for obesity have doubled by 2001[50]; diabetes mellitus has increased ninefold since 1958,[51] and heart disease remains the #1 disease cause of death.[52]

Worst of all, obesity has become widespread among children. Fat kids are referred to as "small fries: the offspring of couch potatoes." Between 1980 and 1994, obesity in American children increased by 100%[53]; currently, one in four children is obese, as reported by Frank Booth and Donna Krupa.[54] Lack of exercise is an important contributory factor to this tragic state of affairs, since—according to the above authors—the average child spends 900 hours a year in school and 1,023 hours watching television. Childhood obesity is particularly dangerous since the child's developing organism is less able to deal with the many complications of gross overweight than that of an adult. Several British researchers have stated that, for the first time in human history, it will be normal for parents to outlive their offspring.[55]

A hugely successful recent movie, produced by Morgan Spurlock and called "Super Size Me," unveiled the truth about the destructive effects of fast food. Spurlock, a healthy 33-year-old man, ate all of his meals at

McDonald's for 30 days to find out what this exclusive diet would do to him. Throughout the experiment, he was regularly examined by gastro-enterologist Dr. Daryl Isaacs, who declared that Spurlock was "an extremely healthy person who got very sick eating this McDonald's diet."[56] At one stage, the doctor even told Morgan Spurlock that his liver had turned into paté and asked him to stop his experiment, but the moviemaker persisted. At the end of the month, Spurlock reported, "I got desperately ill. My face was splotchy and I had this huge gut. [He gained 25 pounds in 30 days.] My knees started to hurt from the extra weight coming on so quickly. It was amazing and frightening."[57] On top of it all, his liver became toxic, his cholesterol shot up from a low 165 to 230, his libido flagged and he suffered from headaches and depression. Within a few days of beginning his "drive-through diet," Spurlock was vomiting out the window of his car, and doctors who examined him were shocked by how rapidly his entire body deteriorated.

Mothers cannot be solely blamed for their children's faulty nutrition and inactivity. Very few mothers receive any nutritional guidance from their pediatrician, who doesn't know much about nutrition either. All they have learned in medical school boils down to the usual "protein, carbohydrates and fats" doctrine, making them unable to recognize the harm done by the children's favorite foods. For instance, the animal products used in fast foods are heat-damaged, poorly assimilated, too high in cholesterol and salt, but deficient in true nutrients—vitamins, minerals and enzymes. As a result, they don't satisfy hunger and a vicious circle is created, leading to overfed but undernourished children. If a child asks for more food after a complete meal, the parent's instinctive reaction is to dish out an extra portion; they don't realize that no additional amount of food will make up for the missing essential nutrients.

The average American diet leaves children hungry and with low energy, so they spend a lot of their free time lounging around, doing nothing. To make up for their low energy, they start to "look for something"; unfortunately, they find it in cola drinks containing caffeine and sugar stimulants, cigarettes full of toxic substances and eventually alcohol and street drugs, giving a brief "high" and leading to addiction.

The same vicious circle affects adults, too. Since the conventional American diet is devoid of live nutrients, the body remains unsatisfied and craves more—not quantity but quality, proper nutrition that it needs to function smoothly and well. Sadly, people don't know or understand this, and they try to satisfy their craving with rich desserts, ice cream, cakes and cookies. These don't satisfy, either, but they do create weight gain, high cholesterol, high blood pressure and eventually diabetes and worse. Obesity is a morbid condition indeed, and can only be overcome by changing to a junk-free, nutrient-rich, plant-based diet.

One doesn't need a degree in nutrition to know that all kinds of sugar are fattening and that the modern Western diet, with its vast range of convenience foods, is over-rich in sugar. However, when it comes to official policy concerning nutrition, such basic facts are often swept aside for commercial reasons, which frequently clash with the interests of public health. One such recent clash concerned the upper safe limit of sugar added to food, as recommended by the WHO. Professor T. Colin Campbell[58] reported on this event in his book, *The China Study* and, with his permission, we quote his account:

"The recommendation on added sugar is as outrageous as the one for protein. When this FNB (Food and Nutrition Board) report was being released, an expert panel put together by the WHO (World Health Organization) and the FAO (Food and Agriculture Organization) was completing a new report on diet, nutrition and the prevention of chronic diseases. Professor Philip James was a member of this panel and a panel spokesperson on the added sugar recommendation. Early rumors of the report's findings indicated that the WHO/FAO was on the verge of recommending an upper safe limit of 10% for added sugar, far lower than the 25% established by the American FNB group. … Politics, however, had early entered the discussion, as it had done in earlier reports on added sugars. According to a news release from the director-general's office at the WHO, the US-based Sugar Association and the World Sugar Research Organization, who 'represent the interests of the sugar growers and refiners, had mounted a strong lobbying campaign in an attempt to discredit the WHO report and suppress its release.' ... According to *The Guardian* newspaper of London, the US sugar industry was threatening to 'bring the WHO to its knees' unless it abandoned these guidelines on added sugar. WHO people were describing the threat as 'tantamount to blackmail.' The US-based group even publicly threatened to lobby the US Congress to reduce the $406 million US funding of the WHO if it persisted in keeping the upper limit so low at 10%. There were reports ... that the Bush administration was inclined to side with the sugar industry. ... So, for added sugars, we now have two different upper 'safe' limits: a 10% limit for the international community and a 25% limit for the US."

This is Professor Campbell's wry conclusion. Clearly, despite official claims, the obesity epidemic hitting the American people is not solely the result of insufficient exercise!

Osteoporosis

Also known as "brittle bones," this progressive loss of bone mass is unfortunately becoming very common. It causes fractures or breaks at the slightest impact, such as a fall or other accident. Fractures are immensely painful and heal slowly—or, in old people, not at all. A serious break, necessitating weeks of bed rest, can lead to infected bedsores and other potentially fatal complications.

More women than men suffer from osteoporosis, so it is assumed to be caused by aging, postmenopausal loss of the female sex hormone estrogen, lack of exercise and smoking. However, we have seen a young man, aged 28, suffering from this condition! The conventional medical treatment prescribes female hormones, vitamin D and regular exercise. The best that these can achieve is to slow down the disease process, not reverse it. Moreover, female sex hormones can cause cancer of the breast, the ovaries or the uterus; the body is unable to utilize the calcium and the synthetic vitamin D. Clearly, this treatment does not restore bone mass.

In the course of worldwide research, it was found that women in Southeast Asia, who regularly bear six to eight children and nurse them all, do not suffer from osteoporosis. In fact, it is virtually unknown in those parts. Referring to this fact, the Physicians Committee for Responsible Medicine (PCRM) reports, "The average calcium intake in Singapore is 389 mg/day, less than half of the recommended daily allowance in the U.S. Yet the fracture rate in Singapore is five times lower than that of the U.S., where the calcium intake is much higher."[59] Further on, the report comments: "Dietary and lifestyle factors that encourage the loss of calcium include: animal protein, sodium, caffeine, phosphorus, tobacco and sedentary lifestyle."[60] In one study, it was found that "eliminating meat from the diet cuts the urinary calcium losses in half."[61] Also, "cutting sodium intake by half can reduce calcium requirements by 160 milligrams per day. Avoiding tobacco has demonstrable effects: smokers have 10% weaker bones than non-smokers."[62]

Despite clear scientific proof[63] that calcium is not the answer to osteoporosis, in January 1997, a new advertising campaign promoting milk consumption was launched, sponsored by the National Fluid Milk Processor Promotion Board. Among other things, the publicity claimed, "With calcium galore, milk is one of the best things around."[64] The ads featured female or male celebrities sporting the new "celebrity milk moustache." The PCRM lodged a complaint with the Federal Trade Commission in Washington, D.C., pointing out that, "Increasing milk consumption is one of the weakest possible strategies for protecting the bones, and to suggest otherwise is dangerously misleading."[65]

The PCRM also stated that, since calcium was needed in the diet, the kind provided by green vegetables appeared to be of greater bioavailability (was better assimilated) than the calcium found in milk. To underline their claim, they added: "Excessive calcium intake does not fool hormones into building much more bone, any more than delivery of an extra load of bricks will make a construction crew build a larger building."[66]

As the evidence accumulates, it becomes increasingly clear that osteoporosis, like so many chronic degenerative complaints, is largely the result of wrong eating habits. Further confirmation comes from best-selling author John Robbins, considered to be a world-class expert on the dietary link with the environment and health. He writes, "One long-term study found that with as little as 75 grams of daily protein (less than three quarters of what the average meat-eating American consumes), more calcium is lost in the urine than is absorbed by the body, establishing from the diet a negative calcium balance."[67]

Every study came up with the same result: the more protein was taken in, the more calcium was lost. John McDougall, MD, one of the nation's leading medical authorities on dietary association with disease, adds: "I would like to emphasize that the calcium-losing effect of protein on the human body is not an area of controversy in scientific circles. The many studies performed during the past 55 years consistently show that the most important dietary change that we can make if we want to create a positive calcium balance that will keep our bones solid, is to decrease the amount of protein we eat each day."[68]

All the above serves as more proof that the Gerson Therapy not only maintains the calcium balance of the body but that it is also able to reverse osteoporosis by restricting animal protein, salt and smoking, while flooding the body with calcium from vegetable sources, along with the proper enzymes to lodge this calcium in the bones. In fact, in numerous patients, bone mass has been increased and the discomfort or pain of osteoporosis has been cleared.

Case History

After stumbling and falling on an uneven pavement, long-term recovered Gerson patient A. C. was sent for an x-ray by her doctor to check whether her hip had been fractured. The hip turned out to be unharmed but osteoporosis was discovered in three places in the spine. The woman doctor, who gave the patient the bad news, offered her a supply of painkillers, which she refused on the grounds of feeling no pain. Instead, she got in touch with Charlotte Gerson, who advised her to drink a liter of freshly made carrot and apple juice and eat some green leaf every day, in addition to her Gerson maintenance routine. Charlotte added, "If those guys tell you that osteoporosis is irreversible, don't believe them."

A. C. did as she was told. Six months later, at her request, her doctor arranged another x-ray, which proved that the condition had not worsened and, in fact, showed considerable improvement. The woman doctor gave her the good news, without expressing any surprise or interest in this unusual development, and offered the patient a supply of painkillers although she had no pain. Some 15 years have elapsed since this incident and, although A. C. is now in her 80s, she isn't showing any sign of osteoporosis.

Teeth

It is a sad fact that the concept of totality, or holism, is poorly understood and not applied to dental health, although teeth are an integral part of the body and can powerfully influence its general condition. Rarely do physicians consider checking the teeth of the patient who presents with various problems, perhaps a tendency to infection, a weakness or some other malfunction of the metabolism that is difficult to diagnose. The reason for this omission is that teeth belong to a totally different area of medicine with which a physician is not concerned.

It is a serious mistake to ignore teeth; worse still, it can become a terrible mistake to treat them incorrectly. Only a few years ago, the dental profession became aware of the problems caused by root canal treatment. This came about because George Meinig, former head of the Root Canal Society, was reading a book written some hundred years ago by Weston Price,[69] and began to understand that it was a grave mistake to drill into root canals, try to clear them, refill the now empty space and assume that this has taken care of the problem.

In his book, Dr. Price relates that he was asked to treat the tooth of a lady who was bedfast with RA throughout her body. He removed the previously root canal-filled offending tooth, cleaned and sterilized it and implanted it under the skin of a rabbit. In five days, the rabbit developed severe RA; in 10 days, the disease killed it. Meanwhile, the patient started to feel better, was able to get up, lost much of her pain and swelling and eventually recovered.

Dr. Price was impressed by this development and decided to research it further. Whenever he removed a damaged tooth, he proceeded in the same way to sterilize and implant it under the skin of a rabbit. To his amazement, whatever disease the patient had suffered from showed up in the rabbit within five days and killed it in 10. This happened dozens, even hundreds, of times with teeth removed from patients suffering from kidney disease, heart disease and other problems. Dr. Price then carried out two more experiments. In one, he implanted a tooth lost by accident from a healthy person under the skin of a rabbit and noted that the rabbit remained healthy and eventually survived for 15 years. Next, he took a tooth from a diseased patient and autoclaved it (i.e., exposed it to steam pressure at 250° F (121° C)). It made no difference: the rabbit still died of the patient's disease.

Having understood the biochemical damage inflicted on the whole body by treating root canals with fillings, George Meinig resigned from the Root Canal Society and wrote a book titled *The Root Canal Cover-Up*,[70] exposing the facts originally discovered and recorded by Price.

Dr. Meinig explains that there are two factors behind the actual damage caused by root canal fillings. One is that removing the nerve of a tooth leaves that tooth dead. No nutrients can enter it via the canules (the equivalent of capillaries in other tissues) nor can metabolic residues be released from it. The second factor occurs due to the fact that the now-empty canules fill with germs and viruses, which then penetrate the jawbone and can in time cause severe infectious bone damage. Toxins from these infections are released into the bloodstream, causing an almost permanent poisoning.

Unfortunately, even deep bone infections with resulting cavitations (hollowed-out bone) do not cause pain, so that frequently the patient is not aware of having a problem. Even a standard dental x-ray doesn't show the bone damage; only the new "panoramic" dental x-rays are able to do that. The only solution is to remove the offending tooth and clear infectious material from the cavitation, which allows the hollowed-out bone to heal.

If a dentist discovers an abscess at the tip of the root of a tooth, he or she will urge the patient to have a root canal treatment done. Do not agree to this procedure. The filling used in the canal eventually shrinks a tiny bit also, allowing germs and viruses to enter, which become conduits for the invaders, causing much trouble. The dentist will assure you that the filling material currently used in the root canal doesn't shrink. However, even if this were true, there remains the problem of the dead tooth, the germ-filled canules and a constant focus of infection active within the organism. Rather than having the root canal treated, regretfully that tooth has to be extracted.

Beside root canals, there are many other dental problems, such as receding gums, gum infections and cavities, which are easily detected and corrected. These should be cleared so that no oral infections can interfere with the healing process. Once we have understood the unbreakable unity of the organism, it becomes clear how an unresolved and ignored dental problem can cause serious damage in some other part of the body.

Mercury fillings should never be used. There is much information and research material[71] proving the damage caused by releasing small amounts of mercury into the system by chewing, drinking and swallowing. These small but continuously released amounts of what is a potent nerve toxin are also absorbed by the lungs and the linings of the digestive system into the bloodstream, leading to severe harm. Despite the mass of scientific research material confirming this risk, some dentists and the American Dental Association vociferously claim that mercury is perfectly safe once installed in the tooth.[72] It is not. These days, there are various minimally toxic inert filling materials available to deal with cavities.

Crowns are another problem. A crown must never be fitted over a mercury filling nor should gold be used if there is any mercury—also known as silver amalgam—present in other parts of the mouth. Between those two metals, a tiny, mild electric current is generated, which is capable of interfering with the enzymes and other factors of predigestion that are active in the mouth. If a crown is necessary, it should be made from other materials, such as plastic or porcelain.

Dental anesthesia needs to be handled with care. When the body is well detoxified, it becomes more sensitive to any toxins, including anesthesia used by dentists to overcome the pain of dental work. It is extremely important that a Gerson patient should tell his or her dentist the following, prior to the use of anesthesia drugs:

- Use no more than one-third to one-half of the normal dose.
- Use no epinephrine in compounding the drug.
- Start the treatment immediately (the effect wears off quickly).

Upon returning from the dentist's office, the patient should take a coffee enema, whether or not one is scheduled for that time. Any additional pain is likely to be cleared by another coffee enema.

Note: If the dentist advises the patient to take a dose of antibiotics, this must not be refused. A dental infection can be very serious and even become life-threatening.

Case Histories

We have several patient reports of dramatic improvements after the removal of root canal-treated teeth. One breast cancer patient using the Gerson Therapy was making slow progress. When her husband began to suspect some dental problem slowing down the healing process, he had her examined by a dentist. Indeed, a cavitation was found and cleared and the infected tooth removed. Subsequently, the remaining breast tumor tissue was rapidly absorbed, and she recovered and remained well for many years.

In another case, a young woman, married to an athlete and hoping for children, conceived readily but suffered three miscarriages in a row. A full examination of her teeth disclosed a far advanced cavitation in her jawbone. When the offending tooth was extracted and the infection in her jawbone cleared up, shortly afterwards she had three normal pregnancies.

A father wrote to us to say that he was impressed by the report, published in the Gerson Institute's *Gerson Healing Newsletter*,[73] on the damage caused by root canal-treated teeth. It caused him to arrange a dental examination for his son who had been suffering from schizophrenia for several years without being helped by the drug treatment he had received. When the young man's teeth were checked and a root canal-filled tooth was removed, he gradually recovered and needed no further medication.

Fibromyalgia

Although this chronic condition is not life threatening, we include it here as another eloquent example of the many kinds of ill health caused by the toxic condition of the body. Fibromyalgia causes severe chronic pain in muscles and soft tissues surrounding joints. Efforts to control it with anti-inflammatories, including corticosteroids, have not been helpful, nor has any effective treatment been found for it so far. Pain-relieving drugs are used to help the patients sleep. According to the conservative estimate of the National Fibromyalgia Research Association, over six million people in the U.S. suffer from this disease.[74]

In our experience, fibromyalgia is basically a toxic condition caused by the combined impact of polluted air and water, poisonous chemical residues in agricultural produce and food additives used in processed foods. There comes a point where the body can no longer excrete these harmful substances. In order not to overload the liver and keep the toxins (enzyme inhibitors) from interfering with the functions of the essential organs, it releases them into the muscles and soft tissues. Once there, the toxic irritants cause pain, which eventually becomes almost unbearable.

Like all conditions resulting from a high degree of toxicity in the body, fibromyalgia yields very promptly to the organic, vegetarian, toxin-free diet of the Gerson Therapy, combined with intensive detoxification via the coffee enemas. We have seen some cases in which it took only a few days to ease and then banish the pain, enabling the patient to resume normal activity. In more advanced cases, aggravated by the use of many pain-relieving drugs, and with bedridden patients, it can take several weeks to obtain lasting pain relief and healing.

Case History

We recall with wry amusement the experience of a seriously ill, mostly bedridden, lady who arrived from Germany at the Gerson clinic in Mexico. She had suffered from fibromyalgia for several years and had eventually found the physician who was regarded as the top authority of that condition. However, that doctor was also suffering from an advanced case of fibromyalgia and was unable to help her. On the contrary, on one occasion, when she called him after a particularly painful, miserable night, he replied to her complaint by saying, "You're telling me!"

LIMITATIONS

It must be remembered that, despite its great healing potential in so many areas of ill health, the Gerson Therapy is no panacea, and there are conditions in which it can heal only partially or not at all. There are sound reasons why the otherwise high-powered twin Gerson methods of hyperalimentation and detoxification don't work under some circumstances. In this chapter, we set them out briefly in two sections: diseases difficult to cure with the Gerson Therapy and diseases not curable by the Gerson Therapy.

Diseases Difficult to Cure with the Gerson Therapy

Brain Cancer

We have seen total, long-term recoveries of brain cancer cases and failures. The problem is not the cancer itself but the location of the tumor.

In the course of a healing reaction, the body almost always produces an inflammation, which in itself is desirable, since inflammation fluid usually destroys tumor tissue. However, it also causes swelling in regular tissue. A brain tumor is enclosed within the skull where there is no room for such swelling to take place. Instead, the "healing inflammation" with its swelling causes serious pressure within the skull, and that is likely to bring on seizures. These have to be handled carefully, reducing the swelling to decrease the seizure activity, thus blocking the healing process. It is hard to find a middle way between allowing inflammation yet relieving severe headaches and seizures. Understandably, the dilemma also worries the patient. There have been several who gave up on the Gerson Therapy and returned to orthodox treatment.

Bone Metastases

Certain cancers can be counted on to produce metastases (spreading of malignancy) into specific tissues. Thus a majority of prostate and breast cancers, if they spread, are found to have migrated to the bone(s). Bone tissue is difficult to heal. While a regular tissue lesion, sewed up, can be relied on to heal within a week to 10 days, a bone fracture will take many weeks and often several months. As bone metastases are painful, the patient must remain determined and strong-minded, knowing that the healing will take a long time.

Open Breast Cancer Lesions

While Dr. Gerson warned that cancers within glands are more difficult to reach, breast cancer generally has responded well to the therapy over many years. The situation changes if and when the breast tumor breaks through the skin. Open lesions possibly leading to infections are much more difficult to heal and require the best possible care and much patience.

Leukemias

There are several kinds of chronic leukemia, usually of the age-onset type, which do not present special problems. However, the rapid-advance childhood leukemias must be stopped rapidly. This is far from easy. For various reasons, such as difficulty in administering the complete intensive Gerson Therapy, the child's resistance or other external problems, the effectiveness of the treatment is hampered and slowed down. When this happens, an acute leukemia can possibly advance too rapidly for the therapy to stop and reverse it.

Multiple Myeloma

Like leukemias, this condition does not belong in the class of solid tumors. It is a disease of the bone marrow, with myeloma cells "forming multiple tumor masses."[75] These infiltrate the surrounding bone—generally the blood-forming long bones of the upper leg—but other parts of the skeleton as well.

The disease occurs more frequently in men than in women by a ratio of 2:1.[76] Since it damages the blood-forming bone marrow, it causes anemia and renal (kidney) lesions. As explained above, it is always more difficult to heal bone lesions, and this applies to multiple myeloma as well. It takes longer and—according to Dr. Gerson's observations confirmed by the latest research[77] on this condition—requires more vitamin B_{12} than other kinds of cancer. Due to the invasion of bone by myeloma tissue, it is also possible for pathologic fractures (weakened bone breaking without external cause) to occur. On the Gerson Therapy, we have seen such fractures heal very slowly.

Long-term Prednisone Treatment and/or Chemotherapy

All drugs are toxic[78]; hence, long-term use causes severe liver damage. Prednisone, a powerful steroid routinely prescribed for multiple sclerosis, lupus, arthritis and many other conditions, depletes the body's defenses and causes considerable organ damage.[79] If this damage becomes excessive due to long-term use, it can be difficult or even impossible to truly heal (i.e., fully restore the liver and other essential organs).

Chemotherapy is much more toxic. While we have seen many reversals of chemo-treated patients' disease, beyond a certain point, the damage caused by powerful chemotherapy is no longer reversible. As a general rule, patients treated for lengthy periods with toxic drugs are more difficult to heal than those who were treated for only a short time or, preferably, not at all.

Diseases Not Curable by the Gerson Therapy

The list of chronic degenerative diseases that are curable by the Gerson Therapy includes hundreds of conditions. However, a very small number of diseases, mainly those affecting the central nervous system, do not respond well, or not at all, to the nutritional healing approach. It has to be understood that the central nervous system, comprising the brain and spinal cord, is so highly specialized that it does not replace lost tissue. For that reason, it is almost impossible to heal serious damage afflicting this area.

Amyotrophic Lateral Sclerosis

Amyotrophic lateral sclerosis (ALS) is also known as motor neuron disease, or popularly as Lou Gehrig's disease. While orthodox medicine considers its cause unknown, in our experience all affected patients had extensive exposure to pesticides. Interestingly, while we were able to obtain healthy young calves' livers and produce liver juice for the treatment of these patients, a number of them showed considerable improvement. Since liver juice is no longer safe, owing to widespread campylobacter infection, ALS patients have made little progress toward healing with the Gerson Therapy, although they deteriorate more slowly than they would without it. We consider that a failure.

Parkinson's Disease

Parkinson's disease (PD) belongs to a group of conditions called motor system disorders, which result from the loss of dopamine-producing brain cells. The four primary symptoms of PD are tremor, or trembling in hands, arms, legs, jaw and face; rigidity, or stiffness of the limbs and trunk; bradykinesia, or slowness of movement; and postural instability, or impaired balance and coordination. As these symptoms worsen, patients have difficulty walking, talking or completing simple tasks.

PD is also known as paralysis agitans, or popularly as "shaking palsy," and usually affects people over the age of 50. The allopathic treatment normally uses dopamines and several other drugs, which help the patient function for a while but do not cure the problem. The Gerson Therapy has also failed to produce a cure.

Alzheimer's Disease

Described as presenile dementia, this condition is caused by the atrophy (wasting) of the frontal and occipital (rear) lobes of the brain. According to *Taber's Cyclopedic Medical Dictionary*, it causes "progressive and irreversible deterioration of intellectual function, apathy, speech and gait disturbance, disorientation and loss of memory."[80] In many cases, it responds reasonably well to the Gerson Therapy, which alleviates and/ or much improves the most severe symptoms. However, only brain cells that are diseased or damaged can be improved and even restored. Those that are dead are gone, so the disease is not cured.

Chronic Kidney Disease

If this has advanced to the point of requiring dialysis, it cannot be reversed. The specific function of the kidneys is to remove the waste products of protein digestion (urea, uric acid and creatinine), as well as excess minerals (sodium and potassium) or other toxic substances from the blood, in order to maintain homeostasis of the system. This is done via a delicate filter system of structures, sacs, the glomeruli; if the latter lose their permeability through inflammation and excess toxins and can no longer function, disease sets in.

However, if disease has damaged kidney function by no more than 80%, and 20% is still active, the condition can be treated and patients can improve and survive. However, if kidney tissue, similar to brain tissue, is dead, it is gone. Therefore, the kidney patient whose condition has been improved on the Gerson protocol can never revert to a so-called normal, average diet. The price of survival is to remain on the Gerson program for life. In brief, kidney disease is treatable and can achieve long-term survival, but it is not curable. Once dialysis has been started, normally when kidney function drops below 10%, the patient should not attempt to go on the Gerson Therapy.

Emphysema

Emphysema is another disease that can be greatly alleviated but not cured. Also referred to as chronic obstructive pulmonary disease, emphysema causes changes in the structure of the air sacs that filter out carbon dioxide for secretion and allow oxygen to pass into the blood. Here, the lung tissue is severely damaged by smoking, air pollution toxins or inflammation, so that it loses its permeability and the exchange of gases is seriously inhibited. The sick tissue can be restored; dead tissue is gone. The patient can probably function normally with only about 50% of functioning lung tissue, but he or she cannot be fully restored.

Muscular Dystrophy

Thought to be a familial (genetic) disease, this condition causes progressive atrophy (wasting away) of muscles and usually starts in childhood, more frequently in boys than in girls. The underlying cause is described as "a disorder caused by defective nutrition or metabolism."[81] In Dr. Gerson's day, it responded favorably to his treatment, but more recently we have not seen good results and have to consider it incurable. In one case, diagnosed as Duchenne's Disease, which usually results in death at an early age, we have seen a more than 20-year-long survival.

TO SUM UP

The Gerson Therapy would be useless and could even cause harm to the following people who should not undertake it under any circumstance:

- Patients on dialysis (the high potassium diet of the Gerson Therapy makes dialysis impossible since it requires sodium)
- Patients with organ transplants (the therapy would cause a rejection)
- Patients with melanoma that has spread to the brain (the only case in which melanoma, eminently curable in any other body part, does not respond)
- Patients with pancreatic cancer if chemotherapy has been administered (pancreatic cancer is curable, but only if not pre-treated with chemotherapy)

REFERENCES

1. *Taber's Cyclopedic Medical Dictionary* (Philadelphia: F. A. Davis Company, 1993).
2. C. P. Rhoads, "Recent studies in the production of cancer by chemical compounds; the conditioned deficiency as a mechanism," *Bulletin of the New York Academy of Medicine* 18 (January 1942).
3. Thomas Thom, et al., "Heart Disease and Stroke Statistics—2006 Update: A Report From the American Heart Association Statistics Committee and Stroke Statistics Subcommittee, *Circulation* 113 (Jan. 11, 2006): 85-151.
4. Joseph M. Price, MD, *Coronaries/Cholesterol/Chlorine* (New York: Jove Books, 1969), p. 37.
5. "Coronary Heart Disease," *MSN Encarta* (http://encarta.msn.com/encyclopedia_1741575718/Coronary_Heart_Disease.html).
6. E. Calva, A. Mujica, R. Nunez, K. Aoki, A. Bisteni and Demetrio Sodi-Pallares, MD, "Mitochondrial biochemical changes and glucose-KCI-insulin solution in cardiac infarct," *American Journal of Physiology* 211 (1966): 71-76.
7. "Heart Attack Treatment Considered," Associated Press, *Bucks County Courier* (Nov. 25, 1998).
8. Ibid.

9. Ibid.

10. Lynn Fischer, W. Virgil Brown, *Lowfat Cooking For Dummies,* 1st ed. (Mississauga, Ontario: John Wiley & Sons Canada, Ltd., April 21, 1997), pp. 235-6.

11. Johanna Budwig, MD, *Flax Oil as a True Aid Against Arthritis, Heart Infarction, Cancer, and Other Diseases* (Vancouver, BC: Apple Publishing, 1994).

12. Lipitor® package insert, Pfizer Phamaceuticals.

13. Ibid.

14. Kash Rizvi, John P. Hampson and John N. Harvey, "Systematic Review: Do lipid-lowering drugs cause erectile dysfunction? A systematic review," *Family Practice* 19 (1) (2002): 95-98.

15. "Heart Disease and Stroke Statistics—2004 Update," American Heart Association (Jan. 1, 2004).

16. "National Diabetes Fact Sheet," Centers for Disease Control and Prevention (www.cdc.gov/diabetes/pubs/estimates.htm).

17. "Type 1 Diabetes," Children's Hospital of Wisconsin (www.chw.org/display/PPF/DocID/22658/router.asp).

18. Ross Horne, *The Health Revolution* (Avalon Beach, NSW, Australia: Happy Landings, Pty. Ltd., 1980), pp. 311-312.

19. Note 1 (*Taber's*), supra.

20. H. J. Roberts, MD, *Aspartame Disease: An Ignored Epidemic* (West Palm Beach: Sunshine Sentinel Press, May 1, 2001).

21. Ibid.

22. Ibid.

23. Harold D. Foster, *What Really Causes AIDS* (Victoria, BC: Trafford Publishing, July 6, 2006).

24. Brazil nuts—50.20 RDA; next highest are mixed nuts—7.14 RDA (no exact measure given).

25. Note 1 (*Taber's*), supra.

26. M. A. Krupp and M. J. Chatton, eds., *Current Medical Diagnosis & Treatment 1983* (Los Altos, CA: Lange Medical Publications, 1983); *see also* D. J. McCarty, ed., *Arthritis & allied conditions, a textbook of Rheumatology*, 9th ed. (Philadelphia: Lea & Febiger, 1979) ("Connective tissue disorders are mostly acquired diseases and the underlying causes cannot be determined in most instances.").

27. T. Colin Campbell and Thomas M. Campbell II, *The China Study: Startling Implications for Diet, Weight Loss and Long-term Health* (Dallas: BenBella Books, 2005), p. 184.
28. "Asthma Explained; the Search for Asthma Relief" (www.asthmaexplained.net).
29. Note 1 (*Taber's*), supra.
30. "Allergy Facts and Figures," Asthma and Allergy Foundation of America (www.aafa.org/display.cfm?id=9&sub=30#prev).
31. Ibid.
32. "Neurology of Attention Deficit Disorder," Neurology and ADHD: Our Attention Deficit Disorder Brain, The ADHD Information Library (www.newideas.net/neurology.htm).
33. Feingold® Association of the United States (www.feingold.org).
34. Bernard Rimland, "The Feingold Diet: An Assessment of the Reviews by Mattes, by Kavale and Forness and Others," *Journal of Learning Disabilities* 16 (6) (June-July 1983): 331-3.
35. Peter R. Breggin, MD, "Report to the plenary session of the NIH consensus conference on ADHD and its treatment" (Nov. 18, 1998).
36. Kelly Patricia O'Meara, "Ritalin Proven More Potent Than Cocaine— Nearly 10 Million Kids Drugged," *Insight* (2001).
37. Simon Gilbody, MD, "What is the evidence on effectiveness of capacity building of primary health care professionals in the detection, management and outcome of depression?," World Health Organization, Regional Office for Europe (December 2004).
38. Carl C. Pfeiffer, MD, *Mental and Elemental Nutrients: A Physician's Guide to Nutrition and Health Care* (New Canaan, CT: Keats Publishing, Inc., 1975), p. 145.
39. Ibid., p. 12.
40. Abram Hoffer, MD, "Megavitamin B-3 therapy for schizophrenia," *Canadian Psychiatric Association Journal* 16 (1971): 499-504.
41. "Death a Risk of Antipsychotics," Associated Press, *Nature* (Oct. 23, 2005), Alliance for Human Research Protection (www.ahrp.org/infomail/05/10/23.php).
42. Note 1 (*Taber's*), supra.
43. National Headache Foundation: Educational Resources (www.headaches.org/consumer/topicsheets/migraine.html). The National Headache Foundation reports that more than 29.5 million Americans

suffer with migraines, with women affected three times more than men ages 15 to 55. In addition, 70% to 80% of migrainers have a family history of migraines. Many migraine sufferers are diagnosed as having a tension headache or sinus headache, resulting in more than 50% of migrainers being improperly diagnosed. Goldberg reports that the incidence of migraine has increased by more than 60% in the past 10 years. The National Center for Health Statistics reports that 30 million workdays and $4.5 billion per year is lost due to migraine headaches. Moreover, research has shown that one in five individuals will experience a migraine in his/her lifetime. *See also* Jerry Adler and Adam Rogers, "The new war against migraines," *Newsweek* (Jan. 11, 1999), pp. 46-52. This article stated that, at the time, there were 25 million Americans who were known migraine sufferers.

44. Topamax® Ortho-McNeil Neurologics, Inc. (www.topamax.com/topamax/index.html).

45. Note 1 (*Taber's*), supra, p. 1342.

46. Ibid., p. 642

47. Ibid., p. 641.

48. Ibid.

49. "Overweight and Obesity: Introduction," DHHS-Centers for Disease Control and Prevention (www.cdc.gov/nccdphp/dnpa/obesity/index.htm) (page last modified: Aug. 26, 2006): "Since the mid-seventies, the prevalence of overweight and obesity has increased sharply for both adults and children. Data from two NHANES surveys show that among adults aged 20-74 years the prevalence of obesity increased from 15.0% (in the 1976-1980 survey) to 32.9% (in the 2003-2004 survey)."

50. "Obesity in children," *New England Journal of Medicine* 350 (2004): 2362-74.

51. "National diabetes fact sheet: general information and national estimates on diabetes in the United States, 2005," U.S. Department of Health and Human Services, Centers for Disease Control and Prevention (Atlanta, GA) (2005) (www.cdc.gov/diabetes/pubs/pdf/ndfs_2005.pdf).

52. "Heart Disease is the Number One Cause of Death," Centers for Disease Control and Prevention, Division for Heart Disease and Stroke Prevention (www.cdc.gov/DHDSP/announcements/american_heart_month.htm).

53. "AOA Fact Sheets: Obesity in Youth," American Obesity Association (www.obesity.org/subs/fastfacts/obesity_youth.shtml).

54. Frank Booth (boothf@missouri.edu).
55. "Research finds fatal flaw in industry's food labelling scheme" (Mar. 1, 2007), Sustainweb (www.sustainweb.org/news.php?id=169).
56. "Super Size Me," Academy Award-winning documentary film by Morgan Spurlock, director (release date: May 21, 2004) (Canada).
57. Ibid.
58. Note 27 (Campbell), supra, pp. 309-10.
59. "Doctor's file complaint over new milk ads," *Nutrition Health Review* (Spring 1995).
60. Ibid.
61. Ibid.
62. Ibid.
63. R. L. Weinsier and C. L. Krumdieck, "Dairy foods and bone health: examination of the evidence," *American Journal of Clinical Nutrition* 72 (2000): 681-689.
64. Note 59 (*NHR*), supra.
65. Ibid.
66. Ibid.
67. John Robbins, *Diet for a New America* (Novato, CA: New World Library, 1998).
68. John McDougall, MD, *The McDougall Program for Women* (New York: Plume, 2000).
69. Weston Price, *Nutrition and Physical Degeneration*, 15th ed. (New Canaan, CT: Keats Pub., 2003).
70. George Meinig, *The Root Canal Cover-Up* (Ojai, CA: Bion Publishing, 1994).
71. Hal A. Huggins, *It's All in Your Head* (New York: Avery Publishing (Penguin Group), July 1, 1993).
72. "Science Versus Emotion in Dental Filling Debate: Who Should Choose What Goes in Your Mouth?," American Dental Association Media Services press release (Chicago) (July 25, 2002).
73. *Gerson Healing Newsletter*, Vol. 14, No. 5 (September/October 1999), p. 9.
74. National Fibromyalgia Research Association (www.nfra.net).
75. Note 1 (*Taber's*), supra, p. 1260.
76. Note 26 (Krupp/Chatton), supra.
77. Carmen Wheatley, in Michael Gearin-Tosh, *Living Proof: A Medical Mutiny* (London: Simon & Schuster, 2002), Appendix, p. 267.

78. Carolyn Dean, MD, *Death by Modern Medicine* (Belleville, Ontario: Matrix Vérité, Inc., 2005); Carolyn Dean, MD, and Gary Null, "Death by Medicine" (www.healthe-livingnews.com/articles/death_by_medicine_part_1.html). For their statistics on the number and cost of annual U.S. adverse drug reaction deaths, *see also* J. Lazarou, B. Pomeranz and P. Corey, "Incidence of adverse drug reactions in hospitalized patients." *Journal of the American Medical Association* 279 (1998): 1200-1205; D. C. Suh, B. S. Woodall, S. K. Shin and E. R. Hermes-De Santis, "Clinical and economic impact of adverse drug reactions in hospitalized patients," *Annals of Pharmacotherapy* 34 (12) (December 2000): 1373-9; Abram Hoffer, MD, "Over the counter drugs," *Journal of Orthomolecular Medicine* (Ontario, Canada) (May 2003). It is reprinted in *Death by Modern Medicine* (supra), Appendix C, pp. 349-58.
79. "Prednisone," MedicineNet.com (www.medicinenet.com/prednisone/article.htm).
80. Note 1 (*Taber's*), supra, p. 510.
81. Ibid., p. 595.

CHAPTER 7

Restoring the Body's Defenses

I look forward optimistically to a healthy, happy world as soon as its children are taught the principles of simple and rational living. We must return to nature and nature's God.

—*Luther Burbank (1849-1926)*

Physicians and the public have exclusively focused on drug therapy to the detriment of at least one of the foundations of good health—appropriate nutrition.

—*Dr. Mary Keith, St. Michael's Hospital, Toronto, Ontario*

B y now, two basic facts will have become clear to the reader:

- Everybody's health and well-being is under constant attack from those factors of modern life that undermine the body's natural defenses and self-healing ability, leading to a multitude of diseases.
- The complex, precision-built nutritional program of the Gerson Therapy is able to undo the harm, restore the organism's damaged defenses and enable the body to heal itself.

In his thinking, Dr. Gerson always made a close connection between the body's defenses and its healing mechanism. Indeed, he invariably saw in his patients that the healing mechanism had been disturbed or severely damaged before the body succumbed to disease. Moreover, he was convinced that the appearance of malignant disease (i.e., cancer) represented the ultimate, most severe kind of breakdown, and that it needed the best expert care and effort to reverse the destructive process and achieve healing.

Perhaps the greatest of Dr. Gerson's many revolutionary insights was his realization that the underlying causes of chronic disease were deficiency and toxicity. This approach differs greatly from that of conventional medicine, which prefers to assign a clear-cut cause to each individual disease but omits the search for the truly basic problems that are common to many. This difference in approach is one of many factors that separate the Gerson protocol from orthodox treatments.

Once the underlying problems are recognized, they can be treated: the deficiency is eliminated with hyperalimentation; the toxicity with systematic detoxification. Despite their vital importance, these methods are simple, straightforward and transparent. Above all, they make sense.

We have already touched on this subject in general terms (see Chapter 3, "Knowing the Enemy," p. 17), but now we need to take a closer look at its practical application.

HYPERALIMENTATION

The answer to deficiency is to give the patient maximum amounts of the best possible foodstuffs. However, seriously ill patients are usually unable to eat much. Their appetite and digestion are poor and their elimination is inadequate. Under these circumstances, the only way forward is juicing, since almost every patient is able—and normally willing—to drink a freshly prepared glass of organic juice every hour. Once that routine is established, the nutrients the body so desperately needs are in constant supply.

A few extremely debilitated patients who cannot cope with the usual hourly 8-ounce glass of juice are given 4- or 6-ounce portions at the beginning of the treatment. To their surprise, after only a few days of juicing and intensive detoxification, they are able to eat three full vegetarian meals a day, prepared from fresh, organic produce, and drink 13 standard size glasses of juice, besides snacking on fruit. Once they reach that stage of hyperalimentation, each patient consumes approximately 20 pounds of food a day.

Critics of the Gerson Therapy, who find the hourly preparation of fresh juices onerous (which it certainly is!), often suggest the use of vitamin and mineral supplements instead. What they don't realize is that the sick body is unable to assimilate and utilize pharmaceutically prepared substances which would simply pass through the organism without doing any good. Only live, fresh, raw vegetables and fruits are absorbed, exclusively in the form of juice, which bypasses the digestive process and is immediately assimilated.

DETOXIFICATION

As soon as the body is flooded with live nutrients, they are rapidly absorbed and force accumulated toxins from the cells into the bloodstream, which in turn transports them to the liver, the body's chief organ of detoxification. However, the patient who embarks on the Gerson Therapy after a lifetime of living on a so-called normal modern diet has already accumulated considerable amounts of food additives, residues of pesticides and other agrochemicals, plus toxins from many sources that block his or her liver. As a result, the liver is unable to deal with the newly arriving toxins driven from the tissues by the live nutrients.

Unless quickly shifted, this logjam of toxins could lead to life-threatening self-intoxication and liver coma, hence the vital role of the rapidly detoxifying and frequent coffee enemas, which are a cornerstone of the Gerson treatment. There are several cancer therapies which use various methods to kill tumor tissue without removing dead toxic material from the liver. In order to allow the liver to discard its toxic load slowly and gradually, the treatment has to be interrupted, which diminishes its impact. However, the Gerson method, with its constant regular detoxification, is able to work continuously, which explains its effectiveness as well as why the coffee enemas are an indispensable part of the protocol. Without them, the additional load of newly released toxins could even cause new liver damage. Whoever wants to embark on the Gerson Therapy must include the required practice of coffee enemas.

CHAPTER 8

Why Does the Gerson
Therapy Work?

T he basic principles of the Gerson protocol are simple and clear and
its practice has been yielding remarkable results for more than 60
years. However, the question remains: Is there any current scientific
research to confirm the methods Dr. Gerson developed partly intuitively, partly through constant study and clinical observation, but without sophisticated research facilities, all those decades ago? Putting it
simply, has anyone discovered just why this therapy works?

The answer is yes. Since Dr. Gerson's death in 1959, a series of eminent scientists and researchers have made discoveries that confirmed
one or another of Dr. Gerson's insights and methods. The sum total of
these piecemeal discoveries explains why his protocol, used in its
entirety, is so effective. We now present a sample of the most striking
scientific endorsements.

In the late '70s, the physicist, mathematician and biophysicist Freeman Widener Cope, MD, wrote in a paper, "The high potassium, low
sodium diet of the Gerson therapy has been observed experimentally to
cure many cases of advanced cancer in man."[1] In another paper, Cope
stated that, in cell damage of any kind, the same responses may occur
in cells throughout the body: "First the cell will lose potassium, second
the cell will accept sodium, and third, the cell will swell with too much
water (cellular edema). When the cell has swollen with too much
water, energy production is inhibited, along with protein synthesis and

lipid (fat) metabolism. *Gerson was able to manipulate tissue damage syndrome, which he recognized clinically in the 1920s, by his dietary management, eliminating sodium, supplementing a high potassium diet with additional potassium amendments and finding a way to remove toxins from the body via the liver.*[2] (Emphasis added.) This is a remarkably concise justification of all of Dr. Gerson's methods, including the strict restriction of protein and fat, which the damaged cell cannot handle, the reason for increased potassium intake and the need for liver detoxification.

In 1988, Patricia Spain Ward, campus historian of the University of Illinois, Chicago, presented an excellent monograph on the Gerson Therapy, under contract to the U.S. Office of Technology Assessment. Although her study is not based on new research, it is worth including for its thoroughness and clarity. Describing Dr. Gerson as "a scholar's scholar and a superlative observer of clinical phenomena,"[3] Dr. Ward reported her observation that patients on a high-potassium, low-sodium diet excreted enormous amounts of sodium in their urine and that, by eliminating animal protein from the diet, this amount was increased. She added, "The medical insistence on large quantities of protein, Gerson showed, was wrong and he stopped the administration of dietary animal proteins for at least six to eight weeks."[4]

Important research justifying Dr. Gerson's withholding of animal protein from his cancer patients was carried out by Robert A. Good, MD, of the University of Minnesota, who is known as "the father of modern immunology." He set up a guinea pig experiment, feeding one group of animals protein-free lab chow, while the other group received the normal variety of food. Dr. Good expected to see failure of the animals' immune system on the protein-free regime, but the opposite happened. The guinea pigs' thymus lymphocytes became tremendously active and remained aggressively so for a long time. Dr. Good realized that he had stimulated immunity by the dietary restriction of animal protein, thus confirming the rightness of the Gerson protocol's identical insight.[5]

Gerson patients do receive adequate amounts of easily absorbed plant proteins contained in the fresh vegetable juices, potatoes and oatmeal that are essential parts of their diet. It is a widespread mistake to believe that only animal foods contain protein. On the contrary, food animals, such as cattle, pigs and sheep, are vegetarians!

The Canadian scientist, Dr. Harold D. Foster, University of Victoria, British Columbia, approached the problem of cancer mortalities from the angle of mineral deficiencies in soils and water supplies. He also carried out an initial computer analysis of 200 cases of so-called "spontaneous" ("a partial or complete disappearance of a tumor in the absence of treatment capable of producing a regression")[6] regressions of a wide variety of cancers.

The result of Professor Foster's painstaking research was that, far from being "spontaneous," most of the regressions were due to a combination of conventional treatments with drastic lifestyle changes and various complementary therapies. Of 200 patients, 10 followed the Gerson diet, and many more used parts of the Gerson protocol (e.g., raw juices and detoxification). Further dietary regimes mentioned in the sample were partly or largely based on the same protocol, raising the percentage of those whose recovery was to some extent due to the Gerson treatment. The most important conclusion Professor Foster was able to draw from his research was that cases of so-called spontaneous regression were far from being spontaneous, and were only categorized as such by orthodox medicine because they were the results of unconventional— alternative and complementary—therapies.

One of the most important techniques of the Gerson Therapy is detoxification via the liver/bile through the use of coffee enemas. Dr. Gerson knew that these dilate the bile ducts, thus allowing the liver to release toxic accumulations. His discovery was confirmed more recently by three scientists—Wattenberg, Sparmins and Lam[7]—from the Department of Pathology, University of Minnesota, who showed that rectal coffee administration stimulates an enzyme system (glutathione S-transferase) in the liver, which is able to remove toxic free radicals from the bloodstream. The normal activity of this enzyme is increased by

600% to 700% by the coffee enema, hence vastly increased detoxification results. Coffee is also rich in potassium, which helps prevent intestinal cramping by boosting the potassium content of deficient smooth muscles in the colon.

In 1990, a remarkable study[8] appeared in a peer-reviewed German medical journal under the title "Experiences with the Use of Dietary Therapy in Surgical Oncology." Its author, Peter Lechner, MD, of the Oncological Outpatient Department, District Hospital, Graz, Austria, reported on a six-year clinical study of a modified version of the Gerson Therapy followed by a group of 60 cancer patients who were also receiving orthodox treatment.

According to Dr. Lechner, this greatly reduced version of the Gerson protocol was used as an adjuvant therapy, not as an alternative to conventional oncological treatments. Moreover, the patients carried out the nutritional therapy in their homes, which made strict supervision impossible. Even so, at the end of six years, Dr. Lechner was able to report the following results:

- Patients generally suffered fewer postoperative complications and adverse side effects of radio- and/or chemotherapy.
- The patients' need for analgesics and psychotropic drugs was less than that of the controls.
- Existing liver metastases progressed more slowly.
- The patients' psychological state was good throughout.
- The malnutrition-caused cachexia (severe wasting), which normally occurs in advanced stages of the disease, could be prevented or was at least greatly delayed in most cases.
- One 77-year-old female patient on the nutritional regime achieved a complete remission without conventional therapy.

In the course of the six-year clinical study, Dr. Lechner and his colleagues were also able to justify Dr. Gerson's use of coffee enemas by following up independent research by C. Djerassi (1959) and Kaufmann (1963).[9] This showed that the two active ingredients of the coffee—cafestol and kahweol—increased up to sevenfold the activity of glutathione S-transferase, which, as we know from the Minnesota research stated above, plays a central role in the elimination of toxins from the liver.

All in all, cautious and restrained though Dr. Lechner's conclusions are, it is clear from his report that even a greatly watered-down version of the Gerson Therapy achieves unexpected and unprecedented good results in the treatment of patients with metastasized malignancies.

The most recent in-depth study of the anticancer components of Gerson's food regime was written by Carmen Wheatley,[10] a member of the Orthomolecular Oncology Group in the U.K. She became interested in the subject through the experience of her friend, Oxford Professor of English Literature Michael Gearin-Tosh, who was diagnosed with multiple myeloma in 1994. His prognosis was poor: six to nine months' survival without any treatment and one to two years with "appropriate" chemotherapy. Professor Gearin-Tosh refused the latter and, after considerable searching, chose the Gerson Therapy, boosting it with meditation, acupuncture and Chinese breathing exercises. He described the process from diagnosis to his then-current state in his brilliant, highly amusing book, *Living Proof: A Medical Mutiny.*[11] (Against expectations, he lived for 11 years and eventually died of blood poisoning following dental work.)

Watching her friend's progress, Dr. Wheatley became intrigued by the fact that Dr. Gerson, apparently intuitively, selected foods for his therapy that have since, some 50 years later, been shown to have anticancer properties. She wrote her findings in an essay titled "The Case of the 0.005% Survivor,"[12] which was peer-reviewed by four eminent physicians and appeared as an afterword in Professor Gearin-Tosh's book.

Dr. Wheatley points out that the Gerson diet contains several foods in which modern research has identified some key cancer-fighting components (e.g., flaxseed oil with its important contents of Omega-3 fatty acids; fruits rich in minerals and bioflavonoids; and vegetables of the cruciferous family, namely cauliflower, cabbages and broccoli, whose anticancer properties are borne out by current scientific nutritional research).[13] She comments, "Gerson's fruit and vegetable diet could be subjected to exhaustive analysis in the light of modern nutritional oncology research. He didn't have any of this scientific knowledge, yet empirically devised a method which ensures that a large range of these products would be delivered to the cancer patient, intact and *in pharmacologically active doses.*[14] (Emphasis added.)

In the rest of her study, Dr. Wheatley reviews further components of the Gerson Therapy—from the value of juicing to the importance of coffee enemas—and finds all of them scientifically justified. In conclusion, let us quote one of her shrewd comments: "Conventional medical methods of treating cancer—chemotherapy, radiation—routinely wipe out an already depressed immune system and do little to restore it. Yet, as Gerson realized, it is the immune system which is needed to fight cancer, and therefore building it up should enhance chances of survival."[15]

As time goes on and the lack of success of much of conventional oncology becomes ever more obvious, research into nutritional therapies is bound to expand and take up its due place in mainstream medicine. Its findings are bound to confirm again and again that the principles and practice of the Gerson Therapy are sound and accurate, offering an eminently logical way to heal disease and maintain health.

REFERENCES

1. Freeman Widener Cope, "A medical application of the Ling Association-Induction Hypothesis: the high potassium, low sodium diet of the Gerson cancer therapy," *Physiological Chemistry and Physics* 10 (5) (1978): 465-468.

2. Freeman Widener Cope, "Pathology of structured water and associated cations in cells (the tissue damage syndrome) and its medical treatment," *Physiological Chemistry and Physics* 9 (6) (1977): 547-553.

3. Patricia Spain Ward, "History of the Gerson Therapy" (1988) under contract to the U.S. Office of Technology Assessment.

4. Ibid.

5. Robert A. Good, MD, *The Influence of Nutrition on Development of Cancer Immunity and Resistance to Mesenchymal Diseases* (New York: Raben Press, 1982).

6. "Lifestyle Changes and the 'Spontaneous' Regression of Cancer: An Initial Computer Analysis," *International Journal of Biosocial Research* 10 (1) (1988): 17-33.

7. V. L. Sparmins, L. K. T. Lam and L. W. Wattenberg, "Proceedings of the American Association of Cancer Researchers and the American Society of Clinical Oncology," *Abstract* 22 (1981): 114, 453.

8. Peter Lechner, MD, "Experiences with the Use of Dietary Therapy in Surgical Oncology," *Aktuelle Ernaehrungsmedizin* 2 (5) (1990).

9. C. Djerassi, et al., "The Structure of the pentacyclic Diterpene Cafestol," *Journal of the American Chemical Society* 81 (1959): 2386-2398; *see also* P. Kaufmann and A. K. Sengupta, "Zur Kenntnis der Lipoid in der Kaffeebohne. III Die Reindarstellung des Kaweals," *Fette, Seifen und Anstrichmittel* (Berlin) 65 (7) (1963): 529-532.

10. Carmen Wheatley, in Michael Gearin-Tosh, *Living Proof: A Medical Mutiny* (London: Simon & Schuster, 2002), Appendix, pp. 267-308.

11. Ibid.

12. Ibid.

13. Ibid.

14. Ibid.

15. Ibid.

PART II

The Complete Guide to the Practice of the Gerson Therapy

What you have read so far introduced you to the philosophy and principles of the Gerson Therapy and explained its approach to health and healing. By now, you should feel at home with the idea that optimum nutrition is not only the key to health and well-being but also the most powerful tool in the fight against disease and suffering.

Now the time has come to get acquainted with the practical side of this unique protocol. The following chapters will lead you step by step through the components that add up to the complete program, as devised by Dr. Max Gerson and practiced over 60 years by thousands of people all over the world. Whatever your interest in the program—whether you hope to heal a serious condition, cope with a minor problem or simply change over to a health-giving lifestyle—this is the way ahead.

There is just one thing to remember: Following the Gerson Therapy in order to recover from a serious illness is a major undertaking that requires determination, endurance and a clear understanding of the program. Also, it is largely a "do-it-yourself" process since, even if you are able to spend time at the Gerson clinic in Mexico, the long, major part of the healing work has to take place at home. This means that you are in sole charge; there is no one to supervise you and make sure that you observe the rules faithfully. However, since you are insightful enough to choose this method of thorough healing, you will also realize that the only person to suffer a setback from even the slightest cheating is yourself!

The necessary self-discipline is made much easier by the immediate improvements most patients experience, even after a few days on the program. These improvements (e.g., better appetite, less pain, more energy and improved sleep) are convincing evidence that the therapy has begun to work and give a powerful boost to the patient's determination.

Trained Gerson practitioners, accredited by the Gerson Institute, are still few in number and therefore hard to find. Please beware of unaccredited therapists who claim to practice the Gerson Therapy—they can harm rather than heal you. Your best chance is to find a sympathetic doctor who is willing to monitor your progress without trying to introduce changes into your routine. Your doctor's main task is to arrange for the blood and urine tests that have to be carried out every four to six weeks at the start of the therapy and less frequently in its later stages. As the test results of Gerson patients often differ from those on a conventional treatment protocol, guidance for interpreting your results is given in Chapter 26, "Gerson Laboratory Tests Explained," p. 269.

CHAPTER 9

The Gerson Household

W hether a patient is able to spend some time at a Gerson facility or decides to embark on the therapy at home, the longest part of the healing process—up to two years or more with malignant disease but much less with other chronic conditions—will have to take place in his or her residence. For the duration of the treatment, the home needs to be turned into a kind of private clinic where everything serves the goal of getting well and nothing is allowed to interfere with that process.

How do we go about that? Quite simply, we bear in mind that the twin pillars of the Gerson program are nutrition and detoxification. Since the ill patient suffering from a chronic disease is both toxic and nutritionally deficient, as a first task the household has to be cleared of all toxic chemicals and damaging materials or appliances. These are present in vast arrays in most modern households. Chemical cleansers, gadgets and labor-saving devices emitting harmful radiation or so-called electrosmog are used daily and taken for granted. We only get rid of them when their dire effects on the body are understood.

As the second pillar of the therapy is to provide the patient with hypernutrition, a suitably equipped kitchen is the all-important center where all foods and juices are prepared daily in large amounts. Let us start by listing the correct equipment for a smoothly running, efficient Gerson kitchen.

REFRIGERATOR

One very large or two average size refrigerators will be needed to store the large quantities of organic produce required. A cool, preferably dark, well-ventilated pantry or laundry room is ideal for storing root vegetables, which don't need refrigeration.

JUICE MACHINES

As freshly made organic juices are one of the most important healing components of the Gerson program, they must be of the best possible quality. It is therefore vital to choose the most efficient juicer—one that will stand up to constant use over two years or so.

There are plenty of models on the market. The simplest and cheapest is the centrifugal type, one of the first to become widely available. It is wasteful, produces deficient, enzyme-poor juice and cannot be used for healing.

Another type is the Champion juicer, which extracts more minerals as well as more fluid. However, it is not satisfactory in itself, since what it produces is not so much juice as a mushy layer of vegetables on top of a watery base. Even so, the Champion juicer can be used, but only as a grinder. The machine comes with a plate that can be placed under the base where the strainer is usually located, releasing the ground-up pulpy material. This pulp has to be put through a hand-operated press, based on a hydraulic jack, to squeeze the juice from the pulped vegetables. The cost of the two items runs at about $600. The Champion juicer is widely available in the U.S. and in several other countries. For the manual press, contact The Juice Press Factory (www.juicepressfactory.com).

Other machines, imported from Korea and made in the U.S., use two interlocking helical blades which grind against each other. They do a better extracting job than the Champion alone and may be used, especially if the patient is not suffering from advanced cancer. However, these "one-process" juicers do not actually conform to Dr. Gerson's instruction to use a two-process method, consisting of a grinder and a press, for obtaining the best juice. These juicers claim to extract more enzymes than the Norwalk (see below), but no mention is made of the equally important mineral extraction. The cost of these machines is between $750 and $900.

The best two-process juicer is the Norwalk Hydraulic Press Juicer, which is also most attractively styled with a stainless steel exterior or a wood grain plastic outer cover. Naturally, in either model, all parts of the machine that come in contact with food are made from stainless steel. The Norwalk is fully automatic, with a simple lever activating the press. Well serviced and guaranteed, it is also the most expensive juicer ($2,195 to $2,295). The stainless steel exterior model also has a lever that adjusts it to the 220 to 240 volt current used in Europe. For information, call 800-405-8423 (outside the U.S., call +1 (760) 436-9684) or visit the Norwalk Juicers California Web site (www.nwjcal.com).

Taking Care of Your Juice Machine

Aside from your normal routine of maintaining maximum cleanliness in the kitchen, it is especially important to keep your juicer clean and free from dried-up juice and/or fibers. Since these are raw, they can easily spoil, dry and attract flies and other insects and germs.

To avoid contamination, the juicer must be cleaned after each use. This should not take up much extra time since those parts of the machine that come in contact with fruits and vegetables are made of stainless steel and are easy to take apart, rinse, dry and reassemble for the next juice.

Use only clean sponges or cloths and reserve them for the juicer alone. Do not use soap or detergent for each cleansing because it is highly important that not even the smallest amount of soap or cleanser remains on the parts that come in contact with the vegetables. If you use a Norwalk juicer, remember to wipe the press plate at the top.

The juice cloths should be rinsed carefully in clean—not soapy—water after each pressing and kept in the freezer until the next juicing. It is best to have separate cloths for the carrot/apple or plain carrot juice and for the green juice.

At night, after all the juices have been made, you may use slightly soapy water for the day's final cleansing; afterwards, rinse thoroughly to make sure that no soapy film remains. Even a small residue of soap getting into the juices could cause the patient diarrhea, cramps or worse. The same applies to the juice cloths. Wash them in slightly soapy water and rinse carefully to get rid of any soapy residue. Keep the cloths in the freezer overnight.

If you use a grinder (i.e., a Champion) and a press operated by a hydraulic system, the same rules apply. Keep both machines scrupulously clean and clear of soap.

STOVE AND OVEN: ELECTRIC OR GAS?

Neither type is ideal. The cooking temperature is easier to control with a gas stove. However, gas burns oxygen, and if the patient spends time in the kitchen, the oxygen-depleted air is likely to prove harmful. The kitchen has to be well ventilated, which may be difficult on cold, winter days. The installation of a room ozone generator in the kitchen/living area is recommended in order to restore a better oxygen level.

Caution: If the ozone level is too high, it could be set on fire by open flames.

Electric stoves or ovens are more expensive than gas to operate in most areas of the U.S. Their advantage is that they are cleaner and don't use up oxygen. However, the cooking temperature, so very important for the correct preparation of vegetables, is more difficult to control on electric stoves.

Microwave Oven

Because of its speed and apparent efficiency, this gadget has spread to countless kitchens in the U.S. and elsewhere, without knowing its serious health hazards. Since many microwave ovens carry an "Underwriter Laboratory" guarantee of safety, the general public is led to believe that these ovens are safe to use. This is not the case.

Research carried out in Switzerland[1] and elsewhere has shown that microwaves cause harmful chemical reactions in food, damaging nutrients, producing unnatural molecules and making natural amino acids toxic. The heat is uneven; it doesn't reach the middle of solid food but instead produces "hot spots." Liquids can overheat and cause severe burns when the food is removed. To make things worse, these ovens emit radiation into the kitchen area even when not in use and "cook the cook."[2] (It is an interesting fact that, for health reasons, microwave ovens were banned in the former Soviet Union as far back as 1976!)[3] If you own one, get rid of it. If it is not removable, unplug it and don't be tempted to use it under any circumstances.

POTS AND UTENSILS

Any contact of food with aluminum causes small amounts (or with some vegetables, such as tomatoes, large amounts) of aluminum to be dissolved and released into the food. This metal is highly toxic; it causes brain damage and is believed to play a role in causing Alzheimer's.[4]

Discard any and all aluminum items and don't allow aluminum foil to come into contact with food. Use stainless steel pots, preferably with heavy "waterless" bottoms, or glass (Pyrex®) or enameled cast iron pots. Stainless steel cooking utensils or wooden spoons are best. Use silver flatware, if available (small amounts of colloidal silver, released from silver forks, spoons and knives are valuable stimulants for the immune system).

Do not use pressure cookers; they work at a very high temperature, which damages nutrients. One of the basic Gerson rules is to cook food very slowly, at a low temperature, to avoid such damage. The glaze used on some crockpots is toxic[5]—best to steer clear of them.

DISTILLERS

Surprising though this may sound, Gerson patients don't drink water. There are two reasons for this. On the one hand, their daily intake of 13 glasses of freshly made organic juices and fluid-rich soup, salads and fruit provide them with all the top-quality nutritious liquid they need. On the other hand, water would only dilute their already deficient digestive juices without supplying any nutrients. However, water is used in the Gerson Therapy in cooking—to make soups, teas and, of course, enemas—and it is vitally important to ensure the purity of this water.

There are various filter systems on the market, including reverse osmosis, which can only be used if the local water supply is guaranteed free from highly harmful fluoride. (See Chapter 5, "Breakdown of the Body's Defenses," p. 29.) The safest way to ensure freedom from impurities, toxic chemicals and, above all, fluoride is to set up a home distiller.

Many kinds of distiller are available in various price ranges. Choice must depend on cost and on the amount of water the household may need. The patient alone will use 2 to 3 gallons in every 24-hour period, and more if other family members also eat Gerson food and/or wish to use enemas.

A distiller needs an electric connection and an extra water faucet, and many patients install theirs in the laundry room or garage. The machine needs to be detached and cleaned every three days. Seeing the sludge left behind will convince anyone of the need to purify water as thoroughly as possible.

Distillation works by heating water to the point of becoming steam, which is run through a tube that causes it to cool and condense back into water. Since minerals, various impurities and additives do not turn into steam, they stay behind, leaving the cooled, condensed steam free from harmful components. However, volatile liquids, such as benzene fractions, also boil away and are condensed back into the purified water. To remove such items, all distillers should contain a small tube of carbon pellets, so that when the condensed water drips back into a fresh container, it passes through the carbon filter, which removes the unwanted volatile items.

It is sometimes claimed by health professionals that distilled water "removes minerals from the body" and shouldn't be used,[6] but they are wrong. The minerals found in water (e.g., sodium or calcium) are generally inorganic and are therefore poorly absorbed or downright harmful. On the other hand, the patient is virtually flooded with the easily absorbed organic minerals contained in the large amount of juices drunk throughout the day; the "loss" of minerals contained in tap water is actually a gain.

CLEANING CHEMICALS

Cleanliness is of course all important in the Gerson household but, as stated before, special care must be taken not to use toxic products. Here are the ones to avoid:

Chlorine

Chlorine is not only bleach but also a powerful disinfectant, able to kill or control all kinds of germs. For that reason, it is present in almost all kitchen cleansers (and in swimming pools and tap water!). Chlorine is harsh and unsafe, able to displace iodine from the thyroid gland, and must be avoided. There are a few kitchen cleansers that do not contain chlorine, so try to find one. You can also produce your own by mixing half malt vinegar with half water and decanting it into a spray-pump bottle to clean glass or polish kitchen surfaces, but keep it off wood. Plain soap and hot water are also recommended.

To remove lime scale, soak a piece of cotton in white vinegar, wrap it around the faucets in your kitchen or bathroom and leave it for 30 minutes. Wash it off with soap and water.

Clean stainless steel pans with olive oil. The result is stunning, but use the oil sparingly and be careful to clean it all off.

Solvents

Paint solvents, grease or glue solvents are all toxic and damaging to the patient. If one has to be used, take it outside and don't allow it to evaporate in the kitchen.

Dishwasher Soap

Most dishwashers are equipped with two wash cycles followed by one rinse cycle. Since the Gerson Therapy does not involve the use of greasy food or baking dishes, it is best to use one wash cycle and ensure that the soap is cleared by using two rinse cycles. In that way, the dishwasher soap should be completely eliminated, with no toxic residue remaining on dishes.

Laundry Soap and Bleach

If the laundry is washed in a washing machine, the same applies to dishwasher soap. You can use any appropriate soap and even add bleach, if needed, as long as it is inside the machine and the patient doesn't smell it. (If the patient can smell it, he or she is getting some into their system.) Make very sure that the laundry is thoroughly rinsed, possibly running a second rinse cycle.

Fabric Softeners

These should be avoided, whether in liquid form or as drying sheets. Either way, they leave a chemical film, which never washes out completely. They are also irritating to sensitive individuals (e.g., asthma sufferers). As a harmless alternative, add 1/4 cup of distilled white vinegar to the wash cycle. This softens your clothes and also gets rid of static cling. If you are washing delicate items (e.g., those marked "hand wash"), use a mild soap and wear rubber gloves.

DRY CLEANING

As this is done outside the home, it doesn't directly affect the patient. However, when dry-cleaned items are brought home, it is wise to leave them outdoors without their plastic covers to let them air out and get rid of any remaining chemicals.

AEROSOLS AND SPRAYS

Do not use any of these. Once the spray is distributed in the air, it is impossible to avoid inhaling it. Obviously, the toxic pesticide sprays are the most dangerous. However, any cleaning chemicals (e.g., window cleaners and oven cleaners) that are sprayed will go into the air and be inhaled.

If a window cleaner is used, pour a little on a cloth and wipe the window clean without spraying.

Oven cleaning is not much of a problem, since the Gerson food is clear of fats and doesn't cause deposits on the oven walls.

THE BATHROOM

Chlorine-containing cleansers should not be used in the bathroom. Disinfect with 3% commercial hydrogen peroxide. Choose mild soaps for personal use and avoid spray deodorizers. Men should use spreadable shaving soaps, not products sold in aerosol cans or sprays. Avoid after-shave lotions and underarm deodorants. (See "Cosmetics" in Chapter 5, "Breakdown of the Body's Defenses," p. 43.) Only use plain, white, unscented toilet paper.

LIVING AREA

Many kinds of toxic damage can be caused inadvertently in the living room. One possible culprit is furniture polish, which contains solvent and must be banished. Carpet cleaning presents another potential hazard. Do not use (or allow cleaning services to use) chemical cleaners, only soapy solutions.

Very serious toxic damage has been caused by new carpeting,[7] most of which is impregnated with toxic pesticides or other chemicals to resist staining. If it is absolutely necessary to install new carpeting, track down nontoxic kinds. Several manufacturers have been sued[8] for their carpets causing allergic reactions in sensitive people and, as a result, nontoxic carpets are now being produced.

An even more dangerous process is termite extermination. Some exterminators use a whole house cover and spread gas throughout the building. When the covers are removed, fresh air is allowed back in, but a lot of poison is left behind in upholstered furniture, carpets and drapes. It takes some six months or so to outgas! There are other nontoxic methods available (e.g., find out about the freezing approach).

Living room areas are often routinely treated to "air fresheners" via sprays or a chemical solid. Do not use either.

WHOLE HOUSE PAINTING

No part of the inside of the house should be painted while the patient is recovering. Walls may be washed down with mild soap; stains can be removed with a nontoxic cleanser. The house may not look perfect but, for the time being, the patient's recovery must be given absolute priority.

OUTDOOR GARDEN SPRAYS/AGRICULTURAL PESTICIDES

Some areas of daily life are beyond the caregiver's control, such as neighbors who spray their gardens with pesticides. If and when this happens, make sure that all windows are closed, and use the room air cleaner and ozone generator to protect the patient. A similar problem is caused by pesticide spraying of agricultural areas in the vicinity. In one such case, the recovering patient had a serious reaction and suffered a recurrence until she moved away (to live with her sister) for the time being, where she recovered again.

REFERENCES

1. Hans Hertel and Bernard H. Blanc, "Microwave Ovens" (Vol. 22, No. 2) and "Microwaves the Best Article Yet," Price-Pottenger Nutrition Foundation, *PPNF Journal* 24 (2) (Summer 2000).
2. Ibid.
3. Ibid.
4. Virginie Rondeau, Daniel Commenges, Hélène Jacqmin-Gadda and Jean-François Dartigues, "Relation between Aluminum Concentrations in Drinking Water and Alzheimer's Disease: An 8-year Follow-up Study," *American Journal of Epidemiology* 152 (2000): 59-66.
5. Dixie Farley, "Dangers of Lead Still Linger," U.S. Food and Drug Administration, *FDA Consumer* (January-February 1998) (www.cfsan.fda.gov/~dms/fdalead.html).
6. P. Airola, *How To Get Well* (Phoenix: Health Plus Publishers, 1974).
7. Cindy Duehring, "Carpet Concerns, Part Four: Physicians Speak Up As Medical Evidence Mounts," Environmental Access Research Network (Minot, ND) (www.holisticmed.com/carpet/tc4.txt).
8. Fluoride Action Network, Pesticide Project, Class Action Suit-PFOA (www.fluoridealert.org/pesticides/effect.pfos.classaction.htm).

CHAPTER 10

Forbidden Foods

A McDonald's "Breakfast for Under a Dollar"
actually costs much more than that. You have to
factor in the cost of coronary bypass surgery.

—*George Carlin*

J ust as some foods, brilliantly combined in the Gerson protocol, are great healers, others are strictly excluded from the patient's diet. In his classic book, *A Cancer Therapy—Results of Fifty Cases,*[1] Dr. Gerson gives a long list of "Forbidden Foods." Actually, "Forbidden Items" would be a more accurate title, since the list is not limited to foodstuffs only. Newcomers to the Gerson program are understandably puzzled by some of these prohibitions, banning foods that are routinely eaten and even considered wholesome by the average "normal" citizen, so let's see why they must be excluded. Rules and regulations are easier to follow if we know the reasons behind them.

In fact, today's list of banned substances is longer than Dr. Gerson's original one. Since he wrote his book half a century ago, many changes have occurred that make healthy living increasingly difficult. The huge development of the food industry—with its vast range of additives, freely used in the ever-wider assortment of convenience foods—has changed people's eating habits for the worse, exposing consumers to the ill effects of what are politely called food cosmetics.

One of the worst—the highly toxic[2] sugar substitute aspartame, sold as NutraSweet, Spoonful, etc.—is contained in some 5,000[3] processed foods found on grocery shelves. Last, but far from least, all processed foods contain salt, the very substance that causes tissue damage syndrome and stimulates tumor growth.[4] (See Chapter 5, "Breakdown of the Body's Defenses," p. 29.)

Added to this, the products of industrial agriculture carry heavy residues of toxic pesticides, herbicides, fungicides, growth promoters, hormones, antibiotics and any one of the thousands of substances allowed to be used by the Food and Drug Administration,[5] which are supposed to be harmless. Indeed, some of these substances tested singly may prove to be harmless but, in combination with others, which is how people consume them in the real world, they add up to a poisonous cocktail. Let's remember that all these chemicals are toxic and damaging to the liver, the very organ which the Gerson Therapy endeavors to heal and restore.

These are the two basic rules for Gerson patients:

- All processed foods, whether they are canned, jarred, bottled, frozen, salted, refined, sulphured, smoked, pickled, irradiated, microwaved or otherwise treated, must be strictly avoided.
- Only fruits and vegetables certified as organic must be used, for they are free of agricultural poisons and are grown in healthy soil, which contains all the necessary vitamins, enzymes, minerals, trace elements and microorganisms that are needed for optimum health.

Admittedly, these days even organically cultivated soil does not contain the same level of useful minerals as it did even 15 years ago, but the great amount of organic food and juices that a Gerson patient is given daily makes up for the deficiencies.

As for the forbidden items, the harmful effects of tobacco and alcohol are too well known to need explanation. Next, sodium (salt) and fats of all kinds, except flaxseed oil, must be avoided. This, of course, brings into the group of forbidden foods many items that contain one or both of these two banned substances (e.g., avocadoes are rich in natural oil, which is fat). If you bear in mind the ban on fats and salt, the following list will make sense without detailed explanations.

To simplify matters even further, let's repeat loud and clear: Only foods that contribute to health and healing are allowed; all else is banned.

FORBIDDEN FOODS AND NONFOOD ITEMS

- All processed foods
- Alcohol
- Avocados
- Berries (except currants)
- Bicarbonate of soda in foods, toothpaste and gargle
- Bottled and canned commercial beverages (soft drinks)
- Cake, candy, chocolate and all kinds of sweets (high sugar and fats; no nutritional value)
- Cheese
- Cocoa
- Coffee for drinking (except as used in the castor oil treatment)
- Cosmetics, hair dyes and permanents (see Chapter 5, "Breakdown of the Body's Defenses," p. 29)
- Cream
- Cucumber (poorly digested)
- Dried fruit (if sulphured or glazed with oil)
- Drinking water (see the section on distillers in Chapter 9, "The Gerson Household," p. 137)
- Epsom salts (also for foot baths)
- Fats and oils (sole exception: flaxseed oil, as prescribed)
- Flour (white and wholemeal; also flour products such as pasta)
- Fluoride, in water and toothpaste (see Chapter 5, "Breakdown of the Body's Defenses," p. 29)
- Herbs (except permitted ones) (see Chapter 12, "Preparing Food and Juices—The Basic Rules," p. 153)
- Ice cream and sherbet (artificial flavors, sweeteners and cream)

- Legumes (only occasional use in latter part of therapy)
- Milk (also defatted or low fat)
- Mushrooms (fungi, not vegetables)
- Nuts (high in fats; wrong configuration of proteins)
- Orange and lemon rind (contains aromatic oils)
- Pickles
- Pineapples (high in aromatics)
- Salt and all salt substitutes
- Soy and all soy products (e.g., tofu, soy milk and flour)
- Spices (high in aromatics)
- Sugar (refined white)
- Tea (black and green if caffeinated; black tea is high in natural fluoride)

Dr. Gerson's total ban on soy and all soy products may sound surprising at first, since soy has the much-publicized reputation of being an ideal vegetarian food (i.e., high in protein and low in fat and cholesterol). It is also consumed in the Far East where cancer incidence is considerably lower than in the West.

However, the truth behind this commercially motivated publicity is very different (soy is very big business in the U.S., where 60% of supermarket foods contain some form of it). In fact, soy is high in oil and contains at least 30 allergy-causing proteins, which can cause severe damage[6] to susceptible individuals. Soy also contains phytic acid, which blocks the uptake of important minerals; enzyme inhibitors, which annul the healing power of the vital oxidizing enzymes contained in the juices; and a clot-promoting substance, which causes red blood cells to clump together—ample justification for the total exclusion of soy from the Gerson protocol.

Please note: Two "home-grown" foods— sprouted seeds and wheatgrass juice—which became fashionable some 20 years ago and are considered wholesome and nutritious, must not be used by Gerson patients. Our experience has shown that, unfortunately, both have harmful side effects.

Sprouts were eaten in large amounts by two Gerson patients at our hospital instead of the usual salads at lunch and dinner. Within a short time, both developed recurrences of their primary diseases (i.e., lupus and cervical cancer) after being symptom-free for months. Other lupus patients, getting sprouts from the hospital kitchen in their salads and juices, stopped responding to the treatment and even got worse.

Shortly afterwards, researchers[7] discovered that sprouts contain immature proteins, called L-canavanine, which suppress the immune system. At the Gerson hospital, sprouts were immediately banned and the earlier problems disappeared at once. All past patients were also advised to stop using sprouts in their diet.

Wheatgrass juice contains many valuable nutrients, but it is difficult to digest, tends to irritate the stomach and can only be taken in 1-ounce portions. Used as a rectal implant, it can cause serious irritation. Besides, the Gerson green juice (consisting of salad greens, chard, a little green pepper, some red cabbage and an apple per 8-ounce glass) (see Chapter 12, "Preparing Food and Juices—The Basic Rules," p. 153) is highly digestible, contains similar nutrients and can be enjoyed in four 8-ounce portions a day without unpleasant side effects—excellent reasons for not using wheatgrass juice.

TEMPORARILY FORBIDDEN FOODS AND NONFOOD ITEMS UNTIL PERMITTED BY GERSON PRACTITIONER

- Butter
- Cottage cheese (salt-free, defatted)
- Eggs
- Fish
- Meat
- Yogurt (and other fermented milk products)

FORBIDDEN PERSONAL AND HOUSEHOLD ITEMS

- Aerosols of all types

- Carpeting (new)
- Chemical cleansers (see Chapter 9, "The Gerson Household," p. 133)
- Chlorine bleach
- Cosmetics (see Chapter 5, "Breakdown of the Body's Defenses," p. 29)
- Ointments
- Paint (fresh)
- Perfumes
- Pesticide sprays
- Wood preservatives

REFERENCES

1. M. Gerson, *A Cancer Therapy: Results of Fifty Cases and The Cure of Advanced Cancer by Diet Therapy: A Summary of Thirty Years of Clinical Experimentation*, 6th ed. (San Diego, CA: Gerson Institute, 1999).

2. Aspartame (NutraSweet®) Toxicity Info Center (www.holisticmed.com/aspartame); *see also* H. J. Roberts, MD, "Does Aspartame Cause Human Brain Cancer?," *Journal of Advancement in Medicine* 4 (4) (Winter 1991).

3. Joseph Mercola, MD, "Can Rumsfeld 'Defend' Himself Against Aspartame Lawsuit?" (www.mercola.com/2005/jan/12/rumsfeld_aspartame.htm); *see also* Note 2 (Roberts), supra.

4. Freeman Widener Cope, "A medical application of the Ling Association-Induction Hypothesis: the high potassium, low sodium diet of the Gerson cancer therapy," *Physiological Chemistry and Physics* 10 (5) (1978): 465-468.

5. Healthy Eating Adviser: Food Additives (www.healthyeatingadvisor.com/food-additives.html) (updated 2006).

6. "Soy Dangers Summarised," SoyOnlineService (www.soyonlineservice.co.nz/03summary.htm).

7. M. R. Malinow, E. J. Bardana, Jr., B. Pirofsky, S. Craig and P. McLaughlin, "Systemic lupus erythematosus-like syndrome in monkeys fed alfalfa sprouts: role of a nonprotein amino acid," *Science* 216 (4544) (Apr. 23, 1982): 415-417.

CHAPTER 11

Happy Foods

Even the highest medicine can cure only eight
or nine out of 10 sicknesses. The sicknesses that
medicine cannot cure can be cured only by foods.

—The Yellow Emperor's Classic of Internal
Medicine *(Chinese, circa 400 B.C.)*

Food is Better Medicine than Drugs

—*Title of book by leading British
nutritionist Patrick Holford*

"**S**o what *is* there to eat?" asks the startled newcomer to the Gerson way of life, after reading the list of forbidden foods in the preceding chapter. That is an important question to ponder. It shows how alienated one can become from a natural way of eating and, above all, from the huge range of available plant foods, rightly called the vegetable kingdom (which, in this instance, also includes fruits). It is a fair guess that the majority of people in the so-called developed world regard vegetables as no more than incidentals that accompany a main course of fish or meat, while fruits are only considered if there is no dessert offered. This is the moment to think again—and to make some delightful discoveries.

151

The fact is that plant foods, which are the basis of the Gerson regime, are superior to animal-based ones. Besides being lighter, more pure and easier to digest and absorb, each one contains a subtle mixture of vitamins, enzymes, minerals and trace elements, which work in synergy (i.e., in cooperation) and supply the depleted organism with valuable nutrients. Only when the nonhealing—in fact, harmful—food items are excluded, the wide range and variety of plant foods become clear. It is their usefulness as well as their beauty that need to be acknowledged.

Try to look at a display of fresh, organic fruits and vegetables with the eyes of an artist. Note the glowing colors and varied shapes of golden carrots, deep red cabbages, creamy cauliflowers with their light green collars, beige pears, multicolored apples and translucent green grapes—the range is vast, and eye appeal adds a great deal to the enjoyment of the produce.

There is another happy surprise that awaits the novice explorer of the vegetable kingdom: the discovery of the true flavor of vegetables and fruits. At first, without salt and pepper, plant foods taste bland—and, frankly, boring—but they are neither. However, a lifetime of excessive use of salt deadens the taste buds of the tongue until they are unable to convey the true taste of any food, and even the salt intake has to be continually increased to have any effect. On the salt-free Gerson regime, it takes a week or so for the paralyzed taste buds to recover. Once that happens, fruits and vegetables suddenly begin to taste more interesting. At the same time, one's sense of smell also becomes more acute and contributes to the enjoyment of every meal.

"Let your food be your medicine, and let your medicine be your food," said Hippocrates, the father of modern medicine, some 2,500 years ago. We might add, "Let your medicine consist of happy foods only!"

CHAPTER 12

Preparing Food and Juices— The Basic Rules

A first-rate soup is more
creative than a second-rate painting.

—Abraham Maslow

A ssuming that your kitchen is now fully equipped for your healing Gerson routine, and that you have banished from your home all forbidden foods and substances, the moment has come to find out about the all-important task of food preparation. The rules are simple, but they must be observed faithfully to secure the best results.

All food must be organic and as fresh as possible. Ideally, we should be able to gather fresh, living food from our own organic gardens; unfortunately, this is not an ideal world and we must compromise. The next best thing is to shop frequently for salad and leaf vegetables in smallish amounts so there is no need to keep them for any length of time. Apples, pears, oranges and root vegetables can be stored for a while without significant loss of quality.

The two most important basic rules of food preparation are the following:

- All foods must be prepared with great care in order to pre-serve nutrients as much as possible. Cooking must be slow, using low heat; high temperatures alter nutrients in vegetables and cause them to be less easily absorbed. Vegetables should not be peeled—valuable nutrients are contained in or immediately underneath their skins—and only washed or well scrubbed. Except for potatoes, corn and whole beets, which have to be boiled in sufficient water, vegetables are cooked with the minimum of water or soup stock (see "Special Soup or Hippocrates Soup," p. 158) or on a bed of sliced onions and tomatoes, which release enough moisture to keep the vegetables from burning. Remember that oxidation, with loss of nutrients, sets in as soon as you cut into a vegetable or fruit; only start chopping when you are ready to cook.

- Food must be tasty, varied and enjoyable to make up for being very different from the so-called normal Western diet. Variety helps to stimulate appetite. It also supplies a wide range of minerals and trace elements needed by the body to heal. Remember the importance of eye appeal! Salads in particular can be made truly tempting by mixing green leaves with chopped tomatoes and multicolored peppers, adding radishes and a smattering of chives. (For further ideas, see Chapter 28, "Recipes," p. 311.)

A small vase of flowers on the dining table can work wonders in making the meal taste even better.

The Gerson diet strikes a fine balance between raw and cooked foods. The ample main meals may suggest to some patients that much of their food is cooked, but this is not the case. Meals begin with huge helpings of raw salad and end with raw fruit, and the daily ration of 13 glasses of freshly made juice is as raw as can be. Cooked foods are necessary. Dr. Gerson's experience showed that patients do not digest well if given only raw foods along with the juices. In fact, cooked foods provide additional variety and enable patients to eat more than they would on an exclusively raw diet. They also supply soft bulk, which promotes the digestion of the raw foods and juices.

The most popular item on the list of cooked foods is the "Special Soup or Hippocrates Soup" (see p. 158) that helps to detoxify the kidneys and is highly comforting, especially in cold weather. All cooked foods serve as a kind of "blotting paper" in the stomach, helping to deal with the constant intake of large amounts of juice. Even so, cooked foods only account for some 3 to 4 pounds of the patient's daily consumption, while raw foods, mostly made into juices, represent some 17 pounds!

THE ALL-IMPORTANT JUICES

Only four kinds of juice are used in the treatment of all categories of patients, except for a few minor exceptions. The basic juices are:

- Apple/carrot juice
- Carrot-only juice
- Green juice
- Orange juice

Occasionally, for special cases, a different juice may have to be substituted. For example, diabetics receive grapefruit juice instead of orange juice, since grapefruit contains less sugar; sometimes a fruit juice, such as apple juice, is given to patients with collagen diseases who should not drink citrus juice.

Apple/Carrot Juice

Use approximately 8 ounces each of carrots and apples. Wash and brush (do not peel), grind to a pulp and place in a cloth supplied with the press-type juicer to press. Serve and drink immediately.

Carrot-Only Juice

Use approximately 10-12 ounces of carrots. Wash and brush (do not peel), grind to a pulp and place in a cloth supplied with the press-type juicer to press. Serve and drink immediately.

Green Juice

Use romaine, red leaf lettuce, endive, escarole, two to three leaves of red cabbage, young inner beet tops, Swiss chard, a quarter of a small green pepper and watercress. Add one medium apple when grinding. Procure as many of these materials as possible. If some of the above items are not available, do not use substitutes, such as spinach or celery. Grind the material to a pulp and place in a cloth for pressing. This juice must be drunk immediately since its enzymes die quickly.

Orange (or Grapefruit) Juice

Use only a reamer-type juicer, electric or hand operated. Do not squeeze the peel of the fruit. The aromatic oils contained in the skin are harmful and would interfere with the treatment.

THE DAILY ROUTINE

The typical average daily menu of the Gerson patient is as follows:

Breakfast

- A large bowl of oatmeal cooked in distilled water and sweetened with a little honey or dried fruit, presoaked (soak overnight in cold water, or pour boiling water over them)
- An 8-ounce glass of freshly squeezed orange juice
- Some additional raw or stewed fruit
- *Optional:* a slice of toasted, unsalted, organic rye bread

Lunch

- A large plate of mixed raw salad with flaxseed oil dressing (see the Flaxseed Oil and Lemon Juice Dressing recipe in Chapter 28, "Recipes," p. 321)

- 8 to 10 ounces of the "Special Soup or Hippocrates Soup" (see p. 158)
- Baked, boiled, mashed or otherwise prepared potato
- 1 to 2 freshly cooked vegetables
- Raw or stewed fruit for dessert

Dinner

- Follows the same order as lunch, but is varied with different vegetables and fruit for dessert

Please note: Either at lunch or dinner, and after the patient has consumed the necessary foods, he or she may eat a second slice of unsalted, organic rye bread. However, bread should not satisfy the appetite or take the place of essential foods.

BASIC RECIPES TO START YOU OFF

For a full range of Gerson recipes, please see Chapter 28, "Recipes," p. 311. The following instructions are only meant to introduce the most fundamental items of the patient's essential daily menu.

Breakfast

For one person, put 5 ounces of rolled oats into 12 ounces of distilled water. Start with cold water, bring to a boil and let simmer for 6 to 8 minutes, stirring occasionally. Meanwhile, squeeze orange juice and add any prescribed medication(s) (see Chapter 14, "Medications," p. 175). Serve the oatmeal with presoaked (soak overnight in cold water, or pour boiling water over them and leave for a couple of hours until plump), unsulphured dried fruit (e.g., apricots, apple rings, prunes, raisins and mango), or use raw or stewed apple or stewed plums, or fresh fruit in season (e.g., peaches, nectarines, grapes or pears) Do not use berries. Up to 2 teaspoons a day of permitted sweeteners (e.g., honey, maple syrup, spray-dried cane juices sold as sucanat (an organic dried cane sugar) and rapadura, or unsulphured molasses) may be used.

Lunch

For the salad, cut up, slice and mix varied lettuces, such as red leaf lettuce, Romaine, escarole, salad bowl and endive. Add to the mixture chopped green onions, radishes, a little celery, some tomatoes, cauliflower florets, slices of green pepper and watercress. For the dressing (see the Flaxseed Oil and Lemon Juice Dressing recipe in Chapter 28, "Recipes," p. 321), mix 1 tablespoon of flaxseed oil (during the first month of the therapy; afterwards, reduce to 2 teaspoons) with apple cider or red wine vinegar, or lemon or lime juice. Add garlic to taste.

"Special Soup or Hippocrates Soup" (see below) is to be eaten twice daily throughout the treatment. To save time and effort, prepare enough for two days (i.e., four portions). It will keep in the refrigerator overnight for the next day.

Special Soup or Hippocrates Soup

1 medium celery root, if available
  (if not, 3 to 4 celery branches (i.e., pascal))
1 medium parsley root (rarely available; may be omitted)
2 small or one large leek (if not available, use 2 small onions instead)
2 medium onions
garlic to taste
  (may also be squeezed raw into the hot soup instead of cooking it)
small amount of parsley
1-1/2 pounds tomatoes (or more, if desired)
1 pound potatoes

Wash and scrub vegetables and cut into slices or 1/2-inch cubes. Put in large pot, add water to just cover vegetables, bring to a boil, then cook slowly on low heat for 1-1/2 to 2 hours until all the vegetables are soft.

Pass through a food mill to remove fibers. Let soup cool before storing in refrigerator.

Please note: Many spices are high in aromatic acids, which are irritants and are likely to counteract the healing reaction. This is why only the following mild spices are permitted, to be used in *very small doses*: allspice, anise, bay leaves, coriander, dill, fennel, mace, marjoram, rosemary, saffron, sage, sorrel, summer savory, tarragon and thyme. In addition, chives, garlic, onion and parsley may be used in larger amounts.

Two herb teas—chamomile and peppermint—are frequently used by Gerson patients. For details, please see Chapter 13, "All About Enemas," p. 161, and Chapter 16, "Understanding Healing Reactions," p. 187.

CHAPTER 13

All About Enemas

To the uninitiated, the coffee enema is the most surprising and apparently bizarre element of the Gerson Therapy. Critics like to attack and ridicule it without bothering to find out its purpose and function. Yet, without this simple tool of detoxification, the Gerson method wouldn't work. Before going into details, let us make clear why this is so.

The moment a patient is put on the full therapy, the combined effect of the food, the juices and the medication causes the immune system to attack and kill tumor tissue, besides working to flush out accumulated toxins from the body tissues. This great clearing-out procedure carries the risk of overburdening and poisoning the liver—the all-important organ of detoxification, which, in a cancer patient, is bound to be already damaged and debilitated. It was this recognition that prompted Dr. Gerson some 70 years ago to incorporate the coffee enema in the program. He realized that, without this additional means of detoxification, the liver was in danger of becoming comatose, which could severely damage or even kill the patient. In this chapter, we fully explain how the coffee enema prevents this.

Generally speaking, any kind of enema introduces a substance into the rectum in order to empty the bowel or to administer nutrients or drugs. It is a medical procedure of great antiquity. Hippocrates, the Greek "father of modern medicine," prescribed water enemas for several conditions some 2,600 years ago. In India, enemas were recommended for inner cleansing by Patanjali, author of the first written work

161

on yoga, in around 200 B.C. According to tradition, the ibis (a sacred bird of ancient Egypt associated with wisdom) used to administer itself an enema with its long curved beak. Closer to our own time, a lady in the court of King Louis XIV of France is reported to have taken an enema under her voluminous skirts, and "Le Malade Imaginaire" (i.e., "The Hypochondriac," in Moliere's play of the same title) enjoyed an enema on stage. It is only in recent times, and mainly in English-speaking countries, that this simple and safe cleansing method had fallen into disuse.

The use of coffee as enema material began in Germany towards the end of World War I (1914-1918). The country was blockaded by the Allies and many essential goods—among them, morphine—were not available, yet trainloads of wounded soldiers kept arriving at field hospitals, needing surgery. The surgeons had barely enough morphine to dull the pain of the operations but none to help patients endure the postsurgical pain; all they could do was to use water enemas.

Although, owing to the blockade, coffee was in short supply, there was plenty of it around to help the surgeons stay awake during their long spells of duty. The nurses, desperate to ease their patients' pain, began to pour some of the leftover coffee into the enema buckets. They figured that, since it helped the surgeons (who drank it), the soldiers (who didn't) would also benefit from it. Indeed, the soldiers reported pain relief.

This accidental discovery came to the attention of two medical researchers—Professors Meyer and Huebner at the University of Goettingen[1] in Germany—who went on to test the effects of rectally infused caffeine on rats. They found that the caffeine, traveling via the hemorrhoidal vein and the portal system to the liver, opened up the bile ducts, allowing the liver to release accumulated toxins. This observation was confirmed 70 years later, in 1990, by Peter Lechner, MD,[2] oncologist surgeon at the District Hospital of Graz, Austria, after running a six-year controlled test on cancer patients following a slightly modified version of the Gerson Therapy. In his report, he quotes independent laboratory results, identifying the two components of coffee that play the major role in detoxifying the liver. (See Chapter 8, "Why Does the Gerson Therapy Work?," p. 123.)

Dr. Gerson became aware of the benefits of enemas early in developing his treatment, and they have remained a cornerstone of his therapy to this day. It is important to realize that, while the patient is holding the coffee enema in his or her colon for the suggested 12 to 15 minutes, the body's entire blood supply passes through the liver every three minutes (i.e., four to five times in all), carrying poisons picked up from the tissues. These are then released through the bile ducts due to the stimulation of the caffeine.

However, in order to leave the body, these toxins still have to travel through the small intestine (25 to 27 feet), through the colon (4 to 5 feet) and out via the rectum and the anus. Naturally, on this long trip, a small amount of the released toxins is reabsorbed into the system and can cause the patient discomfort, especially in the early phase of the therapy, when detoxification had only just started. This is the reason why, in the beginning, five or more enemas are taken daily to keep up the elimination process, and why the more rapid castor oil treatment (see "The Castor Oil Treatment," p. 170) is also part of the program for the average patient.

Important warning: Although high colonics have become fashionable among some celebrities, they must not be used by Gerson patients. Dr. Gerson had stated this very clearly, and we can only reiterate his conclusion. In high colonics, up to 5 quarts of water are forced into the whole length of the large intestine, under pressure that can easily distend it. When the water is released, it washes out the fluids, enzymes, minerals and other nutrients from the colon, together with the friendly bacteria which are vital for good digestion. This can increase the risk of a mineral imbalance. On the other hand, high colonics don't serve the all-important reason for the use of coffee enemas, namely the opening of the bile ducts, which helps the liver to release toxins and cleanse itself. On no account should anyone make the mistake of thinking that high colonics are interchangeable with coffee enemas.

We have presented the history and theoretical background. Now let us see the practicalities.

THE BASICS AND HOW TO USE THEM

The basic components of the coffee enema are the following:

- Organic, medium or light roast drip-grind coffee
- Filtered, or if from a fluoridated source, distilled water
- Enema equipment

The equipment must be carefully chosen, as not all products on the market are suitable. The earliest type—the combination syringe—is a rubber hot-water bottle, complete with appropriate tubing and rectal or vaginal tip. This works well for occasional use or travel but it is difficult to clean. Other rubber bags, not "combination syringes," have a much wider opening, which makes them easier to clean. However, they don't stand up well to constant use.

Most popular among Gerson patients is the plastic bucket, which has an easy-to-read register of ounces. This shows how much of the coffee the patient has introduced into the rectum. The bucket is easy to clean and has only one drawback: if dropped or cleaned too vigorously, it can break and must be replaced.

That risk is avoided by choosing a stainless steel bucket, now available at the relatively cheap price of about $30, including the needed attachments. It is unbreakable and easy to clean, even with very hot water, which shouldn't be used with the plastic bucket. The rubber tubing needs to be replaced occasionally. The only disadvantage of this type is that, not being transparent, one cannot check how far the enema process has progressed.

The standard mixture for one enema consists of 3 rounded tablespoons of organic, medium or light roast drip-grind coffee, and 32 ounces of filtered or distilled water. The procedure is to bring the water to a boil, add the coffee, let it boil for 3 minutes, then turn down the heat and let it simmer (covered) for 15 minutes. Let it cool, then strain it through a cloth-lined strainer. (A piece of clean, white linen or nylon can be used.) Check the amount left after straining and replace the water that has boiled away to restore it to 1 quart.

For patients on the therapy, it is best to prepare the whole day's requirement at once rather than cooking each portion separately every 4 hours. In other words, a coffee concentrate is produced, saving much time and effort. Take a pot which holds at least 3 quarts, put in about 2 quarts of filtered or distilled water, bring it to a boil and add 15 rounded tablespoons of coffee, which will be enough for five enemas, then proceed as above. After straining the liquid, take five 1-quart jars or juice bottles, pour the same amount of the concentrate into each, then add enough water to make up the volume to 8 ounces of concentrate.

The standard mixture for one enema (i.e., 8 ounces of coffee concentrate and 24 ounces of water, making a total of 32 ounces) has to be warmed to body temperature and poured into the enema bucket, having first clamped the tube shut to stop the liquid from running out. Before starting the enema, a small amount of the solution should be released to clear the tube of air. It is a good idea to eat a small piece of fruit to get the digestive system going, especially before the first morning enema. This will provide a little glucose to raise the low blood sugar after a night's sleep.

The more relaxed the patient is, the easier the enema experience will be. That requires comfort. Unless a couch or folding camp bed is available, an enema "nest" is made on the bathroom floor, with a large, soft towel or blanket as its base, covered with an enema mat or a soft polyester shower curtain for accidental leaks or spillage and a pillow or cushion for the head. The bucket is placed at approximately 18 inches above the body, hanging from a hook or standing on a stool. The coffee should not flow in too fast or with too much pressure. About 2 inches of the tube's tip is lubricated with Vaseline® and gently inserted some 8 to 10 inches into the anus, and the clamp on the tube is released to let the coffee flow in. The patient lies on his or her right side with legs pulled up in the fetal position, relaxed and breathing deeply. When all the coffee is absorbed, it should be held in for 12 to 15 minutes, before evacuating.

Many patients enjoy the relaxed comfort of enema time—"upside-down coffee," as some call it—and use it to listen to soothing music, to meditate or to read. One young lady, recovering from a brain tumor on the Gerson program over some two years, first read all the main classics, then switched to philosophy, followed by mathematics, and subsequently became so well read that she won a top scholarship! She also made a full recovery.

Important note: For patients who have been pretreated with chemotherapy, the enema schedule is reduced. It has become evident that such patients must be detoxified more slowly and cautiously so as not to release all the remaining toxic chemotherapy residues too rapidly, which would add up to a dangerous overdose.

HOW MANY? HOW OFTEN?

Most "regular" patients (i.e., those not pretreated with chemotherapy nor very debilitated) are on a four-hourly enema schedule (e.g., 6 a.m., 10 a.m., 2 p.m., 6 p.m. and 10 p.m.), concurrently drinking the prescribed 12 to 13 glasses of juice. This is absolutely essential. Although the enema reaches only part of the colon, it inevitably removes some of the minerals from it and, without the mineral-rich juices, an electrolyte imbalance could result. In general, three juices per enema is a good guideline.

There are times when the four-hourly schedule needs modification, adding extra enemas to the daily routine. Temporarily doing so does not necessitate extra juices. Enemas are excellent pain relievers; if a patient is in severe pain, there is nothing wrong with taking one before the four hours are up. Dr. Gerson also suggested that, in some cases, when very large tumors are broken down and are being absorbed, the patient should take an additional enema during the night—around 2 or 3 a.m.—to avoid waking up in pain, with a headache or even in a semicomatose state in the morning. Some patients even take enemas every two hours to control pain, gas or other kinds of discomfort.

It is important to remember that coffee enemas do not interfere with the normal activity of the colon, producing daily bowel movements. Occasionally, patients worry about that but their fears are groundless. Once the liver and the digestive system are fully restored, normal elimination takes over, even in those who had previously suffered from constipation.

POSSIBLE PROBLEMS

Many patients learn the enema routine without difficulty and enjoy the feeling of lightness and added energy yielded by the practice. Others, however, experience difficulties, which need to be eliminated. Some of the problems that may arise are listed below.

Patients may arrive at the hospital with a massive accumulation of stool in their colon, caused by the use of heavy pain-killing drugs, including morphine. These tend to paralyze peristalsis (the alternate contraction and relaxation of the intestine, by which the contents are propelled onward), causing severe constipation. As a result, these patients are unable to take in a quart (32 ounces) of the coffee solution, let alone hold it in. The answer for them is to take whatever amount they can comfortably accommodate, stop and hold this as long as possible (even if only for a few minutes), then release and take the remaining coffee solution. Again, hold it and release after 12 to 15 minutes. As a rule, after two or three days, when the colon has been cleared of old accumulations, the whole enemas can be taken and held without difficulty.

Some patients may suffer from gas retention, which stops the enema from getting into the colon. When that happens, a small amount—say 6 to 10 ounces—of the coffee can be infused, after which the bucket is lowered to the patient's level, allowing the coffee to flow back into the bucket. This often releases the gas, causing some "bubbling" in the bucket. The bucket is then raised again and, after the clearing of the gas, the enema can continue more easily.

The patient is supposed to take the enema lying on his or her right side in order to help the coffee solution get into the transverse colon from the descending colon. However, as a result of surgery, arthritis or tumors, the right side may be too painful on which to lie. In such case, the patient has to lie on his or her back, with their legs pulled up, and proceed from that position.

If a patient suffers from severe irritation of the colon, a small portion of the coffee concentrate, say 2 to 4 ounces, can be diluted with chamomile tea instead of water. The smaller amount of coffee will still help to detoxify the liver while the chamomile tea soothes the colon. There is no time limit for the use of chamomile tea. In the case of severe diarrhea, an enema of chamomile tea only is used for gentle morning and evening cleansing.

To prepare chamomile tea, put 1 ounce of the dried flower heads into a glass dish, add 1 pint of boiling water, cover the dish and let it stand in a warm place to infuse for 15 minutes. Strain, cool and store it in a stoppered bottle for a maximum of three days. Increase amounts in the above proportion as required. Chamomile is one of the herbs most used in the Gerson Therapy, both as an enema component and as an herbal drink.

Sometimes a patient has been doing enemas for the first few days of the treatment without a problem, but suddenly he or she cannot get more than 8 to 12 ounces into the colon. This may be a symptom of a healing reaction or flare-up, and the solution is to take what is possible, release it and take the rest. Even if the coffee solution has to be infused in three small amounts, it doesn't matter.

Flare-ups are dealt with in detail in Chapter 16, "Understanding Healing Reactions," p. 187. In brief, they occur when so much bile is released that the intestine is unable to contain it all. The bile then overflows and backs up into the stomach. Since the stomach needs to be acid in order to hold and digest food, the highly alkaline bile produces enormous discomfort; the stomach cannot hold food or liquid and the patient vomits. In itself, this type of flare-up is welcome because it clears out a lot of toxic bile but, in the process, the stomach membrane becomes irritated and needs instant relief. To do that, the patient needs to drink as much peppermint tea and oatmeal gruel (see Chapter 16, "Understanding Healing Reactions," p. 189) as possible. At the same time, the coffee enemas are reduced since they are causing the heavy flow of bile. The correct order for the next two to three days is two chamomile enemas and only one coffee enema a day, until the nausea and vomiting clear up. Then the regular schedule can be resumed.

During the flare-up, if the patient vomits and also has diarrhea, the body loses a lot of fluid, so dehydration must be prevented. One way is to use more chamomile enemas instead of coffee. Also, the carrot/apple and green juices can be used as rectal implants. The regular 8-ounce dose of juice is warmed to body temperature by standing the glass in a warm water bath (not on the stove and without diluting it) and gently infused into the rectum. This is not an enema and the patient should hold it until the liquid is absorbed. That may not take more than 10 to 15 minutes of lying still in bed. These infusions can be used with all the juices, even every hour, instead of having them as drinks—particularly valuable at times when, during the flare-up, the patient cannot even bear to look at a juice, let alone drink it.

Please note: Do not infuse orange juice into the rectum.

Another problem occurs when the patient takes in the full 32 ounces of coffee solution but, after 12 minutes, is unable to release it. When that happens, the usual reaction is to take another enema, expecting it to push out the first lot, but that doesn't happen and the patient tends to panic. The reason for the blockage is that the colon spasms, cramps and doesn't release the liquid. Of course, there is no danger in this—the colon could actually hold up to 5 quarts—but that is not the point. If the trouble is caused by cramping, the patient needs to lie down on his or her side, with a warm water bottle on their stomach, and try to relax. If that doesn't put things right, a small amount of castor oil can be applied to the rectum; this usually promotes relaxation and release. However, if the situation lasts a little longer, including the time for the next enema, it helps to put 2 tablespoons of the regular potassium compound (see

Chapter 14, "Medications," p. 175) into each enema for a few days. This will help to release cramps and/or spasms.

Please note: Do not use this method for more than two to three days to avoid irritating the rectum and the colon.

It is only when they are on the regular enema routine that patients realize how much waste material their bodies have stored over many years. Once the organism gets a go-ahead in the direction of self-cleansing, it does release a variety of strange, disturbing accumulations which appear in the enema returns, including a wide range of parasites. Experts claim that some 85% of us harbor parasites in our colon, which are best expelled. So the message is not to panic if the enema returns contain unusual substances; they prove that detoxification and cleansing is progressing well.

THE CASTOR OIL TREATMENT

As we explained above (p. 163), the toxins released from the liver by the all-important coffee enema still have a long way to travel (down the 25- to 27-foot-long small intestine, then through the 4 to 5 feet of large intestine) before they can leave the body via the anus. In the course of this evacuation, it is unavoidable that some of the released toxins get reabsorbed. It takes time—sometimes too much time—to expel from the body the accumulated residues of years of faulty eating, plus the toxic breakdown products of tumors. Time being of the essence on the program, particularly in the case of seriously ill patients, Dr. Gerson saw a real need to speed up the elimination process in order to reduce the reabsorption to a minimum. To achieve this and to clear accumulations in the small intestine, which the enema cannot reach, he added the castor oil treatment to the intensive therapy.

This consists of taking castor oil by mouth, as well as by enema, to speed up and reinforce the release of toxic residues from the intestinal tract. The patient is awakened at about 5 a.m. to take 2 tablespoons of castor oil, followed immediately by 1/2 to 2/3 cup of regular black coffee (not enema coffee or concentrate), sweetened with 1/2 teaspoon of sucanat or other organic dried cane sugar. (Diabetics do not take sugar in this coffee.) People who object to sweetened coffee need to understand that the sugar is necessary to activate stomach peristalsis and counteract low blood sugar. The 6 a.m. coffee enema as well as breakfast are taken as usual. Five hours after the oral administration of the oil—at 10 a.m.—a castor oil enema is taken instead of the normal coffee enema.

The castor oil enema is prepared by using a second enema bucket exclusively reserved for this treatment. Put 4 tablespoons of castor oil into the enema bucket. Add 1/4 teaspoons of ox bile powder and stir well to mix thoroughly. Prepare the regular enema mixture of 8 ounces of coffee concentrate plus 24 ounces of purified or distilled water. Warm to body temperature. Get a cake of mild toilet soap (not detergent) (e.g., Lux®, Camay® or similar), immerse it for a few moments in the coffee and rub some of the soap (but no soap chips or liquid soap) into it. Mix the slightly soapy enema coffee into the castor oil with the ox bile, and stir well to emulsify the solution as much as possible. You may use an electric stirrer, but the somewhat emulsified oil will still rise to the top while you are trying to take the enema. In fact, most patients find it impossible to stir the solution vigorously enough to keep the oil mixed into the coffee on their own; they need a helper to do that. When the coffee plus castor oil is all infused, try to hold the solution for a little while, but you are unlikely to succeed. It doesn't matter; release when necessary. This enema does its work very fast. The castor oil treatment is taken every other day for the first four to five months of the intensive therapy and then slowly reduced.

Please note: Patients pretreated with chemotherapy *must not use the castor oil treatment.*

Patients react to the castor oil treatment in widely different ways. For many, it is just a mild inconvenience due to the powerful cleansing effect of the oil; on castor oil days, it is wise to stay close to the bathroom. Others find the taste and weak smell of the oil off-putting. This can be mitigated by eating a small piece of fruit before taking the oil, or having half an orange handy and sucking it immediately afterwards. Some patients simply add the oil to the cup of coffee, and then use a straw or a glass tube, inserted into the oil, to get it into the back of the mouth, followed immediately by the coffee to chase it down.

This is the only occasion in the Gerson program when patients drink coffee. It is done in order to activate the stomach muscles and move the oil out as fast as possible, so that the patient is not nauseated for hours while the oil remains in his or her stomach but is able to enjoy breakfast and the juices that follow. A few patients have tried to substitute peppermint or some other herb tea for the coffee, but undoubtedly coffee works best and should be taken, even by those who don't normally drink it.

CLEANING THE EQUIPMENT

Like all other tools of the Gerson program, the enema bucket has to be kept clean. Since the anus, rectum and colon are not sterile, the equipment need not be sterilized. After each use, the bucket has to be rinsed with hot, soapy water, running it through the tube as well, and then rinsed again thoroughly to remove the soap. Two or three times a week, it is wise to put a cup of 3% hydrogen peroxide (from the supermarket or drug store) into the bucket with the clamp closed and let it stand overnight to kill any germs or impurities. Rinse it out before the first use in the morning.

Caution: If you keep the plastic tube attached to the bucket, it will eventually become loose and even slip off, treating you to an unwanted coffee shower. Check the fit frequently and, if necessary, cut an inch or so from the loosened end of the tube and replace the tight part. You can prevent accidents by removing the plastic tube every time before running hot water through the bucket, so that it shrinks back to its original size and remains tightly in position.

The bucket reserved for the castor oil treatment is also cleaned as above but with generous use of hot, soapy water in order to get rid of any oily residues. Wipe the inside of the bucket with a piece of absorbent paper to finish the cleaning.

REFERENCES

1. M. Gerson, *A Cancer Therapy: Results of Fifty Cases and The Cure of Advanced Cancer by Diet Therapy: A Summary of Thirty Years of Clinical Experimentation,* 6th ed. (San Diego, CA: Gerson Institute, 1999).
2. Peter Lechner, MD, "Dietary Regime to be Used in Oncological Postoperative Care," Proceedings of the Oesterreicher Gesellschaft fur Chirurgie (Jun. 21-23, 1984).

Medications

F or the general public, "medications" normally mean drugs, used in allopathic medicine in the treatment of disease. In acute cases and emergencies, many drugs are life saving and highly valuable. However, when it comes to chronic conditions, as a rule, the synthetic drugs, which are alien to the body, can merely alleviate (i.e., suppress) symptoms without dealing with the basic cause. This process is often accompanied by severe side effects, which may require more drugs to control.

The medications used in the Gerson Therapy belong to a totally different category. Far from being drugs, they are nutritional supplements consisting of natural substances present in, and needed for, the normal functioning of the various body systems. Being natural, they have no damaging side effects. Their purpose is to make up for the deficiencies of the sick body until it recovers sufficiently to cover all its needs. These substances are so pure that, even if they are incorrectly used by mistake or are in excessive or insufficient doses, they do no harm—with the exception of the thyroid/iodine supplementation, which must be correctly adjusted.

Let us take them one by one and explore their purpose.

POTASSIUM COMPOUND

Dr. Gerson found that the basic problem in all chronic degenerative diseases is the loss of potassium from, and the penetration of sodium into, the cells, now known as the tissue damage syndrome. The average diet in most countries, especially in the developed world, contains far too much salt (sodium), which eventually causes the breakdown of the healthy balance within the body.[1] To correct this, Dr. Gerson added a large amount of potassium (a 10% solution of three potassium salts) to the already potassium-rich, organic vegetarian diet, and observed that this enabled the sick body to release the excess sodium, together with edema, while also reducing high blood pressure and, in most cases, pain.

To prepare the compound, 100 grams of three ready-mixed potassium salts are dissolved in 1 quart of distilled water and stored in a dark glass bottle, or in a clear one kept inside a large brown or black paper bag, to keep out all light. On the full intensive therapy, 4 teaspoons of the potassium compound are added to 10 of the freshly prepared fruit and/or vegetable juices. This dosage is reduced after three to four weeks to 2 teaspoons in each of 10 juices.

In seriously ill patients, it takes many months, even one to two years, to restore normal potassium content to the essential organs. The serum potassium level, as shown in the blood test result, does not reflect the potassium status of the cell. Low serum potassium values may signify healing because the depleted tissues are reabsorbing potassium, while high figures may be found in failures because the tissues lose it.

THYROID AND LUGOL'S SOLUTION

It is a fact—known since Dr. Gerson's day—that most cancer patients are suffering from a low basal metabolism.[2] Much of the problem is caused by the chlorine,[3] widely used in the purification of the water supply and, worse still, by fluoride.[4] Both remove iodine from the thyroid gland, thus reducing its ability to function properly. The thyroid gland regulates the metabolic rate of the organism, acting as its thermostat, being capable of raising temperature and producing fever. It also affects the immune system as well as the proper functioning of all hormone systems.

When thyroid and iodine in the form of 1/2 strength Lugol's solution are added to the patient's intake, the immune system becomes reactivated and healing can begin. The patient's metabolic rate has to be established for a correct dosage, but most cancer patients start with 5 grains of thyroid and 18 drops of Lugol's solution (three drops in each of one orange and five carrot/apple juices) a day, for the first three to four weeks only. Then the amounts are reduced to 2 or 2-1/2 grains of thyroid and 12 drops of Lugol's, and subsequently adjusted according to the Gerson doctor's instruction. Patients suffering from nonmalignant diseases use the less intensive therapy (see Chapter 19, "The Gerson Therapy for Nonmalignant Diseases," p. 205) with much less thyroid and Lugol's solution.

NIACIN

Niacin (common name for nicotinic acid, or vitamin B_3) assists in the digestion of protein and helps to open capillary circulation, thus bringing freshly oxygenated blood (from the constant intake of fresh juices) to all body tissues. By improving circulation, it also works to reduce ascites (abdominal edema) and pain. The dosage is a 50 mg tablet six times daily, taken during meals. This medication often causes the well-known "niacin flush," a temporary reddening of the face and upper chest area, with some itching. This is totally harmless and passes quickly. (Do not switch to nonflushing niacin; it is ineffective.) Niacin should be discontinued during women's periods or in case of bleeding of any kind.

LIVER CAPSULES

The severely toxic and damaged liver of the cancer patient needs maximum assistance to improve its vital functions. The therapy provides this help in the form of liver capsules containing dried, defatted, powdered liver from healthy animals. Two capsules of liver powder are given three times a day with carrot-only juice. According to Dr. Virginia Livingston,[5] the combination of dry liver powder with carrot juice produces abscissic acid, a precursor of vitamin A, which is essential in attacking tumor tissue.

CRUDE LIVER INJECTIONS WITH B_{12} SUPPLEMENT

These injections, which normally contain a small amount of vitamin B_{12}, are an additional substance given to aid in the restoration of the liver. However, since virtually all cancer patients are anemic, additional vitamin B_{12} is needed to help restore the hemoglobin content of the blood, promoting the formation and maturation of red blood cells. It works against different types of anemia and even against degenerative changes in the spinal cord. As seen in animal experiments, this vitamin is able to restore a wide range of tissues damaged by age, chronic illness, surgery, degenerative diseases or various kinds of poisoning. Intramuscular liver extract (3 cc) with added 50 mcg of B_{12}—a tiny amount, a 20th of 1 cc— is given daily for four or more months. Later, the frequency is reduced to every other day; still later—sometimes after as much as a year—to twice a week.

PANCREATIN

This is an extract of various pancreatic digestive enzymes, normally needed to digest fats, proteins and sugar. Gerson patients don't consume those substances; however, these enzymes are vitally important in the digestion and elimination of tumor tissue. The dosage is 3 tablets of 325 mg each four times a day—one after each meal, plus an additional dose in mid-afternoon. For exceptionally large tumors, 2-3 tablets a day of a more concentrated 1,200 mg pancreatin may be added to the patient's medication. Some patients cannot tolerate pancreatin and have to do without it. Dr. Gerson also omitted pancreatin for sarcoma cases.

ACIDOL PEPSIN

These tablets supply digestive stomach juices, badly needed by patients suffering from chronic diseases who tend to have insufficient stomach acid and digestive pepsin. As a result, they have poor appetite and poor digestion. Since the Gerson treatment is based on the patient's optimum intake of food and juices, the stomach needs help for the intake and digestion of food. Acidol pepsin aids protein digestion and the absorption of iron, while helping to eliminate gas and bloating. The dosage is six tablets a day, two to be taken before each meal. No acidol is given in cases of acid reflux, stomach ulcers or other inflammatory or irritated conditions of the stomach.

OX BILE POWDER

This helps to emulsify the castor oil, which is used in the castor oil/coffee enemas. The powder is mixed into the castor oil and stirred before the slightly soapy coffee is added.

FLAXSEED OIL

Also known as food-grade linseed oil, this contains both essential fatty acids—linoleic acid and linolenic acid—and is particularly rich in the Omega-3 series, as discovered by Johanna Budwig, MD.[6] The therapeutic effects of flaxseed oil include the following:

- It attracts oxygen at the cell membrane and transports oxygen into the cell.
- It is able to detoxify fat-soluble toxins and helps to dissolve and remove plaque.
- It is a carrier of vitamin A, which is important for the immune system.
- It removes excess cholesterol, an important function, since patients' cholesterol levels sometimes rise during the initial stages of the therapy.

The dose is 2 tablespoons daily for the first month, then 1 tablespoon daily for the rest of the treatment (limited, similar to medications, and reduced to 1 tablespoon daily after 30 days).

COENZYME Q10

Recently added to the protocol, this coenzyme is valuable in replacing some of the nutrients that were available in the discontinued raw liver juice. It must be administered cautiously at first, since some patients are hypersensitive to this substance. To start, the dose is 50 mg daily for five to seven days, then increased to 100 mg per day, to reach 500 to 600 mg daily.

REFERENCES

1. Freeman Widener Cope, *Physiological Chemistry and Physics* 10 (5) (1978).
2. Kathy Page, "Hypothyroidism and Cancer," supplementary memorandum, UK Parliament Select Committee on Science and Technology (June 2000).
3. Joseph M. Price, *Coronaries, cholesterol, chlorine* (Salem, MA: Pyramid Books, 1971).
4. P. M. Galetti and G. Joyet, "Effect of fluorine on thyroidal iodine metabolism in hyperthyroidism," *Journal of Clinical Endocrinology and Metabolism* 18 (10) (October 1958): 1102-10.
5. Personal communication from Dr. Livingston to Charlotte Gerson (February 1977).
6. Johanna Budwig, MD, *Flax Oil As a True Aid Against Arthritis Heart Infarction Cancer and Other Diseases*, 3d ed. (Ferndale, WA: Apple Publishing, December 1994).

CHAPTER 15

Pain Control Without Drugs

A large percentage of patients arrive at the Gerson hospital in pain or on heavy pain-control medication, including morphine, codeine or the two combined (e.g., in the drug OxiContin®). These drugs are highly toxic[1] and, since detoxifying the body is the basic aim of the Gerson Therapy, every effort has to be made to control the patients' pain without the use of toxic drugs.

The first tool to achieve this is the coffee enema (see Chapter 13, "All About Enemas," p. 161). Removing the accumulated toxins from the liver enables that vital organ to absorb and release more poisons stored in the body, which brings immediate relief to the patient. It does not, however, get rid of the pain altogether, and mild pain-relief drugs (e.g., aspirin, ibuprofen or Tylenol®) might be needed. However, these may not work if the patient had been used to morphine; in such cases, the Gerson doctor will use one or more of the following:

- Castor oil packs
- Clay (mud) packs
- Hyperthermia (hydrotherapy) (artificial fever)
- Laetrile
- Oxygen treatments
- Rebounding
- The "triad" (one aspirin, one vitamin C (500 mg) and one niacin (50 mg))

The following sections give instructions how to apply them.

CASTOR OIL PACKS

Warm castor oil packs help to alleviate muscle and bone pain, spasms and cramping, including those in the liver area or in any part of the body that is painful. They increase circulation, relax muscles and disperse toxicity, and act fast and reliably.

To prepare a castor oil pack, a piece of white wool flannel (cotton flannel is acceptable) is cut into three identical pieces large enough to cover the affected area. The usual size is about 9 x 11 inches. One piece of flannel is placed on a flat surface and covered with a thin layer of castor oil. The second piece goes on top of this and is also spread with the oil. The third piece covers this, making something like a triple-decker sandwich. This basic pack is laid on the skin over the painful area, covered with a slightly larger sheet of plastic to prevent nasty stains on bedclothes or nightwear, and kept securely in position with a bandage or other suitable material. Finally, a mildly warm (not hot) water bottle is placed on top of the pack. This is preferable to an electric heating pad whose electromagnetic output would interfere with the body's own energy field.

The pack can be left in place for several hours, or even all day and all night, provided that the water in the bottle is replaced as it cools. A few patients have felt discomfort as the castor oil pack increased the liver's healing activity. In such cases, the pack was removed and reused another time. The castor oil pack can be saved and reused. Some patients reported the best results from alternating the clay (mud) and the castor oil packs, which is perfectly acceptable.

CLAY (MUD) PACKS

Clay (mud) packs help to relieve "hot" inflammations around arthritic joints and tumors and in other areas of fluid retention. The best clay is montmorillonite (not of marine origin), which also absorbs toxins through the skin. Taken internally in peppermint tea (1/4 to 1/2 teaspoons to a cup), clay even helps to clear diarrhea and general food poisoning. Clay (mud) packs have long been used in many parts of the world. Applied around the head, they are even able to alleviate headaches and seizures.

The clay (mud) pack is prepared by mixing the dry clay powder with enough hot distilled water to make a spreadable paste, neither too runny nor too dry. A layer about 2 to 3 mm thick is spread on a piece of clean, white cloth, placed on the affected area and covered with a piece of plastic and a wool cloth. Secured in position, it can be left in place for two to three hours and removed and discarded when it has become dry. Clay (mud) packs may be used two or three times a day, as required, but must not be placed on an open lesion.

HYPERTHERMIA (HYDROTHERAPY)

When a patient suffers from pain, especially bone pain, or if she or he is uneasy because the expected healing reaction has not taken place, certain procedures can be helpful. One of these is hyperthermia, a warm water treatment. It consists of immersing the patient up to the chin in a tub of unfluoridated water that is considerably warmer than what would be used for a regular bath. When the patient has gotten used to the warmth, the temperature of the water can be cautiously increased by adding more hot water to 102° F (39° C), or even a little above. The purpose of this treatment is not only to increase circulation (which alleviates pain) but also to raise the patient's temperature; in other words, to create a fever.

Malignant tissue is sensitive to an increase in temperature and can be killed by fever. Hence, raising the body temperature to 102° F (39° C) or above is extremely beneficial. We have never seen a fever in excess of 104° F (40° C). True body damage does not occur until the temperature reaches over 106° F (41° C). A nurse or attendant should be present during hot baths for extra safety and to check the water's temperature with a bath thermometer. The patient may be given some hot herb tea to replace fluids lost by perspiration and have a cool (not ice-cold) cloth placed on the forehead for comfort. At the end of the bath, which

183

doesn't usually last for more than 20 minutes, the patient is quickly dried with warm towels and put into a warm bed, allowing his or her body temperature to slowly return to normal.

Hyperthermia should not be used for patients who suffer from cardiac problems, high blood pressure or breathing difficulties or who, due to age, have a weak heart and constitution. It should never be used with fluoridated water.

To enhance the effect of the hyperthermia, some cancer patients are also given an intravenous injection of laetrile some 15 minutes prior to going into the bath. Laetrile, also known as vitamin B_{17}, is derived from apricot pits. It is nontoxic even though it contains a cyanide fraction. This substance is not damaging to normal healthy cells (after all, the full name of vitamin B_{12} is *cyano*cobalamine!) because these cells contain an enzyme—rhodanase—that neutralizes the cyanide fraction. Tumor cells, however, lack this enzyme, hence the laetrile is able to attack and destroy them. It has also been experimentally established that, after a laetrile injection, the temperature of the tumor rises by up to 1°. When the patient's full body temperature is raised by the hyperthermia treatment, this additionally helps to attack and destroy tumor tissue.

OXYGEN TREATMENTS

Two compounds containing extra oxygen are useful tools of pain control. One is hydrogen peroxide (H_2O_2), namely water (H_2O), plus an extra oxygen atom attached to it with a single bond. The other basic compound, oxygen (O_2), can also have an additional oxygen atom attached, resulting in O_3 (ozone). Despite ozone's reputation as an irritant, properly used oxygen treatments are a powerful aid in pain control and healing.

These are the four benefits of the ozone treatment (90% oxygen to 10% ozone):

- It attacks and kills germs and viruses.
- It attacks and destroys tumor tissue.
- It increases oxygenation of the bloodstream.

- It attaches to toxic free radicals and helps the body excrete them.

H_2O_2 (hydrogen peroxide) is easily and inexpensively available in drugstores or even supermarkets. It comes in a 3% solution, which is safe to apply to the skin, or use in a tub of bath water (nonfluoridated), adding some 2 quarts to the tub. It is even more effective to rub the peroxide into the skin after a warm tub bath, to be absorbed through the pores directly into the bloodstream.

It is more difficult to obtain ozone treatment since this requires a special ozone-generating machine, which is generally only available to persons trained in its proper use. There are also machines that generate ozone to mix into the bath water, but these are expensive, require an oxygen tank and are not recommended for use in the patient's home.

REBOUNDING

A small trampoline for gentle rebounding may sound like a surprising choice for pain control, yet it can serve that purpose extremely well. The patient must be told clearly that he or she must not jump vigorously up and down on the trampoline but only raise his or her heels as though they were walking but staying on the spot. This movement causes an increase of weight on the way down and makes the patient feel weightless for an instant on the top of the bounce. This movement stimulates and increases the lymphatic circulation, which in turn helps to overcome blockages and pain. The gentle "walk" on the trampoline may be repeated up to five or six times a day, but each exercise must not last longer than 30 seconds.

THE "TRIAD"

Dr. Gerson used this combination of three tablets successfully in many cases. Once the patient is sufficiently detoxified, the three tablets together act more powerfully than they would separately. This combination, now named the "triad," continues to work well in pain relief as well as in promoting sound sleep.

It consists simply of one regular aspirin, one 500 mg tablet of vitamin C and one 50 mg tablet of the regular niacin, which is part of the patient's normal medication. This combination may be used up to five times a day, every four hours, if needed.

REFERENCE

1. "Drugs and Chemicals of Concern: Summary of Medical Examiner Reports on Oxycodone-Related Deaths," U.S. Department of Justice, Drug Enforcement Administration, Office of Diversion Control (www.deadiversion.usdoj.gov/drugs_concern/oxycodone/oxycontin7.htm)

CHAPTER 16

Understanding Healing Reactions

Healing reactions, also known as flare-ups, are an essential part of the Gerson Therapy. It is important that patients understand their nature and function before embarking on the full treatment, since healing reactions are somewhat paradoxical experiences: although they can produce a number of unpleasant symptoms, they should be welcomed as evidence that the therapy has kicked in and is working well.

Let's see how and when this necessary process is likely to begin. As a rule, after the first few days on the full Gerson program, the patients feel better, suffer less pain, have improved appetite and see reductions in their external or palpable tumors. Naturally, they are greatly encouraged by these positive developments. That is the moment to remind patients that a healing reaction may be on the way, and to explain how it is going to promote detoxification. Without proper preparation, the sudden shift from well-being to its opposite would be hard to bear!

When the body is first turned around from advancing cancer (or other chronic diseases) towards healing, what Dr Gerson called the "healing mechanism" is being activated and the immune system begins to kick in. The body produces a healing inflammation and releases toxins from the tissues, producing a massive toxic load that has to be eliminated from the liver. The process is sometimes accompanied by a healing fever and even spells of depression and panic.

On top of all this, the patient may also experience nausea, toxic stools, lack of appetite and even aversion to food or drink, especially to the green juices. There can also be more gas than usual, plus difficulties with the coffee enemas (due to increased toxic pressure from the liver). Without advance warning, the patients may feel that their condition is worsening. They are weak, nauseated, uncomfortable and sometimes the pain that had been reduced returns to some extent. With the risk of depression, which is one of the possible side effects, patients may even wonder whether the Gerson Therapy is causing their condition to worsen. However, the Gerson doctor or practitioner, who recognizes these symptoms as signaling a welcome healing reaction, is able to reassure patients and dispel their panic.

The first flare-up is usually relatively short, since the body is not yet able to carry out serious healing in its weakened condition and is only just beginning to respond. Even that early start can produce impressive results. Along with the attack on malignant tissue, the body also begins to heal old injuries, fractures, lumpy scars and serious conditions, including long-standing high blood pressure and even age-onset diabetes. This process cannot be held back or stopped since the body is not able to heal selectively! In other words, it does not only heal the present life-threatening disease but also clears up all other damage, whether old or new. That is what the totality of the Gerson Therapy means. Thanks to it, cancer patients have overcome allergies, long-term migraines, arthritis, fibromyalgia and other conditions that have troubled them for any length of time.

How do patients react to a flare-up? Only a general answer can be given based on the reactions of a majority of cases. Since each person is different and has a different medical past with different damages to the body, each healing reaction is also different. It is also impossible to give an exact answer to patients who wish to know how long a flare-up will last. In many cases, the first reaction is mild and only lasts from a few hours to a day or two. The second one is normally longer and somewhat heavier, since the body and its immune system have, to some extent, been detoxified, strengthened with the enzymes and nutrients contained in the raw juices and supported by the medication. As a result, it is able to respond more powerfully.

In most cases, this second flare-up can be expected around the sixth week of the therapy. The third reaction occurs usually around three to three and one-half months into the treatment and is the heaviest one. Please remember that this is not a timetable cast in concrete, only what we have observed in a majority of cases. Reactions are also different in chemotherapy pretreated patients. (See Chapter 18, "Adapting the Therapy for Chemo-Pretreated and Severely Weakened Patients," p. 199.)

What should one do for the patient in a flare-up who is unwell, upset and dismayed? One should not stop the therapy and give no coffee enemas or juices, for doing so would drastically stop the healing process, yet we must help the patient to endure the discomforts of the flare-ups. Here are the best ways:

NAUSEA

If, despite the nausea, the patient is able to drink the juices, by all means continue to provide them. If he or she develops a severe aversion to the green juice, warm it gently (undiluted) to body temperature by standing the container in a warm water bath, pour the juice in the enema bucket and infuse it rectally as a retention implant. This is not an enema and should not be expelled.

The patient should lie comfortably in bed, with legs pulled up in the fetal position, and allow the juice to be absorbed. Patients who are temporarily unable to drink any juices can have them administered rectally (all except the orange juice) and should be encouraged to drink warm oatmeal gruel and plenty of peppermint tea, partly to settle the stomach and also to supply the necessary liquids which would normally be provided by the juices.

To prepare oatmeal gruel, place 1 ounce of oats and 5 ounces of water into a pot and bring to a boil. Let it simmer for 10 to 15 minutes, then strain through a fine tea strainer to remove all solids. Press the oats as far as possible through the strainer in order to obtain a liquid somewhat denser than water. Drink while warm.

For patients severely sensitive to juices during a flare-up, 2 ounces of gruel can be poured into a glass and topped with no more than 6 ounces of juice.

Peppermint tea helps to relieve nausea, digestive discomfort and gas. Peppermint or spearmint is easy to grow in the backyard and spreads quickly. A heaped tablespoon of fresh leaves makes one cup of tea; add boiling distilled water, cover and let it steep for 12 to 15 minutes, then strain. If you use tea bags, make sure they are organic. One tea bag easily makes two cups. If you buy loose leaves, which is preferable, put a tablespoon of leaves in the pot, pour 2 cups of boiling distilled water over them, and proceed as above.

It is a good idea to leave peppermint tea in a thermos on the patient's bedside table, in case he or she gets thirsty at night.

PAIN

Castor oil packs and/or clay (mud) packs can be applied locally. (See Chapter 15, "Pain Control Without Drugs," p. 181.) The patient will also be weakened and should rest in bed. Unless he or she has been given heavy doses of morphine prior to starting the Gerson Therapy, the pain "triad" may be useful, consisting of one aspirin, one 500 mg tablet of vitamin C (ascorbic acid, not sodium ascorbate) and one regular 50 mg tablet of niacin. This triad can be taken every four hours if needed. In cases of prior morphine or other heavy pain medication, it takes time to clear the body of those drugs before the triad can become effective. Keep trying; it will work eventually.

DEPRESSION

Dr. Gerson notes[1] that it is not unusual for the patient to be depressed, temporarily lose hope and even go through lengthy crying jags during a flare-up. Such emotional outbursts run parallel with the body's attempts to detoxify: body and mind cannot be separated. (See Chapter 24, "Psychological Support for the Gerson Patient," p. 251.)

Often, an extra enema helps to ease the upheaval. The patient may even pick a fight with the caregiver for no obvious reason. This is less surprising if we consider the metabolic fact that aggression produces extra adrenalin, which makes the person actually feel better! The caregiver should not be hurt by any unwarranted attacks or accusations. The patient cannot control these outbursts and usually regrets them afterwards. Again, a coffee enema can clear the problem. This part of the healing reaction should be seen as a psychological clearing. Once the flare-up is over, the patient will again be optimistic and forward-looking.

DIFFICULTIES WITH THE COFFEE ENEMAS

See Chapter 13, "All About Enemas," p. 161.

FEVER

This is a welcome response by the immune system, helping to attack the malignant tissue. Do not attempt to stop the fever with aspirin or any other drug. Simply make the patient comfortable, placing a damp cloth wrung out in cool (not ice) water on the forehead. In nearly 30 years, we have never seen the body reach a temperature that could damage the brain or the liver (i.e., in excess of 106° F (41° C)). The highest we have seen was 104.6° F (40.3° C), which is uncomfortable but not serious. Since the body is in charge and the therapy activates healing, the fever is not produced artificially and the body never heals itself to death!

TO SUM UP

The above covers ways to ease the general symptoms experienced by the recovering patient. However, flare-ups can take many different forms.

Case Histories

A lady, recovering very fast from a widespread melanoma, was absorbing tumor tissues rapidly. One day, her son called the hospital and said, "Last night, my mom walked around the house disoriented, talking nonsense and repeating herself, so we put her to bed. However, this morning she didn't really wake up, so we took her to the emergency room at the hospital. There the doctor said that, naturally, her melanoma had spread to her brain and that she was dying. What should we do?"

The Gerson doctor urged him to take her home immediately from the hospital and administer coffee enemas every two hours around the clock. The patient had been absorbing tumor tissue and toxins faster than she had been eliminating them. The toxins were then circulating and reaching her brain but, instead of increasing her enemas, she was put to bed! During the night, more tumor tissue was absorbed, causing her to be semicomatose by the morning. The two-hourly coffee enemas around the clock cleared the problem and she continued her recovery.

Another patient with a very different problem had originally suffered of a carcinoma of his jaw and had part of his jaw and palate surgically removed, but the cancer had spread to his lungs. Within about five days of starting the treatment, he developed violent pain in his right leg, forcing him to be bedfast. Naturally, like any other cancer patient, this person also immediately assumed that his cancer had spread due to the Gerson treatment. However, an x-ray of his leg revealed that an old injury to his shinbone had begun to heal. There was no tumor present, and in a few days his leg was completely healed.

Yet another interesting case was a melanoma patient who had suffered from malaria during World War II and had been taking first quinine and later atabrine for many years before finally stopping it. As a result, he suffered a malaria attack twice a year. One year, he thought he felt an attack coming; however, the usual chills and fever failed to set in. Shortly thereafter, he developed the first tumor which, at surgery, proved to be melanoma. A few months later, another tumor appeared and the patient came to the Gerson hospital.

Within a few days, he developed the chills and fever, typical of a malaria attack. The parasite was still in his body yet, when his immune system failed, he was no longer able to develop a fever. With the help of the treatment, his immune system was reacting again and he experienced a typical malaria attack, with his fever going as high as 104.4° F (40.2° C). The fever broke toward the morning but he had to endure another night with chills and a high fever. The Gerson doctors did not stop or block the fever; they only made him comfortable. By the second morning, the new tumor had virtually disappeared, having shrunk by more than 80%—thanks to the restored immune system. The patient suffered no further malaria attacks.

A middle-aged woman patient with metastasized melanoma also suffered from early stage adult-onset diabetes and disfiguring osteoarthritis in her right hand when she first arrived at the Gerson hospital. Within three weeks, her blood and urine tests showed no sign of diabetes, while her painful crooked fingers stopped hurting and gradually became straight again. A few months later at home, she was wakened one night by an agonizing sharp pain in the right side of her abdomen which, she found, had turned dark red and hot. After her first panic, she realized that these symptoms were clustered around the scar caused by an appendectomy (removal of the appendix) carried out 35 years before. It all blew over quickly, leaving her with a barely visible, painless scar.

These are only a few randomly chosen examples. It must be remembered that virtually every patient has a long history of health problems that become reactivated while clearing up during a healing reaction (e.g., old pneumonias that can cause renewed chest pain and phlegm; old, apparently healed fractures that "act up" during a flare-up while healing completely; increased cholesterol while the plaque within veins and arteries is being broken down and eliminated). The key to recognizing these is that they only last a few days and, afterwards, the patient feels much better. However, if reactions last too long, a blood and urinanalysis test may have to be made, or a thorough check carried out to see if the underlying cause is a severe infection rather than a healing reaction. Occasionally, patients may even suffer from a mineral imbalance and might require an intravenous injection to rebalance their blood.

REFERENCE

1. M. Gerson, *A Cancer Therapy: Results of Fifty Cases and The Cure of Advanced Cancer by Diet Therapy: A Summary of Thirty Years of Clinical Experimentation,* 6th ed. (San Diego, CA: Gerson Institute, 1999), pp. 201-202.

CHAPTER 17

The Full Therapy

T he full therapy is prescribed for general cancer patients who are not severely weakened and have not been pretreated with chemotherapy. The hourly schedule in Table 17-1 covers the first three to four weeks of the treatment. For subsequent reductions, see the annual schedule in Table 17-2.

Notes for Table 17-1

- For an explanation of the medications, see Chapter 14, "Medications," p. 175. Be sure to follow the directions for changes.
- Make a blank schedule to be filled in later as the medications change and the frequency of enemas and of liver injections with B12 are reduced.
- Castor oil enemas are to be taken every other day or as per the Gerson practitioner's order.
- Directions for following the full therapy are given in Chapter 9, "The Gerson Household," p. 133, through Chapter 13, "All About Enemas," p. 161. Please study them carefully.

Notes for Table 17-2

- Depending on test results, thyroid medication may have to be increased or decreased.

Table 17-1

HOURLY SCHEDULE FOR TYPICAL CANCER PATIENT

	Enema	Meal	Flaxseed Oil (tbsp.)	Acidol Pepsin Capsules	Juice (8 oz. each)	Potassium Com-pound (tsp.)	Lugol's Solution (1/2 Strength) (drops)	Thyroid (gr.)	Niacin (mg.)	Liver Cap-sules	Pan-creatin Tablets (.325 g)	Liver and B₁₂ Injection (3cc liver, 1/20 cc B₁₂)
6:00 a.m.	Coffee											
8:00 a.m.		Breakfast		2	Orange	4	3	1	50		3	
9:00 a.m.					Green	4						
9:30 a.m.					Carrot/apple	4	3					
10:00 a.m.	Coffee				Carrot/apple	4	3	1	50			
11:00 a.m.					Carrot					2		Every 2nd day
12: 00 p.m.					Green	4						
1:00 p.m.		Lunch	1	2	Carrot/apple	4	3	1	50		3	
2:00 p.m.	Coffee				Green	4						
3:00 p.m.					Carrot					2		
4:00 p.m.					Carrot					2		
5:00 p.m.					Carrot/apple	4	3	1	50		3	
6:00 p.m.	Coffee				Green	4						
7:00 p.m.		Dinner	1	2	Carrot/apple	4	3	1	50		3	
10:00 p.m.	Coffee											

Table 17-2
ANNUAL SCHEDULE FOR TYPICAL CANCER PATIENT

No. of Weeks	Juices	Meals and Flaxseed Oil	Acidol Pepsin Capsules	Potassium Compound (tsp.)	Thyroid Tablet	Lugol's Solution (1/2 Strength) (drops)	Niacin Tablets	Pancreatin Tablets	Liver and B₁₂ Injection	Coffee Enemas	Castor Oil Enemas
2-3	1 orange 5 apple/carrot 4 green 3 carrot	Regular; Add 2 tbs. flaxseed oil	3 x 2	10 x 2	3 x 1/2	6 x 1	6 x 1	4 x 3	1 daily	Every 4 hours	Every 2nd day
3	same	Regular; 1 tbs. flaxseed oil	3 x 2	10 x 2	3 x 1/2	3 x 1	6 x 1	4 x 2	1 daily	Every 4 hours	Every 2nd day
5	same	same	same	8 x 2	2 x 1/2	6 x 1	6 x 1	4 x 2	1 daily	Every 4 hours	Every 2nd day
4	same	Add 3oz. yogurt	same	8 x 2	3 x 1/2	6 x 1	6 x 1	4 x 2	1 daily	Every 4 hours	Every 2nd day
5	same	6 oz. yogurt	same	8 x 2	3 x 1/2	6 x 1	6 x 1	4 x 2	1 daily	Every 4 hours	2 weekly
4	same	2 x 4 oz. yogurt	same	8 x 2	3 x 1/2	6 x 1	6 x 1	4 x 2	1 daily	3 daily	2 weekly
6	same	same	same	8 x 2	2 x 1/2	6 x 1	6 x 1	4 x 2	Every 2nd day	2 daily	1 weekly
6	same	same, much raw	same	6 x 2	2 x 1/2	6 x 1	4 x 1	4 x 2	2 weekly	2 daily	
6	same	same	same	6 x 2	2 x 1/2	4 x 1	4 x 1	4 x 2	2 weekly	2 daily	
9	same	same	same	6 x 2	2 x 1/2	4 x 1	4 x 1	4 x 2	2 weekly	2 daily	
9	same	same	same	6 x 2	2 x 1/2		4 x 1	4 x 2	2 weekly	1 daily	
7	same	same	same	6 x 2	2 x 1/2	5 x 1	4 x 1	4 x 2	1 weekly	1 daily	

CHAPTER 18

Adapting the Therapy for Chemo-Pretreated and Severely Weakened Patients

Please note: The same modifications apply for both categories.

C hemotherapy drugs were just beginning to be introduced during Dr. Gerson's years of practice and their effects were largely unknown. This explains why no reference to chemotherapy can be found in his classic book, *A Cancer Therapy: Results of Fifty Cases.*[1] The large-scale use of this treatment, based on the theory that strong poisons administered to the cancer patient would kill the malignant cells but allow the healthy cells to recover, only built up in the years following Dr. Gerson's death. By now, it is used almost universally all over the world. Sometimes it is applied as an adjuvant treatment, in combination with other modalities; in other cases, it is prescribed for patients prior to surgery to shrink their tumor, more often than not in terminal cases. If questioned, many doctors admit that chemotherapy can, at best, only extend life expectancy by a few months and certainly does not promise a "cure."

Our aim here is not to discuss the positive or negative results of chemotherapy, which are amply described by Ralph W. Moss[2] and many others. (See Chapter 20, "Things to Remember," p. 209.) We are solely concerned with the changes that need to be made to the Gerson protocol for patients who have previously been treated with toxic chemicals.

When the therapy was first practiced 18 years after Dr. Gerson's death in the first Gerson clinic in Mexico, the doctors were reluctant to admit patients who had received chemotherapy. There was no mention of it in *A Cancer Therapy,*[3] which served as their exclusive guide. Later, as they became more familiar with the treatment and saw its positive effects, they cautiously accepted two chemo-pretreated patients who begged for their help. At that time, realizing the additional damage caused by the highly toxic chemo drugs, the doctors assumed that these patients should also undergo the regular detoxifying treatment to remove the accumulated poisons from their bodies.

Accordingly, they administered the strict intensive protocol, including the castor oil treatment, and were shocked to see that the castor oil began to remove those poisons too rapidly, releasing them into the bloodstream and actually causing the patients to suffer from an overdose of chemo drugs. They had to be transferred to intensive care; fortunately, both survived. This incident quickly taught the doctors not to give chemo-pretreated patients any castor oil, but instead to work out a somewhat reduced treatment program for them in order not to overstress the liver or release toxins too rapidly.

Since then, we have seen a number of such patients making satisfactory long-term recoveries, but the results are achieved more slowly. Also, since the body is much more toxic, owing to its load of synthetic chemicals, the results are also somewhat less reliable. (See Chapter 27, "Case Histories of Recovered Patients," p. 295, for the stories of patients who were unsuccessfully treated with chemo before being sent home to die—yet recovered on the Gerson program.)

Chemo-pretreated patients also produce healing reactions. (See Chapter 16, "Understanding Healing Reactions," p. 187.) These vary in intensity during the first few months. However, as a rule, a major chemo healing reaction occurs after approximately six months on the therapy, which is different from the standard flare-ups experienced by chemo-free patients. The chemo-burdened patient excretes the toxic drugs still stored in his or her organism and suffers disturbances that are similar, though less severe, than the ones caused by the chemotherapy.

They include some hair loss, nausea, mouth sores, pain, reduction in red and white blood corpuscle counts, weakness and changes in the test results. Some patients can actually smell the chemicals being excreted through their skin. Often, the enema returns smell of chemicals. Such a six-month chemo reaction can last up to three weeks, after which time the patient is much improved. The chemo-caused symptoms clear, the blood picture improves once again, the tumors regress more rapidly, hair regrows and energy returns.

After this major clear-out, one important procedure—namely, the castor oil treatment—can cautiously be added to the protocol. The patient is started on the castor oil enema only. Instead of the usual amount (see Chapter 13, "All About Enemas," p. 161), only 2 teaspoons are added to the coffee enema for two to three weeks, up to twice weekly. If the patient does not react too violently, this amount is increased to 4 teaspoons for another three weeks. Again, if this addition is well tolerated, the patient should be given 1 teaspoon of castor oil orally, followed by the usual cup of hot sweetened coffee; then, five hours later, by the castor oil enema twice a week. After this, the amounts are again gradually increased, together with the number of coffee enemas, until the patient is able to take the complete regular castor oil treatment and restore the reduced therapy to its full intensive level, as used by regular patients.

Table 18-1 shows the details of the modified treatment for chemo-pretreated and/or severely damaged patients.

Notes for Table 18-1

- Make a blank schedule to be filled in later as the medications change and the frequency of enemas and liver with B_{12} injections is reduced.
- No castor oil treatments until further notice.
- The exact treatment, specifying the number of juices, enemas, medications, etc., needs to be adjusted by a Gerson trained practitioner.

Table 18-1

HOURLY SCHEDULE FOR CHEMO OR WEAKENED PATIENT

	Enema	Meal	Flaxseed Oil (tbsp.)	Acidol Pepsin Capsules	Juice	Potassium Compound (tsp.)	Lugol's Solution (1/2 Strength) (drops)	Thyroid (gr.)	Niacin (mg.)	Liver Capsules	Pancreatin Tablets	Liver and B12 Injection
8:00 a.m.		Breakfast		2	Orange	2	1	1	50	2	3	
9:00 a.m.	Coffee				Green	2						
10:00 a.m.					Carrot/apple	2	1		50			
11:00 a.m.					Carrot					2		1 daily
12: 00 p.m.					Green	2						
1:00 p.m.		Lunch	1	2	Carrot/apple	2	1	1	50		3	
2:00 p.m.	Coffee				Green	2						
5:00 p.m.					Carrot/apple	2	1		50		3	
6:00 p.m.	Coffee				Green	2						
7:00 p.m.		Dinner	1	2	Carrot/apple	2	1	1	50	2	3	

For easy reference, here is a summary of the items contained in the schedule:

- 10 glasses of 8 ounces each of a variety of juices (e.g., apple/carrot, carrot, green and orange), reduced for severely damaged patients to eight glasses; or to 10 containing 4 to 6 ounces each. For such patients, up to 2 ounces of strained oatmeal gruel can be added to each glass of juice to ease digestion. (See Chapter 16, "Understanding Healing Reactions," p. 187.)
- 18 tsp. of potassium compound (2 tsp. in each of 9 glasses)
- 1-1/2 to 3 grains thyroid
- 5 drops (1/2 strength) Lugol's solution
- 5 tablets of 50 mg niacin (omit if bleeding is present)
- 6 capsules of acidol pepsin
- 6 capsules of liver powder
- 12 tablets pancreatin
- 3 cc liver extract with 50 mcg B_{12} (1 intramuscular injection daily)
- 3 coffee enemas
- 200 to 600 mg CoQ10 starting cautiously with one tablet of 50 mg daily

The meals are unchanged, and include 2 tablespoons of organic flaxseed oil daily for one month, then 1 tablespoon daily for the rest of the treatment.

REFERENCES

1. M. Gerson, *A Cancer Therapy: Results of Fifty Cases and The Cure of Advanced Cancer by Diet Therapy: A Summary of Thirty Years of Clinical Experimentation,* 6th ed. (San Diego, CA: Gerson Institute, 1999).

2. Ralph W. Moss, *The Cancer Industry: Unraveling the Politics* (revised edition of the original *The Cancer Syndrome*) (New York: Paragon House, 1989).

3. Note 1 (Gerson), supra.

CHAPTER 19

The Gerson Therapy for Nonmalignant Diseases

F rom his long clinical practice, Dr. Gerson was able to establish that a patient suffering from a nonmalignant disease had a sick, damaged liver, while the liver of someone with a malignancy was severely toxic (poisoned). Based on this difference, he adjusted the treatment accordingly, creating a less-intensive therapy for nonmalignant conditions. At the same time, he specified that, if patients in the latter category followed a stricter protocol closely resembling the full intensive therapy, they recovered faster.

The less-intensive therapy is less demanding and easier to follow, so that patients on this regime can continue working. This is a great advantage since most people depend on their earned income and cannot leave their jobs for any length of time. Table 19-1 is a typical hour-by-hour schedule for patients on the less-intensive therapy.

Note for Table 19-1

- Make yourself a blank schedule to be filled in later as the medications change and the frequency of enemas is reduced.

Table 19-1

SCHEDULE FOR NONMALIGNANT PATIENT

	Enema	Meal	Flaxseed Oil (tbsp.)	Acidol Pepsin Capsules	Juice	Potassium Compound (tsp.)	Lugol's Solution (1/2 Strength) (drops)	Thyroid (gr.)	Niacin (mg.)	Liver Capsules	Pancreatin Tablets	Liver and B$_{12}$ Injection
8:00 a.m.		Breakfast		2	Orange	2	1	1	50	2	3	
9:00 a.m.	Coffee				Green	2						
10:00 a.m.					Carrot/apple	2			50			
11:00 a.m.					Carrot					2		Every 2nd day
12:00 p.m.					Green	2						
1:00 p.m.		Lunch	1	2	Carrot/apple	2	1	1	50		3	
2:00 p.m.	Coffee				Green	2						
5:00 p.m.					Carrot/apple	2			50		3	
6:00 p.m.	Coffee				Green	2						
7:00 p.m.		Dinner	1	2	Carrot/apple	2	1		50	2	3	

Depending on the patient's condition, it is possible to reduce the number of juices from 10 to eight. These should consist of four carrot/apple juices, three green juices and one orange juice. However, do not reduce it further. Also, patients with collagen diseases (e.g., lupus, rheumatoid arthritis or scleroderma) should not take orange juice. Substitute freshly pressed apple juice, carrot or green juice. It is understood that the food intake, the coffee enemas, the caution to avoid toxins in the home, etc., all apply.

For details on how to pursue the therapy when returning to work, see "Household Help" in Chapter 20, "Things to Remember," p. 209.

Things to Remember

I n this chapter, we present a number of miscellaneous items in support of your efforts to improve and protect your health. Knowledge is power, and the emergence of the so-called "expert patient" around the world is a sure sign that more and more people are willing to take responsibility for their health and well-being. No doubt you are one of them. We hope you will find the following information useful.

ORTHODOX CANCER TREATMENTS

Unlike the noninvasive, nontoxic and holistic cancer treatment contained in the Gerson Therapy, orthodox oncology concentrates on the removal or destruction of the tumor by three means— surgery, radiation and chemotherapy. In the following sections, we give brief summaries of each.

SURGERY

In many cases of cancer, patients are able to avoid surgery by embarking on the Gerson Therapy instead. Occasionally, however, a Gerson doctor will suggest surgery in order to "debulk" the patient's tumor load. It is true that removing a tumor makes it easier for the body to deal with the remaining disease in order to heal. This is because malignancies have a different metabolism from that of normal cells and release toxins into the surrounding tissue as well as into the bloodstream. It stands to reason that this process should be stopped, but surgery has serious negative side effects.

Prior to the operation, tranquilizers are administered to the patient to keep him or her calm and prevent a rise in blood pressure. This is followed by local or general anesthesia for the operation, plus fairly heavy doses of antibiotics. On waking up, the patient is in pain and receives several doses of pain-relieving drugs. In sum, many damaging toxins are introduced into the patient's organism.

In recent times, another problem has emerged. Due to the excessive use of antibiotics and poor hospital hygiene, so-called "superbugs" have come into being, which are resistant to all available antibiotics. As a result, large numbers of patients are infected in hospitals with powerful staph (staphylococcus aureus) bacteria that can't be controlled. Especially for cancer patients who already have a weak immune system, such infections can be life threatening.

Nevertheless, under certain circumstances, surgery is urgent and must be performed quickly to save a life. Such a situation could arise from the development of thick scar tissue that is blocking an organ; it could be bleeding from a large blood vessel, damaged by invading cancer, that has to be stopped; or a patient may be injured in an accident and the damage needs to be repaired urgently. Often, though, surgery does not have to be immediate. For instance, when a patient on the full Gerson Therapy needs to go to the hospital for a nonurgent surgical procedure, there is just enough time to make sensible preparations for the event.

It should be borne in mind that, once a person is well detoxified, his or her body will react much more strongly to drugs, including anesthetics, pain medication and even antibiotics. If a more or less detoxified Gerson patient tries to discuss this concern with the regular hospital surgeon and/or anesthesiologist, they simply will not understand what he or she is talking about. For that reason, it is best to prepare the body to accept the unavoidable drugs by making it temporarily less sensitive, even though unfortunately this means reducing the effectiveness of the therapy. The way to do it is to double the regular daily helping of yogurt, and to serve two or three meals of boiled or broiled fish just prior to entering the hospital. This actually puts a temporary stop to the body's self-healing activity.

After any necessary surgical procedure, it is advisable to leave the hospital as soon as possible. On returning home, the full therapy is resumed, even omitting yogurt for a week or so and stepping up the enemas temporarily to four or more, in order to clear out the toxins that have been introduced. Afterwards, the patient returns to the level of treatment he or she was using before preparing for the hospital visit.

DIAGNOSTIC SURGERY

When a mammogram or MRI (magnetic resonance imaging) discovers a "suspicious" lump or "shadow" in the breast area, the doctor as well as the patient need to know the exact nature of the lump. The physician will usually suggest an urgent biopsy and examination of a tissue sample to ascertain the situation.

The next step is a "lumpectomy" (i.e., removal of the breast lump). If, in the surgeon's experience, this is likely to be malignant, he or she will also examine the surrounding tissue, especially checking the underarm lymph nodes to see if the malignancy has spread. The problem is that when the surgeon starts to dissect the lymph nodes, he or she is likely to take out not just one or two but as many as eight or 10. In orthodox medicine, this is done to give the oncologist the information he or she requires for choosing what is considered appropriate chemotherapy drugs for the patient. However, if the patient has already decided to reject chemotherapy, it is pointless to remove a lot of lymph nodes. To do so would damage their circulation and cause swelling of their arm, due to the accumulation of blocked fluid, and this in turn would lead to severe discomfort and even make the arm virtually useless.

How can this risk be avoided? As a matter of routine, before any surgery, the doctor requires the patient to sign a release, stating that he or she is allowed to do anything deemed necessary or best, under whatever circumstances they may encounter. If the patient agrees to such a general release, he or she may end up having too many lymph nodes removed. Instead, he or she should state in the release that they do not agree to the removal of more than two lymph nodes.

RADIATION

Radiation can be used for medical diagnostic or therapeutic procedures. The earliest exposure of patients to radiation is in the form of x-rays for diagnostic purposes. These are comparatively the least harmful. Other diagnostic tools include computed tomography (CT), originally known as computed axial tomography (CAT or CT scan), which use a large amount of x-rays to produce detailed images from several angles of the patient's body, arm or leg. The only diagnostic tool that does not use x-rays is MRI, which utilizes radio frequency waves and a strong magnetic field to produce clear pictures of internal organs and tissues.

If the initial investigation results in a cancer diagnosis, the patient is advised to have a course of radiotherapy, usually consisting of 30 treatments. Although the technique has been greatly improved in recent years, aiming to limit the radiation solely to the affected area of the patient's body, severe damage in the form of burns can still occur. According to the official allopathic view, radiation burns are virtually impossible to heal, yet the damage is almost entirely reversible by the Gerson technique.

Dr. Gerson's book, *A Cancer Therapy: Results of Fifty Cases,*[1] features a patient (Case #11) who had been pretreated with 88 applications of deep x-rays and was left severely burned. Worse still, his cancer recurred. Interestingly, on the Gerson Therapy, his spreading lung tumors and lymph nodes disappeared faster than the radiation burns. However, he healed completely and lived for almost 50 years in good health.

In cases of oral cancers, radiation treatments are particularly destructive since they cause the salivary glands to dry up. The resulting dry mouth keeps the patient from sleeping and requires constant sipping of water to moisten the dry mouth, yet we have seen patients' mucous membranes reverting to normal after radiation damage in less than two weeks on the therapy.

In general, Gerson doctors rarely use radiation treatments. There is only one specific case in which they can be useful, namely in easing the extreme pain of bone cancers or bone metastases, which are difficult to control and heal more slowly than malignancies in soft tissues. In order to help the patient, a very few (sometimes just three to five) radiation treatments are used to stop the advance of the tumor and alleviate the pain. Radiation is preferable to pain management with drugs, which—being toxic—interfere with healing. Since radiotherapy makes drugs unnecessary, the bone can heal and the pain does not return.

CHEMOTHERAPY

Since about 1960, chemotherapy has been one of the main tools of orthodox cancer therapy. It has many varieties, but they all have one thing in common: they are highly toxic. The purpose of using them is to kill cancer cells and thus eradicate malignant tumors. However, no form of chemotherapy exists that doesn't also kill healthy cells.

The way these toxic chemicals are supposed to work is by interfering with the metabolism of malignant cells and stopping their rapid division. They do this, but there are other cells and tissues in the human body that also divide rapidly—namely the bone marrow, which, among other things, produces the white blood cells essential to immunity, the mucous membranes of the intestinal wall and the hair follicles. These are seriously damaged by the chemotherapy's toxins, resulting in reduced immune function, nausea, vomiting, intestinal bleeding, mouth ulcers and loss of hair. Eventually, the damage becomes much worse. Patients report loss of memory and children have learning difficulties. Heart, lung and kidney damage have been reported, together with a much higher incidence of infections.

Chemotherapy drugs are subject to constant innovations, often motivated by financial considerations. One of the latest drugs, Gemzar®, which had originally been accepted for the treatment of lung and breast cancer, has now also been cleared for use in advanced ovarian cancer. There is no evidence to show that this drug extends life. On the other hand, it worsens the side effects of previously used chemotherapy drugs; however, it is very expensive. Recent reports state that one course of Gemzar treatment, consisting of six doses given over six months, costs about $12,600.

Chemotherapy can claim a few triumphs, achieving true cures, but these are limited to rare and special cancers, such as women's cancer of pregnancy (choriocarcinoma). A type of lymphatic cancer known as Burkitt's lymphoma, found mostly in certain areas of Africa, has also been cured in some 50% of cases.[2] An additional area of success has been the control of many acute childhood leukemias, where some 50% of child patients survived over five years.[3] Testicular cancer is also claimed to be curable, and indeed a good number of recoveries are on record.[4] Unfortunately, these successes only refer to rare kinds of malignancy. The most common types, such as breast, prostate, lung cancer and, more recently colon cancer, have not shown a good response, even though chemotherapy is almost always administered in such cases.

A telling and alarming summary of the use of chemotherapy in late cases was given as long ago as 1972 by Dr. Victor Richards in his book, *Cancer—the Wayward Cell: Its Origins, Nature, and Treatment*. In his book, Richards states that, while even palliation (pain relief and mild tumor shrinkage) occurs only "for brief duration in about 5 to 10% of the cases, chemotherapy serves an extremely valuable role in keeping patients oriented toward proper medical therapy, and prevents the feeling of being abandoned by the physician. ... These potentially useful drugs may also prevent the spread of cancer quackery...."[5]

Deploring the use of chemotherapy, Ralph W. Moss writes in his book, *The Cancer Industry: Unravelling the Politics*, "In Richards' view it is worthwhile to risk putting patients through possible nausea, vomiting, dizziness, hair loss, mouth sores, and even premature death simply in order to keep them 'oriented toward proper medical therapy' and away from 'cancer quackery.'"[6] In other words, it is worthwhile to stop patients from looking for help other than what is provided by orthodox medicine. In most chemotherapy drug packages, the warning states that this very drug is known to cause cancer.[7]

The seriousness of chemotherapy's toxic effects may be best seen in an oncology nurses' manual. It warns nurses who only prepare the drugs for administration that they may experience "significant risk" of damage to the skin, reproductive abnormalities, hematologic (blood system) problems and liver and chromosomal lesions. Nurses are also instructed "to never eat, drink, smoke, or apply cosmetics in the drug-preparation area."[8]

BREAST IMPLANTS

These are the choice of some breast cancer patients, mainly for cosmetic reasons, but they can have serious health consequences. Of course, it is understandable that postmastectomy patients wish to make up for the loss of one or both breasts. However, there are risks in the procedure, depending on what materials are used for it.

The worst choice is a silicone-filled pad, which has been known to burst and release the silicone into the surrounding tissues. In one case, we have seen this cause serious toxicity in the entire chest area, as well as migraine headaches and extreme weakness, to the point where the patient became bedfast. The Gerson treatment cleared most of the trouble. The patient got rid of the migraines, regained her energy and was able to function normally.

If other fillers are used, bursting is less of a problem, except that the implant is still a foreign material, which the body attempts to reject. It cannot do so, since the implant remains firmly in place; this in turn causes constant irritation, which is particularly dangerous for patients who had mastectomies for breast cancer. Weighing the pros and cons of implants, it stands to reason that cosmetic considerations are less important than the avoidance of a recurrence.

HOUSEHOLD HELP

The only serious drawback of the Gerson treatment is that it is highly work-intensive, almost the equivalent of a full-time job. Much time, energy and sustained effort is needed to produce 10 to 13 8-ounce glasses of freshly made juice a day, every hour on the hour, besides preparing three daily meals and coffee concentrate for enemas, plus securing the constant supply of large amounts of organic produce needed for the smooth running of the program. The produce needs to be washed and prepared for juicing and cooking, salads and vegetables have to be made ready as near mealtimes as possible in order to safeguard their freshness and, of course, all of this is accompanied by the constant washing of dishes. Moreover, this daily routine, taking up nearly eight hours, must continue nonstop seven days a week.

Obviously, seriously ill patients, or even less ill ones, cannot cope with such a demanding schedule. Irrespective of their condition, patients must rest if they are to heal. This cannot be repeated too often, for many people—especially members of the patient's family—are not clear about this. Healing, the body's heroic effort to defeat disease, requires energy; a sick person's already diminished energy must be reserved for that.

In other words, a whole person is needed to fulfill the therapy's requirements. In many cases, a spouse or some other family member is willing and able to do the work, but the intensity of the nonstop tasks will soon exhaust a single person. In this case, a kitchen helper has to be hired and trained. In fact, it is best to have two helpers, each one working several days a week.

Choosing the right helper is important. It is unwise to engage a nurse trained in allopathic medicine, since he or she might not approve of the nutritional regime and could try to add items of their choice. Likewise, a "gourmet cook" would probably find the Gerson way of food preparation difficult to handle. The ideal choice would be a kind and open-minded person willing to be trained in the exact requirements of the job. Some patients have found it helpful to approach their church to provide volunteers. The best way is to arrange for several volunteers to schedule continuous assistance, so they take turns if one or the other is unable to attend.

Since the hourly preparation of juices with all the other tasks keeps the helper busy, a cleaner may also be needed once or twice a week. As pointed out earlier (see Chapter 9, "The Gerson Household," p. 133), no toxic cleaning materials are to be used in the patient's home.

After eight to 12 months on the therapy, the patient is usually in a much better condition and can take on a number of food preparation tasks, including juicing. However, if this extra effort brings on new symptoms or excessive fatigue, outside help must be brought in. Some people, particularly the breadwinner, are able to return at first to part-time work and later to a regular job.

There is one important condition: the patient must never eat lunch in a restaurant. He or she needs to eat the usual Gerson lunch at home, together with the freshly made green juice (which cannot be taken along to work), and have some rest plus the midday enema. The carrot/apple juices can be taken to work in the morning, in a glass-lined thermos flask; another thermos full of juice needs to be ready for the patient to drink during the afternoon. Then, on returning home, the balance of the green juices can be taken, along with the missing enemas, followed by rest. This arrangement only works if there is a person at home able to prepare all the therapy items needed by the patient.

THE TROUBLE WITH SUNSHINE

Sunshine can be a source of good health; it can also be a killer. The difference lies in the degree of exposure we choose. The human body needs vitamin D, which helps to maintain several organ systems and is essential for forming and maintaining healthy bones. However, very few foods are naturally rich in vitamin D (some commercial foods are fortified with synthetic versions of the substance), so we need vitamin D, which is produced in our skin exposed to sunlight.

The trouble is that the ultraviolet (UV) rays contained in sunlight can cause severe damage to cells. This partly explains why the widespread fashion for deep tanning has been accompanied by the doubling of skin cancer cases in the last few decades.[9] Even those who don't lie for hours practically naked on a sunny beach, but instead have an outdoor job, may develop skin cancer, since 30% to 50% of UV rays reach us even on a cloudy day.

Gerson patients must take great care to avoid sunburn, which causes immediate harm in the form of blisters, reddening and discomfort, but can also produce long-term damage with dry, wrinkled skin as its mildest and melanoma as its worst effect. The first rule is to keep out of sunshine between 10 a.m. and 3 p.m. in the summer and in hot climates year-round. It is still possible to enjoy brightness from a shady spot, but not close to water, which reflects back sunshine powerfully. Even at other times of day, it is important to be well covered when outdoors. Light, white, long-sleeved cotton shirts, full-length pants and wide-brimmed hats or white caps with visors give necessary protection.

Healthy children need to be able to play outdoors and swim in summer, but they are even more sensitive to sunburn than adults. Unfortunately, 90% of commercial sunscreens and sunblocks contain a chemical called octyl methoxycinnamate, which is toxic and doubles its toxicity when exposed to sunlight.[10] As the skin absorbs 60% of everything applied to it, obviously such preparations cannot be used by children. However, effective nontoxic sunscreens containing natural ingredients, such as green tea, are available and can be tracked down with a little effort.

COMPLEMENTARY THERAPIES

These days, there is a bewildering array of complementary treatments offered and the question arises whether Gerson patients should use any of these. The simple answer is that anything which promotes healing and does not clash with the requirements of the therapy is permissible and potentially helpful. However, there is no margin for error, so let us see which techniques are safe to use.

Reflexology or Zone Therapy

This dates back to ancient Egypt, China and India. It is based on the principle that the feet and hands are a mirror image of the body and that, by applying pressure to certain points—especially on the feet—corresponding parts of the body are affected. The purpose of the treatment is to break up congestion, blockages and patterns of stress and restore homeostasis, the body's internal equilibrium. Reflexology does not claim to diagnose or cure, but it has a good record of improving general well-being. It must be used gently and cautiously with cancer patients, avoiding reflex points that correspond to affected areas of the body.

Reiki

This is a Japanese technique for stress reduction and relaxation that promotes healing. Its practitioners claim that there is an invisible life-force energy that flows through us and keeps us alive. If this energy becomes low, we fall sick and suffer from stress. In order to heal, the Reiki master channels the energy through his or her hands into the patient's body. There is no need for massage, only for very gentle touch. Although the patient feels very little, the treatment is truly holistic, affecting body, emotions, mind and spirit. Because of its nonspecific nature, Reiki is able to help in any disease and works well with other medical or therapeutic techniques. The word itself consists of two parts: *Rei* means higher power and *Ki* stands for life-force energy, so the implication is that Reiki is a spiritually guided way of restoring universal life-force energy in those who need it.

Acupuncture

This originated in China some 2,000 years ago and has been known and increasingly practiced in the U.S. since 1971. Its essence is the stimulation of certain anatomical points on the body by penetrating the skin with thin metal needles and manipulating them by hand or electrical means. This is claimed to regulate the nervous system, activate the body's own painkilling biochemicals and strengthen the immune system. Acupuncture has a proven record of good pain control and of hastening recovery from surgery. It can impart a sense of well-being and boosts depleted energy. Acupuncture needles, which cause minimal pain, were approved by the Food and Drug Administration for use by licensed practitioners in 1996.[11] Today, this ancient technique is used in the U.S. by thousands of physicians, dentists and other practitioners for the prevention or relief of pain, and members of the American Academy of Medical Acupuncture use it on cancer patients in many hospitals and clinics.

Yoga

Yoga first emerged in India some 5,000 years ago. It has several varieties, including hatha yoga, a physical discipline consisting mainly of stretching and breathing exercises, which has grown in popularity in the West since the mid-20th century. Being noncompetitive, gentle and accessible to people of all ages and levels of ability, yoga is an ideal exercise for Gerson patients who wish to improve their flexibility, stamina and muscle tone. Yoga postures, known as asanas, help to achieve balance and poise. The breathing exercises are soothing and relaxing and increase the supply of oxygen to the organism—a great advantage, since cancer cells can only thrive in an anaerobic (i.e., oxygen-free) setting.

Please note: Patients suffering from lung cancer or emphysema should only undertake breathing exercises under the supervision of a trained yoga teacher, whose help would also be valuable to all beginners.

Massage

Massage for Gerson patients must be limited to the mildest, gentlest kind, involving barely more than soft stroking. Deep manipulation is strictly counterindicated because cancer patients' muscles are normally weakened and vigorous handling could easily damage them. The only kind of massage Dr. Gerson recommended for cancer patients consisted of a twice-daily skin rub before meals with a mixture of 2 tablespoons of rubbing alcohol and 2 tablespoons of wine vinegar in 1/2 glass of water. This method stimulates the circulation, opens the capillaries and leaves the patients feeling refreshed and invigorated.

REFERENCES

1. M. Gerson, *A Cancer Therapy: Results of Fifty Cases and The Cure of Advanced Cancer by Diet Therapy: A Summary of Thirty Years of Clinical Experimentation,* 6th ed. (San Diego, CA: Gerson Institute, 1999), p. 295.
2. "Non-Hodgkin Lymphomas," The Merck Manuals, Online Medical Library (www.merck.com/mmpe/sec11/ch143/ch143c.html); *see also* Ralph W. Moss, *The Cancer Industry: Unravelling the Politics* (revised edition of the original *The Cancer Syndrome)* (New York: Paragon House, 1989).
3. Hiromu Muchi, MD, Hiroko Ijima, MD, and Toshio Suda, MD, "The Treatment of Childhood Acute Lymphocytic Leukemia with Prophylactic Intrathecal and Systemic Intermediate-Dose (150 mg/m^2) Methotrexate, *Japanese Journal of Clinical Oncology* 12:363-370 (1982); *see also* Note 2 (Moss), supra.
4. Lawrence H. Einhorn, "Curing metastatic testicular cancer," *Proceedings of the National Academy of Sciences* 99 (2002): 4592-4595; *see also* Note 2 (Moss), supra.
5. Victor Richards, MD, *Cancer—the Wayward Cell: Its Origins, Nature, and Treatment* (Berkeley: University of California Press, 1972).
6. See Note 2 (Moss), supra.
7. Ralph W. Moss, *Questioning Chemotherapy* (Brooklyn: Equinox Press, 2000) ("Chemotherapy Can Cause Cancer: The strangest thing about chemotherapy is that many of these drugs themselves are carcinogenic. This may seem astonishing to the average reader, that cancer fighting drugs cause cancer. Yet this is an undeniable fact.")
8. Ibid.
9. "Tanning Beds May Increase Skin Cancer Risk," American Cancer Society News Center (May 16, 2005).
10. Rob Edwards, "Sinister side of sunscreens," *New Scientist* (Oct. 7, 2000).
11. "Get the Facts: Acupuncture," National Center for Complementary and Alternative Medicine (http://nccam.nih.gov/health/acupuncture).

CHAPTER 21

Watch Out:
Pitfalls Ahead!

To err is human—and, as humans, we can make mistakes in any area of life—but when seriously ill people undertake a potentially life-saving program, such as the Gerson Therapy, even a minor blunder or oversight could cause a major setback. This way of healing demands a total transformation—not only of lifestyle but also of how the patients understand the principles of sickness, health and healing, and how they respond to their bodies' needs. This understanding is all the more important because the therapy forbids a great many things that are normal parts of the Western lifestyle, and patients need to know the reason behind the strictures in order to accept them wholeheartedly.

There is also the matter of observing the rules of the therapy, even without an authority figure to check or chide the patient as there would be in a conventional medical setting. It takes maturity and inner strength to be one's own supervisor and stay on the straight and narrow path, but the rewards are enormous and make it all more than worthwhile.

SAVE UP YOUR ENERGY!

Let's take a close look at the possible mistakes, temptations and trip-wires that a patient is likely to encounter, especially in the early stages of the Gerson protocol. Ironically, the first pitfall is the great improvement in the patient's condition that sets in during the first few weeks on the full therapy, especially if these are spent at the Gerson clinic in Mexico.

When such patients return home—and this holds true especially for women—they look and feel better and are often free from pain, so the family assumes that they can once again rely on the patients to take up all "normal" duties and serve them. This is particularly heavy on the wife/mother, who probably feels guilty anyway for "letting down" the family by being ill and having very real needs of her own; guilt may drive her back into her normal routine. Male patients normally have a more relaxed attitude on coming home, but even they want to start to work, take exercise or deal with chores around the house.

Neither behavior is acceptable. As stated before, patients need a great deal of rest. Their bodies are working hard to detoxify and heal, and that is more important than any domestic activity. Actually, in most cases, although patients look remarkably better, they do feel tired and even weak for the first two to three months of the therapy, unable to indulge in much activity. Instead of listening to their bodies' message, some patients actually force themselves to be up, make their own food and juice (a six- to eight-hour daily job!) and exhaust themselves. That is a serious mistake, almost guaranteed to undermine the good effects of the program.

A similar problem arises, three to four months into the therapy, when the initial tiredness goes and energy returns to such an extent that patients feel virtually normal. They want to be fully active again and make up for "lost" time." Women launch themselves into major house-cleaning by washing curtains, scrubbing floors and attacking mountains of ironing; men clear out the garage and, according to the season, either shovel snow or cut the lawn, or even repair the roof, just to prove that they are fully functioning once more. The urge is understandable but must be resisted. Superficial improvements (e.g., increased energy) do not equal healing. Rest and more rest are still essential to avoid a sudden downturn.

One of Dr. Gerson's important rules was that patients should be in bed no later than 10 p.m.—not reading or watching television or listening to the radio—but sleeping, if possible, or at least at complete rest. The time before midnight is particularly valuable for the body's self-repairing and restoring work and must not be curtailed.

BENDING THE RULES

Admittedly, the dietary rules of the Gerson Therapy are pretty strict and, while most patients quickly get used to them, there are some who long for their now-forbidden favorite foods (never mind that those had probably contributed to their health breakdown!). These patients tend to think that surely having a "little extra" on the side every now and then can't possibly do much harm, and would even raise their morale and improve their mood.

This is wrong on all counts. First of all, how much is "a little" and how often is "every now and then"? Furthermore, once the strict adherence to the protocol is broken, it's easy and tempting to break it again … and again. Also consider that, since in this treatment the body receives instructions and messages via precisely calculated nutrients, each of which affects all the others, to disturb the process with occasional additions of salty, fatty, chemical-laden junk food sounds like a disastrous idea.

Often, it is not the patient but well-meaning visitors—friends and relatives—who suggest breaking the diet and having "a nice big steak to build you up!" They are the ones who question how a grown person can survive, let alone heal, on all that "rabbit food" and, even if the patient manages to ignore their advice, a certain irritation ensues. Please remember that people who criticize the Gerson protocol, including otherwise helpful and well-meaning health professionals, do so out of ignorance and incomprehension and, for that reason, can be safely ignored. It's best to ask your visitors and friends to please respect your choice of treatment and support and encourage you—or else leave you alone. Ask those who suggest changes to the therapy, "How many terminal patients have you saved with your advice?"

BEING FIRM WITH FRIENDS

Of course, it's nice to have visitors to break up the necessary monotony of juices, meals and enemas, but only under certain conditions. One rule is never to allow anyone in the house who is suffering from a cold, however mild, a cough or a flu-like symptom. It takes nine to 12 months before the patient's immune system grows strong enough to deal with a cold or, worse still, the flu; an infection of that kind could lead to complications that might even endanger the patient's life.

If a friend or relative thoughtlessly turns up while suffering from a cold or any other infectious condition, the patient must retreat to his or her bedroom and have no contact whatsoever with the visitor. That level of firmness is very difficult when children and especially grandchildren visit. The patient wants to love and hug them, even if they are sneezing and spluttering, but it is not to be. Moreover, if the patient's spouse gets a cold, he or she has to sleep in another room.

BEING FIRM WITH FRIENDLY DOCTORS

A friendly allopathic doctor willing to support a Gerson patient is a great asset if he or she agrees to prescribe the necessary blood tests and urinanalyses. The problem arises when he or she reads the test results. If any item is out of the normal range, the doctor suggests that the patient take some drug or medication "to bring it to the normal level." That, too, can be a serious mistake. The abnormal value will clear up on the Gerson Therapy, but allopathic drugs can cause damage.

For example, we know of a doctor who noticed a somewhat low iron level in the patient's blood and prescribed an iron medication. The trouble is that iron supplements are toxic,[1] which automatically rules them out for Gerson patients. In time, with all the green juices, liver medication and vitamin B_{12}, the blood readings will return to normal without drugs. (See Chapter 26, "Gerson Laboratory Tests Explained," p. 269.)

Drugs can be life saving in acute illnesses and emergencies but, when it comes to chronic diseases, such as cancer, they only provide symptomatic relief at best and can cause serious harm at worst. Keep this in mind if and when you are told by a well-meaning doctor that chemotherapy works faster and better than carrot juice. Keep your cool and stick with the carrot juice.

FLARE-UPS AND MOOD SWINGS

Healing reactions or so-called flare-ups are regular events on the Gerson Therapy. (See Chapter 16, "Understanding Healing Reactions," p. 187.) These episodes can be frighteningly intense; at the same time, the patient may also suffer from depression and a black mood. If the family panics, the patient may end up in the emergency room of the nearest hospital, where the doctors are kind and concerned and give the patient a shot or a pill to stop the symptoms. Unfortunately, they also stop the healing, which has caused serious problems in some cases. The fact is that the average allopathic doctor has probably never heard of a healing reaction, does not understand its symptoms and function and therefore can't be expected to handle it correctly. The proper way to deal with a flare-up is clearly set out in Chapter 16 and should be followed closely.

Psychological problems and mood swings are dealt with fully. (See Chapter 24, "Psychological Support for the Gerson Patient," p. 251.) Here, we only want to acknowledge the power of occasional fits of negativity, when the patient not only feels physically unwell—with nausea, sweating, headache, horror of food and juices and possibly fever—but is also mentally and emotionally crushed. The toxins cruising through the central nervous system and the brain are to blame, but all the patient feels is an urgent wish to stop the therapy, break out of all the restrictions and run away. This is a passing phase. It is wise to find out about it in advance so that, when it arrives, the patient is more or less prepared and snaps out of it faster.

WATER WARNING

Don't underestimate the importance of ensuring the purity of all the water used in your home. The worst offender is fluoride (see Chapter 5, "Breakdown of the Body's Defenses," p. 29), so make sure that your water supply is free from this harmful chemical. If it is not, you must take special precautions. Unlike chlorine, fluoride is not eliminated by boiling the water! The only way to get rid of it is by distillation. (See Chapter 9, "The Gerson Household," p. 133.)

However, fluoride is also present in the water used for the daily shower. Although a shower needn't take many minutes, even brief exposure to warm water opens the pores, so that any undesirable component in the water gets quickly absorbed. There are two solutions to this problem:

- Take a sponge bath, instead of a shower, in a gallon of warmed distilled water poured into a basin or sink.
- Install a camping shower in the bathroom and fill it with warmed distilled water. Full description, various models and prices of this appliance are available on the Internet.

MIND WHAT YOU READ

Knowledge is power and the well-informed patient is likely to make the right choices. However, the big and growing range of so-called health books and diet bibles is a dangerous area full of contradictory theories and advice. Open-minded patients keen to learn new things read as many health books as they can find and end up confused. Although most nutritional methods are at least in part based on the Gerson Therapy, none is complete or free from its author's prejudices and subjective ideas.

The chances are that if you read 10 health books, you are likely to get 12 different opinions. Sadly, people who added to the Gerson protocol some "anticancer" substances they had read about didn't do well at all. Please wipe the slate clean. If you have decided to use the Gerson Therapy, inform yourself about it as thoroughly as you can and stay with it. After all, it has the longest and best track record.

CUTTING CORNERS

No one can deny that the Gerson Therapy is labor-intensive; at times, it can feel truly overwhelming. When that happens, patients and/or their caregivers may feel tempted to ease things a little bit by changing the routine (e.g., by preparing all the day's juices in one go and storing them in the refrigerator, instead of making them fresh every hour on the hour as prescribed). This undermines the treatment and guarantees failure since the all-important enzymes in the freshly made juices have a lifespan of some 20 minutes. After that time has elapsed, the minerals, trace elements and most vitamins may survive in the juices, but the living enzymes and their healing power will have been lost.

Another temptation occurs when some ingredient of the Gerson program becomes hard to obtain, and the patient decides that something else will do just as well in the short term. Extreme caution is needed in such a situation. For instance, if organic carrots are not available, under no circumstances should nonorganic ones be used for juicing (or eating). Commercially grown carrots are saturated with agrochemicals; scrubbing and peeling them will not remove the poisons. As an emergency measure, organic bottled carrot juice may be used on its own or mixed with organic bottled apple juice, but it should be understood that this substitution must only be a short-term solution and not a matter of routine.

One of the worst examples of substitution concerned a woman patient suffering from a collagen disease, who was doing well on the Gerson program until her supply of organic carrots dried up completely. Rather than search for another source, she and her husband decided to substitute orange juice for the elusive carrots, and so she began to drink up to eight glasses of freshly pressed orange juice a day. This would have been harmful to any Gerson patient; in this case, it was disastrous since citrus fruits are counterindicated in all collagen diseases. Her condition deteriorated drastically.

P.S.

Thomas Jefferson wrote, "The price of freedom is eternal vigilance." Well, the price of getting well is the same: eternal vigilance to avoid pitfalls, resist temptations and decline unasked-for advice from well-meaning outsiders who don't understand what you are doing. However, you know what you are doing and why, and that is all that matters.

REFERENCE

1.   Anna E. O. Fisher and Declan P. Naughton, "Iron supplements: the quick fix with long-term consequences," *Nutrition Journal* 3 (2) (Jan. 16, 2004).

CHAPTER 22

Frequently Asked Questions

T he Gerson Therapy is so fundamentally different from the usual pill-popping, symptom-centered approach of orthodox medicine that newcomers to this method of healing find some of its details puzzling. It is important to explain the reasons behind the rules; once understood, they prove to be eminently logical. Here is a random selection of the most frequently asked questions with the appropriate answers.

Q: *Why not steam vegetables for a short while, then use the water at the bottom of the pan in the soup, rather than cook all the life out of the vegetables over a long time?*

A: Dr. Gerson was very specific about using the lowest possible heat for cooking vegetables. High heat—steam is hotter than boiling water— changes the colloidal structure of the nutrients, particularly the proteins but also the minerals, and makes them hard to absorb and assimilate. Dr. Gerson even suggested putting a heat disperser under the pan to keep the heat just high enough to simmer the food slowly until well done.

This method does not "cook the life out of the food." The only nutrients that are damaged are the enzymes, which die in temperatures above 140° F (60° C), but patients get a huge supply of enzymes in the fresh raw juices to make up for that loss. The lower heat preserves protein and mineral structures and some vitamins.

Suggesting that the water remaining in the pan should be used acknowledges that the good nutrients, especially the minerals, have been leached out into the water, leaving the cooked vegetables without nutrients! This explains why steamed vegetables have very little taste. Another reason for cooking food slowly at the lowest possible heat is to provide the patient's intestinal tract with "soft bulk" (well-done fiber) to cushion all the raw foods and juices the patient has to consume.

Q: *What about using a B-complex supplement to keep the B vitamins in balance since we use fairly large amounts of B_3 and B_{12}?*

A: Dr. Gerson states in his book[1] that patients were damaged when he administered vitamins B_1 and B_6 to them. The Gerson protocol, with its huge number of juices and fresh foods, is very well balanced and has no need for supplements.

Q: *When can organic soy products be introduced into the diet?*

A: The short answer is never. Soy products of all kinds (e.g., tofu, flour or sauce) contain a substance that blocks absorption of nutrients, besides having a high fat content. A great deal of research has proven the toxicity of soy, even when grown organically. The hype claiming soy's usefulness in preventing breast cancer has turned out to be unsubstantiated and the opposite of truth: soy is likely to stimulate malignancy.[2]

Q: *Proper food combining, not mixing starch and fruit, is supposed to be healthy. Why isn't it used on the therapy?*

A: Food combining is probably useful if applied to the average American diet, which is high in animal proteins and sodium (salt). Since all Gerson foods are vegetarian and all vegetables contain a certain amount of starch, it is neither necessary nor possible to separate those two substances.

Q: *Why not supplement vitamins C and E, which help to boost the immune system? Surely one glass of orange juice a day isn't enough?*

A: It is a general misconception that only orange juice contains vitamin C. This is not so. The juices used in the Gerson program are richer in vitamin C than orange juice, and patients consume them in huge quantities every day. Raw salads and fruit increase the intake even further. Dr. Gerson insisted that no additional vitamins should be given to patients. Besides, we have found that pharmaceutically produced synthetic vitamins and minerals are poorly absorbed and can even be harmful.

Q: *Potatoes and tomatoes both belong to the deadly nightshade family and are banned from many dietary regimes. Why are they the most used foods on the therapy?*

A: They are not! The most used items are carrots, apples and greens for juicing. Potatoes are extremely nutritious, high in potassium as well as in protein and easily digestible (much more so than rice). Tomatoes are also valuable as they contain vitamins and minerals, including lycopene—a powerful antioxidant that has been extensively researched in recent years and is reputed to boost immune competence.[3] Other vegetables belonging to the nightshade family, such as green peppers and eggplants, are also used in the diet and have never shown any toxic effects.

Q: *How many flare-ups or healing reactions can a patient normally expect?*

A: There is no "normal" number for these. The body produces them as long as it needs to heal. As a rule, the first healing reaction sets in some six to eight days after starting the intensive treatment; the second one comes usually after about six weeks; the third, which is often the most severe, is generally observed after three to three and one-half months. In patients pretreated with chemotherapy, we further expect a so-called chemo reaction after some six months on the therapy. These timings are not fixed and only suggest that the patient can expect healing reactions at certain intervals, which can vary widely in individual cases.

Q: *Are headaches a good sign?*

A: Certainly not. They may be a symptom of flare-ups, when the body is releasing its overload of toxins. In that case, an additional coffee enema should be taken to speed up the process of detoxification. In some rare cases, the toxicity is so high that an enema does not relieve the headache and one or more additional enemas are needed. In almost all patients, as healing progresses, headaches disappear forever, even if they had been a problem for many years. If headaches recur after the therapy has ended, the chances are that exposure to toxins or unsuitable food has occurred and must be avoided in the future.

Q: *When do patients begin to feel better and have more energy?*

A: Almost all patients, including extremely ill ones, feel better after the first week on the therapy. Pain diminishes, appetite returns and sleep improves; in some cases, even tumors recede or become softer. All this adds up to a great psychological boost. It also signals the moment when the patient has to be warned about an impending healing reaction, bringing with it days of feeling unwell. A true rise in energy may occur in three to six months, depending on the age and condition of the patient. At that point, it is most important that the patient continues to rest and doesn't launch into multiple activities! The new energy must be used for healing and nothing else. There will be plenty of time later to build muscles and make up for lost exercise time. Trying to do so too soon can result in a serious setback.

Q: *How much of their increasing energy can Gerson patients use for exercise? Surely they needn't save it all up for healing?*

A: It all depends on the patient's condition, but it's wise to use great caution in all cases. To start with the worst scenario, for the terminally ill patient, total and complete rest (i.e., no exercise) is essential in the first few months. Such patients frequently experience a decline in energy after arriving at the Gerson hospital and assume that this is due to the lack of (animal) protein. Of course, this is incorrect. Gerson food is high in easily assimilated plant-based proteins, which amply cover the patients' nutritional needs.

The initial weakness is caused by the various healing processes: the release of toxins from the body tissues and the destruction of tumor tissue that circulates through the bloodstream before being excreted. Clearly, the body is working flat out to start healing itself and needs every ounce of energy it can muster. In such patients with advanced disease, exercise should be entirely banned for at least three to five months. After the sixth month, the patients normally experience a surge of energy. At that point, it is more important than ever to limit exercise, for misusing the newfound energy would seriously curtail the continuing healing process.

We suggest no more than five-minute walks to start with, and only in mild weather (i.e., not in summer heat nor in winter blasts of icy wind!). After three to four weeks, exercise can be cautiously increased to 10 minutes. It is also possible to start using a mini-trampoline, but only to the extent of raising and lowering the heels a dozen times without moving the body, and later doing a little stationary walking.

Recovering patients can gradually step up their exercise program with the proviso that, if they become seriously tired and unable to recover after a rest, the duration of the exercise must immediately be reduced to the last level that was comfortable. Gentle hatha yoga exercises can also be tried. However well the patient feels, it is never wise to abandon healing in favor of exercise. After complete recovery, it is easy to rebuild muscle strength.

Q: *Why is it so important for patients to avoid getting a cold? Surely even a mild flu won't do us much harm?*

A: We have to assume that patients who have developed cancer have a seriously damaged, weakened immune system. If it weren't so, there could be no cancer! With the intensive Gerson Therapy, the immune system will be restored in time. However, that time could well mean a whole year and, until then, colds and flu caused by viral infection remain dangerous since the recovering immune system is not able to deal with them easily.

Furthermore, viruses invade healthy cells and change their genes in the same manner as cancer tends to change the genetic structure of normal cells. These changed genes are called oncogenes. If the patient contracts a viral invasion before the immune system is sufficiently restored, a dangerous and potentially life-threatening situation arises, which must be treated with ozonation, extra immune boosters, possibly selenium and more. Therefore, prevention is obviously vastly preferable. Don't allow anyone, with colds or flu, especially children anywhere near the patient!

Caution: Even if the patient recovers well from a cold or flu, it is possible that tumor tissue recurs and grows.

Q: *I know that the purpose of the coffee enema is not to promote evacuation but it does that anyway, especially on the five-a-day routine. Why must I also take that ghastly castor oil?*

A: Seriously ill cancer patients usually carry a huge toxic load of tumor tissue. As this load is attacked by the recovering immune system and gets excreted, large amounts of toxins are released into the bloodstream, collected by the liver and released into the small intestine for eventual evacuation. Most people don't realize that the transit from the release by the liver/bile system to the anus can take many hours, even with the regular five daily enemas. During that time, it is unavoidable for the body to reabsorb some of those toxins.

Castor oil is needed to remedy that situation. The oil rapidly clears the entire intestinal tract, not just the colon, and especially the small intestine where the reabsorption would take place. The same cleansing effect would also benefit noncancer patients who, due to so-called civilized living, are carriers of large amounts of toxic substances other than tumor tissue. They may well recover without the castor oil enemas, but using the additional detoxifying by orally taken castor oil speeds up healing.

Q: *Can I do this therapy at the same time as receiving chemotherapy treatment?*

A: It seems a contradiction to poison the body on the one hand with chemotherapy drugs and on the other to detoxify it at the same time with coffee enemas, juices, etc. So sharp is the contrast between the two approaches that patients, who come to the Gerson Therapy after chemotherapy has failed to help them, have to go on a reduced form of the Gerson program for at least six months to allow for the gradual detoxification of the body. You may, however, support your body during chemotherapy by switching to the Gerson diet and having no more than three glasses of freshly made juice and one enema a day, as long as you realize that you are not doing the Gerson Therapy.

Q: *If this therapy is so effective, why isn't it recognized by the medical authorities?*

A: As is well known, the present orthodox medical system is dominated by the huge and powerful pharmaceutical companies. They even control, via substantial donations to medical schools, what is being taught to medical students: drugs, drugs and more drugs to suppress symptoms. Drugs never heal, with the result that chronic degenerative diseases are termed "incurable."

The Gerson Therapy cuts totally into drug use, and therefore drug sales, by healing the body of its true underlying problems: the disturbances in the entire metabolism, the diminished immune system and the damaged essential organs. Thus, the whole body can be healed, "cured" of the underlying problems and health is restored. The problem is that the big pharmaceutical companies cannot make money out of natural, organic food, such as a sack of carrots, so they fight the nutrition-based therapy as long as they can. They know that the public is beginning to understand what is going on.

Q: *There are so many different kinds of cancer. How can the same therapy be right for all of them? What about specialization?*

A: It is true that, when the body is severely damaged by toxins, steady irritation, genetic causes or any other reason, it is normally the weakest part that breaks down. This allows the wild cell growth, which equals cancer, hence the wide variety of malignant disease. However, the Gerson Therapy works on the entire organism. It restores the body's defenses so that it becomes able to attack and destroy malignant tissue, which is actually foreign to it. The healthy immune response kills and removes this "foreign" tissue, no matter what its name, origin or location! Of course, precise minor adjustments are made in the program, according to individual needs, but, beyond that, specialization is a mistake. The bottom line is still the need to heal all the body systems along with the immune system, including the mineral balances, the hormone system, the essential organs—everything—and only that ensures true healing.

Q: *Can the Gerson Therapy be used on small children? How is it scaled down to suit them?*

A: Yes, small children respond extremely well, such as in Case #15 in *A Cancer Therapy: Results of Fifty Cases,*[4] where the patient was an eight-month-old boy. Of course, since then we've had many successes, with patients ranging from toddlers to teens. Medication is scaled down more or less according to their weight, but they are well able to take juices, even from a nursing bottle, and generally don't need coffee enemas before the age of two to three years.

Q: *What is the earliest age a baby can be given carrot juice?*

A: There are some babies who are allergic to every type of milk: mother's milk when the mother is ill, goat's milk and soy milk and formula. Such babies have been raised on nothing but organic carrot juice, starting at a few weeks old. The juice gives them all the nutrients they need and they grow up totally well and healthy.

Q: *Some people are terrified of needles. Why can't they take the liver extract with B$_{12}$ by mouth?*

A: People who are afraid of needles are surprisingly not afraid of putting every kind of poison into their bodies, including nicotine, alcohol and all sorts of toxic painkillers and other drugs. The problem is that, when they are terminally ill, the body is so severely depleted that oral administration is insufficient to make up for the deficiency to stop cancer growth.

The other problem is that we already use liver powder, which is not enough, and B_{12}, which is needed to enhance the production of healthy red blood cells, is poorly absorbed in almost all people. For proper absorption of B_{12} orally, the body needs the so-called "intrinsic factor," which very few people have, so they must get B_{12} faster and more efficiently by intramuscular injection.

By the way, if the injection is correctly delivered into the "gluteus medius" (as Dr. Gerson instructed) and not into the "gluteus maximus" (as most doctors and nurses wrongly do), it is entirely painless.

Q: *Beet is generally considered a very healthy vegetable. Why is it not used in the juices?*

A: Beet is a healthy vegetable and it is all right to use it as such. Dr. Gerson avoided it for juicing because it is very sweet (beets are used in sugar production). Also, it is a powerful cleanser, and patients already undergoing systematic detoxification should not be given any extra cleansing substance. However, small amounts used occasionally as a vegetable will not do any harm.

Q: *These days, even organic produce is lower in nutrients than it used to be. Shouldn't patients be given extra vitamins and minerals?*

A: It's true that organic produce is not as rich as it used to be. However, synthetic vitamins and minerals, which the pharmaceutical industry uses in its supplements, are almost always poorly absorbed. Moreover, some are outright damaging,[5] such as vitamins A and E and several of the B vitamins. Vitamins A and E are found in fish oils and soy oil. These have to be avoided since the fatty substances stimulate tumor growth. The only B vitamins that are important to use are B_3

(niacin) and B_{12}. The others disturb the metabolism; Dr. Gerson found that they cause damage to the patient.

Even if organic foods are lower in nutrients, with 13 glasses of freshly made juice a day, the patient's body is thoroughly flooded with vitamins and minerals in their living, active form that even the sick body is able to assimilate—and they are being given in truly huge amounts to replenish the sick, damaged organs. Pharmaceutical vitamins and minerals, even so-called "organic" ones from plant sources, are usually not or are only poorly absorbed so that some go into the system and others do not. This causes new imbalances.

Q: *Why can't a cured patient after a year or two start eating a normal diet?*

A: In theory, a "cured" patient could start to eat a "normal" diet, but what is normal? Does this mean canned, bottled, chemically preserved, artificially flavored and colored, frozen food? Most patients no longer want to eat this type of food and know that it is not healthy or indeed "normal." They are also unwilling to return to the very foods that caused their disease in the first place! The next question is: What exactly is a "cured" patient? How do we know if the organs are fully restored, or whether the immune system can function despite the input of toxic artificial food? Will the defenses be lost or weakened again? How soon?

There is more and more information showing that meat and all animal products (i.e., cheese and all dairy produce, fish, poultry and eggs) are heat damaged, making proteins largely damaging to the human body rather than providing it with healthy nutrition.[6]

Q: *What lifestyle changes should a recovered patient introduce?*

A: The patient must bear in mind that household chemicals (e.g., cleansers, bleaches, solvents, polishes and paints) are toxic[7] and must be avoided. Also, many—in fact most—cosmetics applied to the skin enter the bloodstream, are toxic[8] and should be excluded. Especially harmful are underarm gels, creams or sticks to block perspiration.[9] Healthy perspiration is odorless. The body attempts to detoxify through perspiration; blocking it forces the toxins back into the lymphatic system. (See Chapter 5, "Breakdown of the Body's Defenses," p. 29.)

Q: *How long will I have to do the therapy? How long until the tumor is gone? How long until the pain is gone? How long until I can exercise? How long until I can eat (whatever)?*

A: Questions beginning with "how long" cannot be answered with any certainty. It all depends on the questioner's individual circumstances and condition. How large is the tumor? How far has it spread? How old is the patient? How much damage has he or she suffered from drugs or surgery, or inflicted on himself or herself with junk food, smoking and other self-destructive habits? How faithfully will the patient and family follow the therapy, day in and day out, for whatever time is necessary?

No precise answer in terms of weeks or months is possible, but there is an overall answer that my son Howard learned in the U.S. Navy. When faced with the possibility of hanging on to the bridge of a submarine that temporarily submerged due to a high swell, he asked, "How long will I have to hold my breath?" The incredulous senior officer, after pausing for a few seconds to assess this neophyte, simply said, "As long as it takes!"

Q: *Carrot juice is high in sugars. From several sources, we hear that carrot juice feeds tumors. Is that true?*

A: All fruit and many vegetables contain complex carbohydrates, which are not actual sugars but instead form the basis of human nutrition. Contrary to the false claims of some practitioners, carrot juice does not feed tumors. If it did, the Gerson Therapy would kill every cancer patient!

The truth is that carrot juice plays a very important part in healing. Rather than harming patients, it supplies them with plenty of beta carotene, which is converted in the body to vitamin A, and many other vitamins. Moreover, as one of the most complete sources of minerals, it contains most of the essential ones in an easily absorbed form. Carrot

241

juice is even high in plant proteins and, as a result, represents an excellent provider of total nutrition and healing.

Q: *With all the enemas being used in the course of the two years on the therapy, will I become dependent on enemas forever?*

A: Certainly not! Please bear in mind that the purpose of the enemas is not to clear stools from the intestines; indeed, they only reach part of the colon and don't interfere with evacuation. This explains why some Gerson patients are able to pass normal stools between enemas. If constipation was a problem before embarking on the therapy, once the liver and intestines are fully restored, the patient develops "regular" bowel movements.

The enema routine need not threaten the recovered "regularity." In most cases, when the therapy has come to an end, normal evacuation takes over without a hitch. In exceptional cases, when this does not happen, at worst the patient will have to take a half-strength enema daily as a morning routine. To quote Dr. Gerson's emphatic rule, "Never let the sun set on a day when you haven't moved your bowel!"

Q: *Since this therapy bans animal products, where do I get my protein?*

A: It is a mistake to believe that all protein is of animal origin. On the contrary, most vegetables contain adequate amounts of protein that are easily absorbed, well digested and assimilated. Thanks to these qualities, it produces healing, rather than feeding tumor tissue, bringing on arthritic conditions, damaging kidneys and giving rise to other health problems caused by the heavy consumption of animal protein. Carrot juice, a mainstay of the Gerson program, is high in protein; so are potatoes, oatmeal and most vegetables.

It is no accident that the strongest and largest land animals (e.g., elephants, bulls, orangutans and bison) are vegetarians and obtain their protein from grasses, plants, leaves and fruit.

REFERENCES

1. M. Gerson, *A Cancer Therapy: Results of Fifty Cases and The Cure of Advanced Cancer by Diet Therapy: A Summary of Thirty Years of Clinical Experimentation*, 6th ed. (San Diego, CA: Gerson Institute, 1999), Appendix II, p. 418.
2. G. Matrone, et al., "Effect of Genistin on Growth and Development of the Male Mouse," *Journal of Nutrition* (1956): 235-240.
3. "Tomatoes, Tomato-Based Products, Lycopene, and Cancer: Review of the Epidemiologic Literature," *Journal of the National Cancer Institute* 91 (4) (Feb. 17, 1999): 317-331.
4. Note 1 (Gerson), supra, p. 306.
5. Ibid., Appendix II.
6. T. Colin Campbell and Thomas M. Campbell II, *The China Study: Startling Implications for Diet, Weight Loss and Long-term Health* (Dallas: BenBella Books, 2005).
7. "Toxic Household Products," University of California, Santa Barbara Tenants Association (http://orgs.sa.ucsb.edu/tenants/hot_topics_files/safe%20chemicals.pdf).
8. Molly M. Ginty, "FDA Failing to Remove Toxic Chemicals from Cosmetics" (posted Jun. 1, 2004), Health & Environment, Organic Consumers Association (www.organicconsumers.org/bodycare/fda060104.cfm).
9. K. McGrath, "An earlier age of breast cancer diagnosis related to more frequent use of antiperspirants/deodorants and underarm shaving," *European Journal of Cancer Prevention* 12 (6) (December 2003): 479-485.

CHAPTER 23

Life After Gerson

B y now, it should be clear that recovering from a life-threatening disease on the Gerson Therapy is a difficult journey—a long and hard
process, demanding courage, patience and perseverance—and certainly
worth every ounce of effort. Besides defeating the potential killer, this
way of healing is also a great investment in a long and healthy future.
We have many recovered patients on record who enjoy excellent health
and vitality well past the age that is generally assumed to bring on all
manner of illnesses and all-round physical and mental decline. Not
many therapies can claim to be lifesavers and powerful rejuvenators!

Coming off the therapy at the right time has to be handled with care.
Determining the right time is a tricky issue. To stop too soon, before all
the essential organs are restored, is a great mistake, likely to lead to a
recurrence. In Dr. Gerson's time, rebuilding the body's defenses after
cancer took some 18 months; today, that is no longer enough. The
world is infinitely more toxic and people are more seriously damaged
than they were half a century ago. As a result, cancer patients need two
full years to recover on the therapy. Even that may not be enough for
those who have been pretreated with chemotherapy prior to starting the
Gerson protocol; it is difficult to set a time limit for them. (See Chapter
18, "Adapting the Therapy for Chemo-Pretreated and Severely Weakened Patients," p. 199.)

Patients suffering from nonmalignant diseases which respond well to
the Gerson Therapy (see Chapter 19, "The Gerson Therapy for Nonma-

lignant Diseases," p. 205) can be fully healed in a year or 18 months, on a less demanding protocol than the one prescribed for cancer patients.

While coming off the treatment too soon is dangerous, staying on it for too long doesn't seem to do any harm. Stopping the therapy has to be a gradual process. Provided all is going well, juices, enemas and medication are slowly and gradually reduced (as set out in Table 17-1, "Hourly Schedule for Typical Cancer Patient," p. 196; Table 17-2, "Annual Schedule for Typical Cancer Patient," p. 197; Table 18-1, "Hourly Schedule for Chemo or Weakened Patient," p. 202; and Table 19-1, "Schedule for Nonmalignant Patient," p. 206). By the end of two years, patients may manage on eight juices and one enema a day or, if the bowel function is regular on its own, one or two enemas a week. If this reduced program feels comfortable, with no headaches, no constipation and no new symptoms, juices may be cut down to five or six a day and enemas dropped altogether. As a "health insurance," it is wise to drink a few freshly made organic juices every day—indefinitely.

EATING WISELY

Changing over from the strict dietary rules to a more permissive regime also needs care. During the treatment, the body has gotten used to the best possible nutrition: fresh, pure, tasty, organic vegetarian food that is easily digested and provides all the necessary nutrients for health and fitness. It would be a grave mistake to switch from such a wholesome diet to the so-called normal variety—heavy with meat, poultry, cheese and chemically rich convenience foods—and risk a serious upset.

In our experience, recovered patients with their "clean" systems don't feel tempted by such foods even if, during the long treatment, they did fantasize about some "forbidden fruit." On the saltless Gerson regime, their taste buds have recovered from the paralysis caused by the highly salty foods of the past; now they find anything salty unpleasant and even offensive. (This is similar to former smokers who find it impossible to stay in a smoky room, let alone start smoking again.)

Of course, once a recovered patient is in a truly good condition with their systems working well, it is all right to attend a banquet, a wedding or a birthday celebration and "binge" a little. Afterwards, digestive enzymes should be taken for a few days, accompanied by a daily enema, to get rid of the mess and feel good again. Please don't discard your enema bucket. "Upside-down coffee," in Gerson parlance, helps if you have a headache, a toothache or even an incipient cold or a general malaise. Also, hang on to your Norwalk or other juicer instead of switching over to bottled juices; they won't help keep you well.

Patients who had been very seriously ill must take extra precautions to preserve their newfound health. We suggest that, however long they have been off the therapy, they should go back on the full intensive program for two weeks, twice a year. (Spring and fall, the times of seasonal changes, are best for this purpose.) During those two weeks, they should drink 10 to 13 juices a day, eat only freshly prepared organic foods, avoid animal proteins and take three or more enemas daily. If this return to the strict Gerson protocol produces a healing reaction, which these patients would recognize at once, the body is obviously clearing up some fresh damage and the strict program should be extended for another two weeks. If, however, no new symptoms pop up, the patient is doing well and can stop the "refresher course" after two weeks.

THE ART OF MAINTENANCE

Originally, Dr. Gerson suggested that recovered patients should maintain their good health by ensuring that 75% of their diet consisted of "protective" foods—namely, organic fruits and vegetables high in nutrients, vitamins, minerals and enzymes—to keep the immune system in prime condition. The remaining 25% of food was to be "at choice." Unfortunately, this division is no longer applicable since the freely chosen foods would be far too damaging. We therefore have to urge former patients to stay with 90% of "protective" foods and have at most 10% of their intake consist of freely chosen items.

Even so, they should never return to fast foods, junk foods containing pesticides, food additives and other toxic stuff, and most certainly not items such as hot dogs, spiced meats and sausages laced with preservatives or cheese—the very foods that contributed to the breakdown of their health in the first place. However, if some serious dietary indiscretion occurs, it is wise to go back on the full therapy for a few weeks and clear up the body rather than risk long-term damage. Obviously, great care must be taken with alcohol; very occasionally, a little wine may be enjoyed, but only if it is organic. Commercially produced wines, made from frequently sprayed grapes, are to be avoided.

If you know what to avoid and what to hang on to, maintenance quickly becomes an easy and pleasant routine. The answer to the question, "Is there life after Gerson?," is a clear and resounding yes!

Essential Extras

T o complete your experience of using the Gerson Therapy for the best possible results, the following chapters contain a mixture of advice, information and encouragement specially chosen to speed you on your way. Until now, we have largely concentrated on the care and healing of the body. However, body, mind, emotions and spirit cannot be separated; they are parts of a greater whole and must be treated as such.

Accordingly, we have included ample information on the psychological needs of Gerson patients and on simple techniques for overcoming stress and tension. An important chapter explains in detail how you can monitor your progress by learning to analyze the results of your periodic blood and urine tests from the therapy's angle, which is not identical with the allopathic method of assessment.

Finally, you will find the stories of many former Gerson patients who have recovered from a wide variety of often terminal cancers and gone on to lead active, healthy lives. To encourage you to do the same and enjoy a varied menu of tasty Gerson dishes, we offer a real treasury of tried and tested recipes, selected with enthusiasm and love.

CHAPTER 24

Psychological Support for the Gerson Patient

By Beata Bishop

Beata Bishop is an experienced psychotherapist and counselor. As a recovered Gerson patient, since 1983 she has worked with a large number of people suffering from cancer and other serious degenerative diseases.

G erson patients and others interested in the therapy often wonder why, apart from one or two passing references, the psychological aspect of healing does not figure in Dr. Gerson's epoch-making book.[1] The reasons for this apparent omission are simple. For one thing, Dr. Gerson wrote his book solely from the point of view of the physician-scientist, excluding all other considerations. For another, psycho-oncology, a branch of psychology specializing in the care of cancer patients, did not come into being until the early 1960s, after Dr. Gerson's death. However, by now it has become an important specialty in its own right that needs to be included in any healing protocol claiming to be holistic.

Holistic medicine is based on the insight that body and mind are two sides of one coin. They sicken together and must be healed together; whatever affects one will affect the other. This is particularly relevant to the Gerson Therapy, whose powerful effects extend beyond the body to the patient's nonphysical self as well.

While detoxifying the body, the combined impact of the juices, the food and the coffee enemas reaches the brain and the central nervous system, causing strong emotional reactions, mood swings and uncharacteristic behavior in the unsuspecting patient. For that reason alone—and it is not the only one—the psychological side of the healing journey must be properly understood and adequately handled. Neglecting it poses the risk of some repressed psychological problem sabotaging the therapeutic process.

Since body and mind interact and influence each other every moment of our lives, it makes sense to try to ensure that both are in good condition. The therapy works on the body, but what about the psyche, the inner world of emotions and drives? Is it really important that they, too, should be in good health? The answer is yes, and here is why.

There is now solid scientific evidence to prove that our moods, emotions and general outlook have a direct and measurable impact on our immune system. The proof comes from psychoneuroimmunology (PNI), a new medical specialty, which has been rapidly developing since the late 1970s, thanks to a better understanding of brain chemistry and of the subtle connections that exist on the cellular level of the organism. Put briefly, the limbic system of the brain and the central nervous system releases certain hormones that fit into receptor sites located throughout the body, causing them to release other hormones. The quality of these hormones determines whether the immune system is boosted or weakened, switched on or off; that quality, in turn, depends on our emotions, prevailing mood, beliefs and self-image.

A positive, hopeful, determined attitude strengthens immune competence, while despair, negativity and fear weaken it. A traumatic event or lasting depression can overwhelm our cells and disturb their normal functioning. In that light, our every thought and feeling can be seen as a biochemical happening. According to neuroscientist Candace Pert MD,[2] co-discoverer of endorphins, "Cells are conscious beings that communicate with each other, affecting our emotions and choices." It is equally true that our emotions and beliefs affect the activity of our cells.

FEAR IS THE ENEMY

As a recovered Gerson patient and practicing psychotherapist, I know the devastating emotional impact of a cancer diagnosis. It is a major trauma, which evokes powerful emotions: panic, shock, rage or hopeless resignation and numbing despair. To make things worse, there is also a sense of isolation, as if having cancer excluded one from the rest of humanity and from normal, everyday life. The overriding and over-whelming feeling is fear. I know this profound fear from my own experience and that of the many patients with whom I have worked over the past 23 years. Although there are many other life-threatening diseases, probably none of them is able to induce the same abject, debilitating fear as cancer.

There are good reasons for this. One is the growing incidence of the disease. Most people know someone who has died of cancer after much suffering, having endured drastic treatments with horrendous side effects but no hope of a cure. To find oneself suddenly confronted with the same fate is truly terrifying for all those who see a cancer diagnosis as an automatic death sentence. There is a nonrational fear, too, that interprets cancer as an intruder, an evil alien that has breached our defenses, is growing and spreading beyond our control and will eventually kill us. Panic-stricken patients are in no state to realize that tumors don't come from outer space but from their own malfunctioning organisms, where "law and order" on the cellular level have broken down.

The shock of the diagnosis is usually made worse by the average physician's way of announcing it. Doctors are not trained in the art of communication. They hate to give bad news and protect themselves by becoming withdrawn, remote and cold, at the precise moment when the sick person would most need human warmth and support. If the patient then spends time in an average hospital, the sense of dependence, loss of autonomy and privacy will make the prospects look even bleaker. The patient becomes a passive sufferer, with no say in what is being done to him or her. In the telling phrase of the brilliant thinker and author, the

253

late Ivan Illich, "Modern medicine turns the patient into a limp and mystified voyeur in the grip of bio-engineers."[3]

These observations apply to cancer patients diagnosed and treated in a conventional medical framework. As almost all patients come to the Gerson Therapy after that system had failed them, it is important to recognize their depressed or scared state and do something about it at once. Ordinary human empathy and caring demand we try to dispel their fear and hopelessness. Just as importantly, in the light of PNI's findings, there are sound medical reasons for urgently relieving the patients from their huge emotional burden and steer their negative orientation towards a positive outlook. "No attempt should be made to cure the body without the soul," wrote the Greek philosopher Plato nearly 2,400 years ago—a powerful endorsement of the body-mind link in healing from an unimaginably remote past.

If something deep down in the patient's inner world does not want to live, even the tried and tested Gerson program cannot do its best. That "something" may have nothing to do with the cancer diagnosis. It could be an almost forgotten early emotional wound, a severe loss, a deep resentment or some unfinished business with a loved or hated person. We may even be dealing with someone who conforms to the so-called "cancer-prone personality," as defined by Lawrence LeShan,[4] pioneer researcher of the body-mind link in malignant disease. LeShan, also known as "the father of psycho-oncology," has observed over several decades that certain personality traits seemed to predispose some people to cancer. These traits include low self-esteem, difficulty in expressing anger or aggression, an urge to please others and ignore their own feelings and needs and inhibited emotions. The true self of such people has been banished behind a false self, probably developed quite early in life to ensure parental approval and maintained in adulthood, too, when it was no longer necessary.

Of course, this personality profile does not apply to all cancer patients, although, in my work with sufferers, I have often come across similar character traits. Together or separately, they suggest a dispiritingly negative outlook on life, which a cancer diagnosis can turn into black despair, and PNI tells us what that means in terms of reduced immune competence.

It has been observed that cancer often appears 18 months or two years after some adverse life event, such as divorce, bereavement, a financial crisis or loss of a job or of an important relationship. Experience with clients has shown me that those events only represented for them the last straw, and they had long existed in an impossible existential situation which apparently could neither be borne nor changed. LeShan and Carl Simonton, MD,[5] call this setup a life trap, which they describe in detail.

My case material bears out its power and the fact that those who feel unable to break free eventually reach a stage when they don't care whether they live or die. As many of them put it, "Something snapped inside me." I suspect it was the last strand of their frayed will to live.

THE ROLE OF STRESS

I am often asked whether stress can cause cancer. I don't think it can, certainly not by itself, but it can be the ultimate extra burden that pushes an already weakened, barely functioning immune system over the edge so that it can no longer dispose of the irregular maverick cells that every healthy organism produces in vast numbers every day. Yet, without the eternal vigilance of a well-functioning immune system, there is nothing to stop a few of those irregular cells initiate a malignant process.

We are dealing with the mysterious interaction of biochemistry and emotions, which we have only begun to explore and understand. There is already enough orthodox clinical—as opposed to anecdotal—evidence to prove that inner attitudes can make a big difference to survival.

For example, British researcher Stephen Greer[6] interviewed a group of women three months after they had undergone mastectomies to find out how they were coping. He found four distinct types among them: a fighting spirit, denial, stoic acceptance and hopelessness. After five and

10 years, 80% of the fighters, but only 20% of the hopeless, had survived. These rates had nothing to do with medical prognoses.

In the U.S., David Spiegel, MD,[7] invited 36 women with metastasized breast cancer to attend weekly meetings for a year where they could share worries and sorrows, encourage each other and make their mental attitude positive. A control group of 50 women attended no such meetings. Spiegel only wanted to discover whether the group meetings enhanced the members' quality of life, which it certainly did. However, he was amazed to find that they also lived twice as long as the members of the control group.

Another interesting insight comes from U.S. oncologist Bernie Siegel, MD,[8] author of several best-selling books that have helped to extend public understanding of the body-mind link in health and sickness. He claims that 15% to 20% of cancer patients consciously or unconsciously want to die, no doubt to escape a difficult life trap; 60% to 70% wish to get well but are passive and expect the doctor to do all the work. 15% to 20%, however, are exceptional in that they refuse to be victims, they research their disease, don't obey the doctor automatically but instead ask questions, demand control and make informed choices. In Dr. Siegel's words, "Difficult or uncooperative patients are most likely to get well." Apparently, they have a more warlike immune system than docile patients.

FIRST AID FOR THE MIND

There are simple ways to dispel the newly diagnosed patient's sense of hopelessness and isolation. The first step is to demystify the disease and discuss it openly, in a natural voice, without avoiding the dreaded word "cancer." One of the very first advantages which the intending Gerson patient experiences is the calm assurance with which his or her problem is approached, with the clear message that yes, it is possible to be healed and not just put into remission (which is the best orthodox medicine has to offer).

What the patient needs is a safe space in which to release stormy emotions and to be heard with total unhurried, nonjudgmental attention—something that time-starved doctors and nurses cannot give. It is a mistake to try to comfort and console too soon or offer cheerful assurances. To do that would simply stop the patient from expressing his or her true feelings. They must be given free flow.

Once that has happened, I ask a vital question: "Do you want to live?" If the answer is "yes," I ask, "Do you want to live unconditionally?" Another firm "yes" settles the matter, while a hesitant "yes, but ..." hints at an undecided individual, possibly stuck in a life trap. If I ask what the rest of the sentence might be, I often get something like, "If things go on as before, I'm not sure I want to live."

That "but" needs careful exploration to make sure that it will not undermine the healing work. The 18 to 24 months of the patient's life prior to the diagnosis can yield valuable clues. Did some major stress or trauma drive the patient to alcohol, drugs or other destructive habits which caused significant liver damage? Gentle questioning often allows us to identify some life trap. The next task is to show that there is a way out other than dying.

It helps to build a therapeutic partnership with the patient, in which he or she has an important role to play. This is easy with the Gerson Therapy, which cannot succeed without the patient's active cooperation. If a patient tells us that 85% of people with his or her condition die within three years, we suggest joining the 15% who don't. (I recall with admiration the fragile, little woman riddled with cancer who, when told that she had six months to live, brightly replied, "Oh good, I have six months to get well!" ... and get well she did, on the Gerson program.) I like the way LeShan approaches the task of shifting the mood from negative to positive. His basic questions are, "What is right with you? What are your special ways of being, relating, creating? What is blocking their expression? What do you need to fulfill yourself? Above all, what do you want to do with your life?"[9]

Once these basics have been clarified, it is time to point out the enormous potential open to the patient, if only he or she will act—not just react—and start making personal decisions. Much can be achieved in a short time. The main tool of the therapist is his or her personality and calm, reliable presence. Often, this is the only solid support in the patient's confused, chaotic world. Other tools, such as teaching relaxation techniques, simple meditation and creative visualization focused on self-healing, should also be used by trained counselors or therapists. (See Chapter 25, "Overcoming Stress and Tension," p. 263.)

CLEARING THE FIRST HURDLE

Many patients come to the Gerson Therapy as a last resort, after the failure of conventional medical treatments which have left them with deep disappointment, loss of trust and a lot of severe after-effects. To embark on the Gerson program is for them a final gamble, an end-of-the-line decision. Others choose the Gerson path at an earlier, less serious stage of their disease, with fewer irreversible changes in their bodies but with a poor prognosis.

Either way, they embark on an unfamiliar treatment, much of which sounds bizarre at first. Moreover, they are aware of having stepped outside the limits of orthodox medicine, leaving behind the network of doctors, consultant, hospitals and referrals—an entire system which has been unable to heal them yet still carries an aura of great power. Some may have been rudely dismissed by their physicians simply for daring to consider an "unproven" alternative therapy. Others face pressure and doubts from family members and friends who refuse to accept that a weird-sounding therapy may possibly succeed where modern high-tech medicine has failed.

This kind of pressure can be debilitating for the patient, who probably also suffers from some niggling doubts, so the next urgent task is to make clear how and why the Gerson Therapy works. Most people are familiar with the workings of allopathic medicine, where there is a pill for every ill and you either recover or die, but at least things happen fast. Here, however, the patient faces two years of unremitting effort, strict discipline and a total change from a so-called normal lifestyle—all of which sounds pretty scary, especially because there is no guarantee of success at the other end. This is when the cognitive approach works best. It needs no medical background to understand why rebuilding the immune system is a better idea than knocking it out with radiation and a cocktail of poisons. Once the simple but powerful logic of the Gerson program is grasped, the patient is reassured and willing to proceed as an equal partner and ally of the doctor or counselor.

HELP COMES FROM THE BODY

One of the most striking results of the Gerson program is the immediate improvement in the new patient's general condition. Pain diminishes, appetite begins to return and sleep improves within the first few days on the program. This in itself boosts the mood of the patient who, over the preceding months, if not years, had only experienced deterioration in his or her condition and a fading of hope. Now the opposite has begun to happen and it immediately changes the atmosphere. (Visitors to a Gerson clinic are astonished by its relaxed atmosphere and the patients' good mood; mealtimes are usually loud with laughter as opposed to the heavy, sad air of the average cancer hospital.) Obviously, this changed mood and the accompanying sense of relief also begin to have a helpful effect on the immune system.

However, the healing journey has only just begun, while the need for psychological support is far from over. The patient is faced with a total change of lifestyle, diet and daily routine for a minimum of two years (less in the case of nonmalignant conditions). Inevitably, it takes a lot of determination and discipline to stick to the schedule. Equally inevitable, boredom and monotony take their toll after a while. The patient feels restricted and deprived of most social pleasures and, at times, gets sufficiently fed up and wants to quit the therapy. When that happens, it is best not to contradict the patient's grumbles but, on the contrary, agree that the process is demanding, restricting and monotonous. Point out the good results so far, and ask tactless questions such as, "Would

259

you rather have chemotherapy?" or "All right, you quit—and then what?" and wait for the answer. Above all, remember: this, too, will pass.

Boredom can be relieved by providing relevant reading material, tapes and DVDs. Once individuals have gotten a taste of natural medicine, they are keen to find out more about it. Networking with other Gerson patients or choosing a fresh hobby or study that can be fitted in between juices, enemas and meals also works well.

Interim goal-setting is another good way to break up the monotony: What would the patient want to achieve in one week, one month and three months? The goals have to be realistic and modest and celebrated when they are achieved. The ones that did not work out can be rephrased or postponed but not written off as failures.

PROBLEMS ON THE PATH

Food can be a tricky issue for some. Many people take to Gerson food at once and enjoy it; others do not. When they vigorously express their dislike, or even refuse to eat certain essential foods, they are driven by their deep, emotional attachment to certain kinds of food, however unhealthy. Normally, these are the foods their mother gave them in childhood, when food equaled love, even if it was low-grade junk. Now, at a fraught time—even though these people accept the rightness of the Gerson diet—on a deep, nonrational level, they reject it. The answer is to remind the patient that the food on offer is—literally—medicine, that the diet is not forever and that accepting it now is an essential investment in the future. I have found it helpful to make a contract with the patient who undertook to stick to the diet meticulously for two weeks and explore its varied flavors. As a rule, quick improvement followed and extending the contract was easy.

Firmness is needed when patients wish to bend the dietary rules by committing small lapses or having occasional "treats." The only answer is no, for what exactly is small and how often does an occasional exception occur? Once the rules are broken, the safe boundaries of the therapy are damaged and the consequences can be serious. Even so, the rules must be enforced with tact and affection, otherwise we as carers or therapists end up in the role of the overstrict parent, with "thou shalt not" written all over us.

There is also the problem of flare-ups or healing reactions, which can be extremely unpleasant yet must be welcomed, since they mean that the body is responding to the treatment. The practical measures for dealing with flare-ups are fully set out in Chapter 16, "Understanding Healing Reactions," p. 187. By way of psychological support, the likely symptoms of flare-ups must be explained in advance so that the patient doesn't panic when they set in.

Here, too, our calm, reassuring presence is the best we can offer, especially when physical symptoms are accompanied by behavioral changes. The body can't detoxify without causing psychological detoxification as well. Toxins passing through the central nervous system cause strange reactions and out-of-character behavior (e.g., anger, irritability, violent mood swings, aggression and unfair accusations). The patient's usual civilized behavior is swept aside by drives and emotions that have been repressed, probably since childhood.

The adult self is temporarily pushed aside by a raging inner child until it takes over again amid profuse apologies. (A client of mine called such incidents "the Gerson Rage" and, as she could sense when a flare-up was in the offing, she told the family that whatever she would do or say in the next few hours or days, she still loved them dearly.) This, too, has to be prepared for and not taken personally. It is part of the process. In whatever capacity we work with the patient, we remain calm, caring and unchanged, waiting for the inner upheaval to pass.

By the time the patient has been restored in body and mind, and it comes to the winding down of the Gerson Therapy, the final task is to ensure that the process runs smoothly. Some patients who used to ask, "Is there life after Gerson?" are now reluctant to let go of the routine. They need a slow, patient "weaning." Besides, there is the maintenance routine (see Chapter 23, "Life After Gerson," p. 245), to which they should adhere for the rest of their lives, to safeguard their restored health. (At the time of this writing, I've been happily doing that for 24 years and have no intention of stopping.)

There are others who have to be discouraged from rushing back into the disastrous eating habits that had contributed so much to their disease. As a rule, any such temptation is short-lived. Their detoxified, cleared, optimally nourished organisms shrink away from the so-called normal food they had been dreaming about during the therapy (i.e., food heavy with fat, painfully salty and harsh with synthetic flavors). If their brains don't object to junk food, their taste buds will.

In my experience, after recovery, there is no way back into the pre-disease state. Living with the holistic Gerson Therapy changes you—not only in your lifestyle and eating habits but also in your set of values, priorities and general outlook. You have been reborn without the need to die first, and you may spontaneously decide to help others on the same path by way of repaying a debt to life.

REFERENCES

1. M. Gerson, *A Cancer Therapy: Results of Fifty Cases and The Cure of Advanced Cancer by Diet Therapy: A Summary of Thirty Years of Clinical Experimentation,* 6th ed. (San Diego, CA: Gerson Institute, 1999).

2. Candace Pert, *Molecules of Emotion: The Science Behind Mind-Body Medicine* (New York: Simon & Schuster, Inc., 1997).

3. Ivan Illich, *Medical Nemesis: The Expropriation of Health* (New York: Pantheon Books, 1976).

4. Lawrence LeShan, *Cancer as a Turning Point* (New York: Plume, 1994).

5. Carl Simonton, MD, S. Matthews-Simonton and James L. Creighton, *Getting Well Again* (New York: Bantam Books, 1992).

6. Stephen Greer, "Mind-body research in psycho-oncology," *Advances* 15 (4) (1999).

7. David Spiegel, MD, "Effect of psychosocial treatment on survival of patients with metastasized breast cancer," *The Lancet* (Oct. 14, 1989): 888-891.

8. Bernie Siegel, MD, *Love, Medicine & Miracles* (New York: Harper Perennial, 1998).

9. Note 4 (LeShan), supra.

CHAPTER 25

Overcoming Stress and Tension

In the previous chapter, it was explained how the mind and body interact every moment of our lives. In other words, our moods, emotions and general outlook have a measurable and direct impact on our physical processes and, above all, on the immune system—that all-important tool of the healing journey.

A hopeful, trusting, determined state of mind strengthens immune competence; fear, despair, anger and negativity weaken it. There is also the harmful effect of stress, keeping the entire organism in a state of high tension. Yet, the body—that wonderful organism with its own intelligence—only functions well when it is relaxed, free from tension and able to follow its inner rules and rhythms. Obviously, the Gerson program will also work best for the relaxed, unstressed patient. After all, it is not enough to eat the best possible food and drink the most health-giving juices; they also have to be digested and absorbed properly. It is no secret that anxiety and worry can wreak havoc with digestion.

Keeping mind and emotions on an even keel, banishing stress and fear must be part of the Gerson patient's daily routine. Fortunately, there are some simple, enjoyable methods that make this possible. In this chapter, we present a full range. Please try them and see which suit you best.

MINDING THE BODY

Posture can have a huge impact on how we feel, just as how we feel is often betrayed by our posture. When we are happy, we walk on air. When we are miserable, our head goes down, our shoulders move up and our back curves forward and slumps—all of which compress our innards and add to the gloom. That will never do.

Learn to keep your spine straight but not rigid, both standing and sitting. (Please freeze for a moment and check what your spine is doing.) Sit with both feet on the ground and don't cross your legs; doing so impedes the circulation and twists the spine. Walk from the hips and avoid leaning forward, as if you were pushing a grocery cart. You can't get ahead of yourself! Think of your head as the hook of a coat hanger, with your body hanging from it loosely and comfortably. The shoulders are a particularly tension-prone part of the body. They tend to move forward and up, whenever we feel stressed, as if wanting to protect the chest. A side effect of this unconscious move is that anxious people seem to have short necks. In the memorable words of a yoga teacher, opening up your chest means saying yes to life.

Make sure your shoulders are where they belong. Stand up straight, draw both shoulders up as far as they will go, right up to the earlobes, and then drop them as if they had become redundant. Where they land is their natural position. Please memorize it for future use.

It is also helpful to keep your neck supple and relaxed (and make it longer!) by regular exercise. Turn your head slowly from left to right and back. Drop your head gently forward and backward, keeping your lower jaw loose. Rotate your head first clockwise, then counterclockwise, repeating each movement five times. If at any time you feel you are tensing up and no one can see you, imagine that you are a rag doll in a strong breeze and move accordingly.

Hands are also tension-prone. They tend to curl into fists as soon as we feel anxious or angry. In old Western films, you could tell that things were getting dangerous when the hero's knuckles turned white. Actually, anybody's knuckles can turn white from fear and this is what needs to be avoided. Train yourself to keep your fingers splayed when your hands are at rest. That prevents the tensing up of the arms, which would lead to further tension rushing through the body. If at first you fail and all you have are fists, imagine that you have washed your hands and have no towel, so that you need to shake both hands vigorously from the wrists. As you do that, feel the tension dropping away from your fingertips.

Breathing deserves our full attention. Breath is the basic condition of life. We can live for quite a while without food and for a much shorter time without water, but life without breath ends in a few moments. Most of us neglect this vital function until we learn otherwise and switch from shallow to deep abdominal breathing. This way, routinely used by singers, speakers, practitioners of yoga and athletes, boosts the body's oxygen intake and has a calming effect.

The method is simplicity itself. With each in-breath, push out your stomach so that the breath can fill your lungs to full capacity. With each out-breath, pull in your stomach hard, squeezing out the stale air. Find your own rhythm and practice this method several times a day until it becomes your natural way of breathing. If at first it is a bit difficult, imagine that, in your abdomen, there is a beautiful balloon, which you inflate with each in-breath and deflate by letting the air out. You will be surprised what a difference better breathing makes to your well-being.

MATTERS OF THE MIND

Your mental attitude can be your best ally—or your worst enemy—and the same applies to your imagination, depending on how you use it. Positively used, your thoughts and ideas can help you to reprogram your entire outlook, your moods and your feelings so that they promote health and healing instead of dragging you down. Energy follows thought!

There are several ways to achieve the best possible state of mind. All of them depend on your ability to relax as fully as possible so that no tension interferes with what you are trying to do. The simplest way is to lie on your back on a comfortable but not too soft surface, with your hands loosely resting by your sides. Close your eyes. Start breathing slowly, deeply, from the abdomen. With each in-breath, imagine drawing in brilliant light, which fills you with peace, strength and energy. With each out-breath, imagine releasing all tiredness, tension, pain or anxiety in the shape of dirty, dark smoke. Let your head and your body become very heavy so that the floor carries your weight. Check through your body, starting with your toes and working your way up to the top of your head, for traces of tension or stiffness, and release them. Make sure your jaw is relaxed and your tongue lies easy against your upper palate. Stay with this feeling of peace, release and relaxation for a little while.

This basic letting-go is the key to all kinds of inner work, including meditation, prayer, visualization and affirmations. Practiced at least twice a day, free from disturbance, noise and interruptions, it will make a great difference to your mental state, which in turn will affect your body.

Meditation is a simple way to still the ever-busy brain and enter a place of profound stillness and peace which, for a short while, lets us escape from everyday reality. It needs practice; the brain is hard to discipline and keeps bringing in thoughts, fragments of ideas and all kinds of mental rubbish. At first, you may find that even 30 seconds of stillness is quite an achievement. Don't give up! There are ways to improve the situation.

One way is to get hold of intruding thoughts, identify them, imagine tying a big balloon to each one and watch them float away. Another way is to improve concentration by counting from one to four, seeing in your mind's eye the numbers, shining bright and beautiful against a dark curtain, and repeat the counting 10 times. You can also place a clock at eye level and fix your entire attention to the second hand going round and round so that nothing else matters. Gradually—but with perseverance—you'll find it easier to achieve spells of thought-free awareness, leading to an extraordinary sense of restfulness and peace.

Switching off the brain for a little while also enables us to hear our so-called inner voice—the voice of intuition and wisdom. Whatever our belief system, and whether or not we are religious, we all have an inner life and a set of values by which we live. Often, it is at a time of crisis, caused by a serious health breakdown, that we turn inward and review our position in life. Naturally, Gerson patients are totally free to choose their own way in this field; we are all different and must respect our differences. However, it is the experience of many doctors, counselors and other health professionals that patients who believe in a higher reality, who are able to pray and put their faith in God, fare better than those who don't. Prayer, coming from the heart, with trust in the ultimate rightness of things, can be a great support on the rocky path of recovery.

Visualization uses the imagination to reprogram not only the mind but, to a certain extent, the body. It works through images, bypassing the thinking-talking brain, and those images come from the same deep area of the psyche as the ones we meet in our dreams. The purpose of visualization is to prescribe, so to speak, what we want to achieve: defeating disease, rebuilding health, recovering and living a full life. Using visualization in the context of cancer was first developed in the 1970s by the American radiation oncologist Carl Simonton, MD. *Getting Well Again*,[1] the book he wrote with his then-wife, psychologist Stephanie Matthews-Simonton, has appeared in many editions and several languages.

The essence of the Simonton technique is to find one image for the disease and another one for the treatment, and see how the latter attacks and gradually demolishes the former. For instance, in the state of deep relaxation described above, the Gerson patient may visualize his or her tumor as a big blob of black mud, and the juices as powerful bursts of golden liquid that attack and gradually clear away the mud. Read cold from the page, this may sound odd; practiced as it is meant to be, it can be a powerful experience.

Here is a simple visualization exercise for daily use: See yourself in a perfectly beautiful place, real or imaginary, where you feel safe, secure and happy. Make yourself comfortable in imagination, in whatever way feels right for you: gently swaying in a soft hammock, walking in a perfect garden or sitting happily with a loved one. Choose your own setting outside time and space and be refreshed by its peace and beauty.

Now see yourself as you wish to be: healthy, fit, strong and active, doing the things you most enjoy, able to give and receive love and feeling at home in the world. Surrender to this image, become it and anchor it in your mind and heart, then slowly return to mundane reality but bring with you the memory of the experience. It does make a difference. Actually, a similar technique is used by successful sportsmen and sportswomen who, before an important event, visualize themselves doing extremely well in their chosen area.

Imagination is powerful. Used well, it stimulates and tunes the body. It is free, nontoxic and has no harmful side effects, which makes it the ideal supplementary tool for Gerson patients.

REFERENCE

1. Carl Simonton, MD, James L. Creighton and Stephanie Matthews-Simonton, *Getting Well Again* (New York: Bantam Books, reissue edition April 1, 1992).

Chapter 26

Gerson Laboratory
Tests Explained

G erson patients are able to monitor their own healing process by having regular laboratory tests of their blood and urine. Patients on the intensive therapy, and chemo-pretreated persons on the adjusted version, should have these tests every six to eight weeks; those on the modified protocol for nonmalignant diseases may only need them every three months.

Ideally, laboratory tests should be arranged and analyzed by a Gerson-trained health professional. If no such practitioner is available, it is still possible to access these important tools of follow-up. Patients need to find a conventionally trained allopathic physician who is willing to order laboratory tests for them (against the payment of a fee). Without the prescription of a licensed health professional, no tests can be carried out.

Once the test results are available, you need to be able to interpret them in order to check your progress. This chapter contains detailed explanations of every item found in any standard laboratory report. If you read it as a lay person, you are bound to find the unfamiliar technical terms bewildering. Fortunately, you don't need to work your way through them. The laboratory reports set out clearly the normal range for each item, marking the ones where yours diverge from the norm. Look them up in this chapter and then ask your doctor for his or her interpretation. As a rule, combining the medical opinion with the information contained below will allow you to understand the physiological processes going on in your organism.

However, let us reiterate the warning already given earlier (see Chapter 21, "Watch Out: Pitfalls Ahead!," p. 223): a well-meaning allopathic doctor not trained in the Gerson protocol may suggest that you take certain drugs or change your diet. Please listen to his or her suggestions but realize that to follow them would clash with the rules of the Gerson program and slow down or even stop your progress.

SERUM CALCIUM LABORATORY TEST

The laboratory test for serum calcium is a measurement of the levels of calcium in the blood. Knowing these levels helps a health professional to interpret the patient's physiological status regarding neuromuscular activity, enzyme activity, skeletal development and blood coagulation.

Calcium (Ca^+) is a predominantly extracellular ion (a cation) derived from the calcium absorbed in food through the gastrointestinal tract, provided sufficient vitamin D is present in the food eaten. Excess quantities of calcium ions in the blood are excreted in the urine and feces, while insufficient calcium concentrations can deplete the storage areas of bones and teeth in order to restore low blood levels. Daily ingestion of 1 gram of calcium is necessary for normal calcium balance. For Gerson patients, this should not be given in the form of supplements. Juices and foods contain more than adequate amounts of calcium.

Serum calcium testing aids in diagnosing arrhythmias, blood-clotting deficiencies, acid-base imbalance and disorders of the neuromuscular, skeletal and endocrine systems. Normal adult serum calcium levels range from 8.9 to 10.1 mg/dL (atomic absorption is 2.25 to 2.75 mmol/L). Serum calcium levels for children are higher than for adults.

When the level of Ca^+ is too high, a condition of hypercalcemia results, which can indicate one or more of the following pathologies: hyperparathyroidism, Paget's disease of the bone, multiple myeloma, metastatic carcinoma, multiple fractures and prolonged immobilization. Elevated serum calcium may also be due to inadequate excretion of calcium and may result in kidney disease and adrenal insufficiency.

In contrast, low calcium levels (known as hypocalcemia) may come from hypoparathyroidism, total parathyroidectomy or malabsorption. Decreased serum Ca^+ levels may arise from calcium loss in Cushing's syndrome, kidney (renal) failure, acute pancreatitis and peritonitis.

Hypercalcemia may bring on deep bone pain, flank pain from renal calculi and muscle hypotonicity. Its beginning symptoms are nausea, vomiting and dehydration, leading to stupor and coma, and may end in cardiac arrest.

Hypocalcemia may produce peripheral numbness and tingling, muscle twitching, facial muscle spasm (Chvostek's sign), carpopedal spasm (Trousseau's sign), seizures and arrhythmias.

SERUM PHOSPHATES LABORATORY TEST

The laboratory test for serum phosphates is a measurement of the blood levels of phosphates to show the state of body energy, carbohydrate metabolism, lipid metabolism and acid-base balance. Phosphate ion (P^+) is the dominant cellular anion, which is essential for bone formation. Testing for its blood level aids in the diagnosis of acid-base imbalance plus renal, endocrine, skeletal and calcium disorders.

In a normal adult, serum phosphate levels range from 2.5 to 4.5 mg/dL (0.80 to 1.40 mmol/L) or from 1.8 to 2.6 mEq/L. Children show a higher range that can rise to 7 mg/dL (2.25 mmol/L) during spurts of increased bone growth.

Phosphates are absorbed through the intestines from dietary sources in the presence of vitamin D. Excess quantities are excreted through the kidneys, which act as the regulating mechanism. Due to the fact that calcium and phosphate interact in a reciprocal relationship, urinary excretion of phosphates increases or decreases in inverse proportion to serum calcium levels.

Abnormally high concentrations of phosphates in the blood (hyperphosphatemia), which can come from drinking an overabundance of carbonated beverages, set up a pathological process of bone loss, tooth demineralization, poor healing of fractures, hypoparathyroidism, acromegaly, diabetic acidosis, high intestinal obstruction and renal failure.

Depressed phosphate levels in the blood (hypophosphatemia) may result from malnutrition, malabsorption syndromes, hyperparathyroidism, renal tubular acidosis or treatment of diabetic acidosis. In children, such hypophosphatemia can suppress normal growth.

SERUM SODIUM LABORATORY TEST

This test is a measurement of the blood levels of sodium to determine body water distribution, osmotic pressure of extracellular fluid, neuromuscular function and acid-base balance. The sodium ion (Na^+) is the major extracellular cation, and it influences both chloride and potassium blood levels.

Sodium is absorbed by the intestines and is excreted primarily by the kidneys; a small amount is lost through the skin by sweating. This mineral aids the kidneys in regulating body water, for decreased Na^+ promotes water excretion and an increased level promotes water retention (edema).

Testing for Na^+ helps to evaluate fluid electrolytes, acid-base balance and certain disorders of the kidneys, adrenals and neuromuscular system. The sodium blood test also determines the effects of drug therapy, such as diuretics on the body. For an adult, serum sodium levels normally range from 135 to 145 mEq/L (mmol/L). For Gerson patients, a level of 127 is still acceptable.

Sodium imbalance comes from either a change in water volume intake or variation in how much sodium is consumed. Elevated serum sodium levels (hypernatremia) may be caused by inadequate water intake, diabetes insipidus, impaired renal function, prolonged hyperventilation, severe vomiting or severe diarrhea. Sodium retention also comes from consuming excessive salt. The signs and symptoms of hypernatremia are thirst, restlessness, dry mouth, sticky mucous membranes, flushed skin, oliguria, diminished reflexes, hypertension, dyspnea and edema.

Ingesting too little sodium mineral for serum Na^+ (hyponatremia) is rare and doesn't even occur on the low-sodium Gerson Therapy dietary program. There is always some sodium coming from food. Still, hyponatremia can occur, and its indications appear as apprehension, lassitude, headache, decreased skin turgor, abdominal cramps, tremors or convulsions. It can be brought on by profuse sweating, gastrointestinal suctioning, diuretic therapy, diarrhea, vomiting, adrenal insufficiency, burns and chronic renal insufficiency with acidosis. If you do have testing for serum sodium performed, make sure to get a simultaneous urine sodium determination.

SERUM POTASSIUM LABORATORY TEST

The laboratory test for serum potassium, a quantitative analysis, is the measurement of blood potassium for regulation of homeostasis, osmotic equilibrium, muscle activity, enzyme activity, acid-base balance and kidney function. Potassium (K^+) is the body's major intracellular ion (a cation); small amounts of it are also found in the extracellular fluid.

Since the kidneys excrete nearly all the ingested potassium, a dietary intake of at least 40 mEq/day (mmol/d) is essential. A normal diet usually includes 60 to 100 mEq/day of this mineral. In the blood, normal K^+ levels range from 3.8 to 5.5 mEq/liter (mmol/L).

Vital to maintaining electrical conduction within the cardiac and skeletal muscles, K^+ is affected by variations in the secretion otadrenal steroid hormones and by fluctuations in pH, serum glucose levels and serum sodium levels. A reciprocal relationship exists between K^+ and Na^+; the substantial intake of one causes a corresponding decrease in the other. Although the body naturally conserves sodium, potassium deficiency may develop rapidly and is quite common because there is no efficient method for conserving potassium.

The serum potassium laboratory test is used to evaluate clinical signs of either potassium excess (hyperkalemia) or potassium depletion (hypokalemia). It also monitors kidney function, acid-base balance and glucose metabolism, and evaluates arrhythmias, neuromuscular disorders and endocrine disorders. Hyperkalemia is common in patients with excessive cellular K^+ entering the blood, as in cases of burns, crushing injuries, diabetic ketoacidosis and myocardial infarction (MI). It will also be present where there is reduced sodium excretion from renal failure that causes an abnormal Na^+-K^+ exchange and in Addison's disease, due to the absence of aldosterone, with consequent K^+ build-up and Na^+ depletion.

Note: Although elevated serum potassium is uncommon in Gerson Therapy patients, if it does occur, supplemental potassium should be reduced or temporarily discontinued. The Gerson-trained physician in charge should immediately be consulted.

The signs and symptoms of hyperkalemia are weakness, malaise, nausea, diarrhea, colicky pain, muscle irritability progressing to flaccid paralysis, oliguria and bradycardia. An electrocardiogram (EKG) reveals a prolonged PR interval; wide QRS; tall, tented T wave; and ST depression. Indications of hypokalemia are decreased reflexes; rapid, weak, irregular pulse; mental confusion; hypotension; anorexia; muscle weakness; and paresthesia. The EKG shows a flattened T wave, ST depression and U wave elevation. In severe cases of hypokalemia, ventricular fibrillation, respiratory paralysis and cardiac arrest could occur.

SERUM CHLORIDE LABORATORY TEST

The laboratory test for serum chloride, another quantitative analysis, is a measurement of blood levels of the chloride ion (Cl^-), the major extracellular fluid anion. Interacting with Na^+, Cl^- helps maintain the osmotic pressure, blood volume, arterial pressure and acid-base balance. Chloride is absorbed from the intestines and is excreted primarily by the kidneys.

By evaluating the body's fluid status, the serum chloride laboratory test detects two types of fluid imbalance: acid-base (acidosis and alkalosis) and extracellular cation-anion. Normally, serum chloride levels range from 100 to 108 mEq/liter (mmol/L). Maintaining a normal amount of chloride in the blood reflects acid-base balance by its inverse relationship to bicarbonate. Excessive loss of gastric juices or other secretions containing chloride may cause hypochloremic metabolic alkalosis or excessive chloride retention. Ingesting it may lead to hyperchloremic metabolic acidosis.

Elevated serum chloride levels (hyperchloremia) can come on from severe dehydration, complete renal shutdown, head injury (which produces neurogenic hyperventilation) and primary aldosteroism. Manifestations consist of stupor, rapid and deep breathing and weakness that leads to coma.

A state of low chloride levels in the blood (hypochloremia) is associated with reduced blood sodium and potassium levels coming from prolonged vomiting, gastric suctioning, intestinal fistula, chronic renal failure or Addison's disease. Congestive heart failure, or edema resulting in excess extracellular fluid, can cause dilutional hypochloremia. The indications are hypertonicity of muscles, tetany and depressed respirations.

LACTIC DEHYDROGENASE LABORATORY TEST

The laboratory test for lactic dehydrogenase (LDH) is a measurement of five specific isoenzymes which catalyze the reversible conversion of pyruvic acid present in all muscles of the body into lactic acid. Many common diseases (e.g., MI, pulmonary infarction, anemias, liver disease, kidney disease and erythrocytic damage) cause elevations in total LDH, and the LDH laboratory test is useful for differentiating between them.

The five identified isoenzymes in LDH are LDH^1 and LDH^2 appearing in the heart, red blood cells and kidneys; LDH^3 in the lungs; and LDH^4 and LDH^5 in the liver and skeletal muscles. Testing for these enzymes is especially appropriate for the delayed measurement of creatine phosphokinase, associated with MI, and for monitoring patient response to some forms of chemotherapy. Total LDH levels normally range from 48 to 115 U/L. Normal distribution of the five isoenzymes is as follows:

LDH¹	17.5% to 28.3% of total
LDH²	30.4% to 36.4% of total
LDH³	19.2% to 24.8% of total
LDH⁴	9.6% to 15.6% of total
LDH⁵	5.5% to 12.7% of total

Since a vast number of illnesses involve the enzymes of LDH, this laboratory test for LDH is broadly employed for establishing diagnoses.

ASPARTATE TRANSAMINASE/SERUM GLUTAMIC-OXALOACETIC TRANSAMINASE LABORATORY TEST

The laboratory blood examination for aspartate transaminase and serum glutamic-oxaloacetic transaminase (AST/SGOT) is a measurement of specific amino acid residues left behind by nitrogenous portions of the metabolized amino acids. Aspartate aminotransferase (AST) is found in the cytoplasm and mitochondria of many tissue cells, primarily in the liver, heart, skeletal muscles, kidneys, pancreas and red blood cells.

AST is released into blood serum in proportion to cellular damage, and its detection (together with creatine phosphokinase and lactate dehydrogenase) indicates MI. The test also helps in the diagnosis of acute liver disease. It monitors patient progress in healing. AST adult serum levels range from 8 to 20 U/L. Normal values for infants are four times higher.

Maximum elevations of AST are associated with viral hepatitis, severe skeletal muscle trauma, extensive surgery, drug-induced liver injury and passive liver congestion. Levels ranging from 10 to 20 times normal may indicate severe MI, severe infectious mononucleosis and alcoholic cirrhosis. Moderate to high levels, ranging from 5 to 10 times normal, indicate Duchenne muscular dystrophy, dermatomyositis and chronic hepatitis, along with prodromal and resolving stages of diseases. Low to moderate levels of two to five times normal may show hemolytic anemia, metastatic liver tumors, acute pancreatitis, pulmonary emboli, alcohol withdrawal syndrome, fatty liver and the first stages of biliary duct obstruction.

SERUM BILIRUBIN LABORATORY TEST

The laboratory test for serum bilirubin, the main product of hemoglobin catabolism, is a measurement of bile pigment which indicates the state of health of the liver and gallbladder. After being formed in the reticuloendothelial cells, bilirubin is bound to albumin and then transported to the liver, where it is conjugated with glucuronic acid to form bilirubin glucuronide and bilirubin diglucuronide. These two compounds are then excreted in bile. Measurement of indirect or prehepatic (unconjugated) bilirubin helps to evalute hepatobiliary and erythropoietic functions.

The serum bilirubin laboratory test showing elevated levels often indicates liver damage in which the parenchymal cells can no longer conjugate bilirubin with glucuronide. Indirect bilirubin then reenters the bloodstream. Also, an elevated reading alerts the health professional to the possibility of severe hemolytic anemia. This test aids in the differential diagnosis of jaundice, biliary obstruction and dangerous levels of unconjugated bilirubin.

Normally in an adult, indirect serum bilirubin measures 11 mg/dL or less, and direct serum bilirubin less than 0.5 mg/dL. Neonates have total serum bilirubin ranging from 1 to 12 mg/dL; if elevated, to 20 mg/dL (for them, it indicates neonatal hepatic immaturity or congenital enzyme deficiencies). An exchange blood transfusion may then be required.

If readings of bilirubin are elevated for adults, the test advises about the possibility of autoimmunity or transfusion reaction, hemolytic or pernicious anemia or hemorrhage and hepatocellular dysfunction, perhaps from viral hepatitis. Obviously, elevated levels of direct conjugated bilirubin usually show biliary obstruction with overflows into the bloodstream. Intrahepatic biliary obstruction may come from viral hepatitis, cirrhosis or chlorpromazine reaction. Extrahepatic obstruction may come from gallstones, gallbladder cancer, pancreatic cancer or bile duct disease.

SERUM GAMMA-GLUTAMYL TRANSPEPTIDASE LABORATORY TEST

The laboratory test for serum gamma-glutamyl transpeptidase (GGT) is a measurement of obstructive jaundice in neoplastic liver disease and is also useful for the detection of excessive alcohol consumption. The GGT enzyme is sensitive to drug use and detects alcohol ingestion; therefore, it is used to determine compliance with alcoholism treatment. It also helps in the diagnosis of obstructive jaundice and liver cancer.

The normal range for GGT varies with age in males but not in females. For men ages 18 to 50, it varies between 10 and 39 U/L. Older males show a GGT range from 10 to 48 U/L. The normal range in women is 6 to 29 U/L. Elevation signals a cholestatic liver process.

Note: The immune-stimulating effect of the Gerson Therapy frequently causes a rise in GGT blood levels.

ACID PHOSPHATASE LABORATORY TEST

The laboratory test for acid phosphatase is a measurement of the prostatic and erythrocytic isoenzymes to detect cancer. Active at a pH of 5, the two phosphatase enzymes appear in the liver, spleen, red blood cells, bone marrow, platelets and prostate gland.

Successful treatment for prostate cancer decreases acid phosphatase levels. Its normal values range from 0 to 1.1 Bodansky units/mL; 1 to 4 King Armstrong units/mL; 0.13 to 0.63 Bessey-Lowry-Brock units/mL; and 0 to 6 U/L in SI units. Normal range of radioimmunoassay results is 0 to 4.0 ng/mL.

An elevated prostatic acid phosphatase test indicates Paget's disease, Gaucher's disease, multiple myeloma or a tumor that has spread beyond the prostatic capsule. If metastasized to bone, the high acid phosphatase level accompanied by a high alkaline phosphatase shows increased osteoblastic activity.

ALKALINE PHOSPHATASE LABORATORY TEST

An enzyme that is most active at pH 9.0, alkaline phosphatase (AP) influences bone calcification and the transport of lipids and metabolites. The AP laboratory test measures combined activities of those AP isoenzymes found in the liver, bones, kidneys, intestinal lining and placenta. Bone and liver AP are always present in adult blood serum, with liver AP most prominent—except during the third trimester of pregnancy when the placenta originates half of all AP.

The AP laboratory test is particularly sensitive to mild biliary obstruction and indicates liver lesions. Its most specific clinical application is in the diagnosis of metabolic bone disease and the detection of skeletal diseases characterized by osteoblastic activity and local liver lesions causing biliary obstruction, such as tumor or abscess. It furnishes supplemental information for liver function studies and gastrointestinal enzyme tests and assesses the response to vitamin D treatment in rickets.

The normal range of serum alkaline phosphatase varies in accordance with the laboratory method employed, but the usual total AP levels range from 30 to 120 U/L in adults and from 40 to 200 U/L in children. Since AP concentrations rise during active bone formation and growth, infants, children and adolescents normally show levels three times higher than adults. Additional normal ranges for AP are 1.5 to 4 Bodansky units/dL; 4 to 13.5 King-Armstrong units/dL; 0.8 to 2.5 Bessey-Lowry-Brock units/dL; 30 to 110 U/L by SMA 1260.

High AP blood levels indicate skeletal disease, intrahepatic biliary obstruction causing cholestasis, malignant or infectious infiltrations, fibrosis, Paget's disease, bone metastases, hyperparathyroidism, metastatic bone tumors from pancreatic cancer and liver diseases before any change in blood serum bilirubin levels.

Moderate rise in AP levels shown by this laboratory test may reflect acute biliary obstruction from liver inflammation in active cirrhosis, mononucleosis, osteomalacia, deficiency-induced rickets and viral hepatitis.

ALANINE TRANSAMINASE, SERUM GLUTAMIC-PYRUVIC TRANSAMINASE LABORATORY TEST

Alanine aminotransferase (ALT), one of the two enzymes that catalyze a reversible amino group transfer reaction in the Krebs citric acid (tricarboxylic acid) cycle, is necessary for tissue energy production. (The second enzyme is aspartate aminotransferase.) Elevated serum ALT indicates acute hepatocellular damage before jaundice appears. The alanine transaminase, serum glutamic-pyruvic transaminase (ALT/SGPT) laboratory test makes use of spectrophotometric or colorimetric methods, which detect and evaluate treatment progress for hepatitis, cirrhosis without jaundice, liver toxicity and acute liver disease. It also distinguishes between myocardial and hepatic tissue damage.

ALT values range from 10 to 32 U/L in men; from 9 to 24 U/L in women; and twice those levels in infants. When they are very high—up to 50 times normal—viral or drug-induced hepatitis must be suspected. There may also be other liver disease with extensive necrosis.

Moderate to high levels of ALT may indicate infectious mononucleosis, chronic hepatitis, intrahepatic cholestasis, early or improving acute viral hepatitis or severe hepatic congestion due to heart failure. Slight to moderate ALT elevations may appear with any condition that produces acute cellular injury in the liver, such as active cirrhosis and drug-induced or alcoholic hepatitis. Marginal elevations possibly show acute MI or secondary hepatic congestion.

An interfering factor for the ALT/SGPT laboratory test is the taking of opiate analgesics, such as morphine, codeine and meperidine.

TOTAL SERUM CHOLESTEROL LABORATORY TEST

This quantitative serum analysis measures the circulating levels of free cholesterol and cholesterol esters, and reflects the amount of cholesterol compound appearing in the body tissues. Both absorbed from the diet and synthesized in the liver and other body tissues, cholesterol is a structural component in cell membranes and plasma lipoproteins. It contributes to the formation of adrenocorticoid steroids, bile salts, androgens and estrogens. A diet high in saturated fat raises cholesterol levels by stimulating absorption of lipids, including cholesterol, from the intestine; a diet low in saturated fat lowers them. Elevated total serum cholesterol is associated with an increased risk of atherosclerotic cardiovascular disease.

Thus, the total serum cholesterol laboratory test assesses the risk of coronary artery disease (CAD), evaluates fat metabolism and aids in diagnosing kidney disease, pancreatitis, liver disease, hypothyroidism and hyperthyroidism. Total cholesterol concentrations vary with age and sex. Its common range is from 150 to 200 mg/dL.

A desirable level of blood cholesterol is below 175 mg/dL and levels from 180 to 230 mg/dL are considered borderline or at high risk for CAD. A level in excess of 250 mg/dL (hypercholesterolemia) indicates high risk of cardiovascular disease, incipient hepatitis, lipid disorders, bile duct blockage, nephrotic syndrome, obstructive jaundice, pancreatitis and hypothyroidism. They require treatment.

Hypercholesterolemia can occur from taking adrenocorticotropic hormone, corticosteroids, androgens, bile salts, epinephrine, chlorpromazine, trifluoperazine, oral contraceptives, salicylates, thiouracils and trimethadione.

Low serum cholesterol (hypocholesterolemia) is associated with malnutrition, cellular necrosis of the liver and hyperthyroidism. Cholesterol often drops below normal in the Gerson program because patients are eating an extremely low-fat diet.

LIPOPROTEIN/CHOLESTEROL FRACTIONATION LABORATORY TEST

To assess the risk of CAD, the lipoprotein/cholesterol fractionation laboratory test is conducted. By centrifugation or electrophoresis, it isolates and measures the cholesterol in blood, which appears as low-density lipoproteins (LDL) and high-density lipoproteins (HDL). It is known that a lower HDL level in the population gives rise to a higher incidence of CAD. Conversely, higher HDL levels produce a lesser amount of CAD.

Note: Since the Gerson Therapy uses a minimal amount of fat, it often lowers the risk of CAD, but it does provide an adequate supply of certain polyunsaturated essential fatty acids and fat-soluble vitamins that cannot be synthesized in adequate amounts for optimal body function.

Normal HDL cholesterol ranges from 29 to 77 mg/100 mL of blood, and normal LDL cholesterol ranges from 62 to 185 mg/100 mL. Too-high LDL levels increases the risk of CAD, while elevated HDL generally reflects a healthy state. It might also indicate chronic hepatitis, early-stage primary biliary cirrhosis or too much alcohol consumption.

SERUM TRIGLYCERIDES LABORATORY TEST

Triglycerides are the body's main storage form of lipids (constituting 95% of fatty tissue) and the serum triglycerides laboratory test provides a quantitative analysis of these. It identifies hyperlipemia in kidney disease and CAD. Expected triglyceride values vary according to age (see Table 26-1).

Test abnormality suggests that other measurements are needed. High triglycerides indicate the risk of atherosclerosis or CAD. Mild to moderate levels show biliary obstruction, diabetes, kidney disease, endocrinopathies or overconsumption of alcohol. Decreased levels are rare but may show malnutrition or a betalipoproteinemia.

Note: On the Gerson diet, flare-ups and healing reactions are shown by elevated triglycerides.

SERUM PROTEIN ELECTROPHORESIS LABORATORY TEST

The major blood proteins of the body, albumin and four globulins, are measured in an electric field by separating them into patterns according to size, shape and electric charge at pH 8.6. Comprising more than 50% of total serum protein, albumin prevents leakage of capillary plasma by oncotic pressure (the pressure exerted by plasma proteins on the capil-

Table 26-1
Triglyceride Values

Age	Mg/dL	nmol/L
0-29	10-140	0.1-1.55
30-39	10-150	0.1-1.65
40-49	10-160	0.1-1.75
50-59	10-190	0.1-2.10

Table 26-2
Normal Blood Serum

Total serum protein	6.6 to 7.9 g/dL
Albumin fraction	3.3 to 4.5 g/dL
Alpha^1 globulin fraction	0.1 to 0.4 g/dL
Alpha^2 globulin	0.5 to 1.0 g/dL
Beta globulin	0.7 to 1.2 g/dL
Gamma globulin	0.5 to 1.6 g/dL

lary wall) and transports the many water-insoluble substances, such as bilirubin, fatty acids, hormones and drugs. Of the four globulins— alpha^1, alpha^2, beta and gamma—the first three act as carrier proteins for transporting lipids, hormones and metals through the blood; the fourth, gamma globulin, acts in and upon the immune system.

As indicated by its label, the serum protein electrophoresis laboratory test uses electric current to measure the total serum protein and albumin-globulin ratio to convert them into absolute values. These values help to uncover the presence of liver disease, blood dyscrasias, kidney disorders, gastrointestinal illnesses, neoplastic (benign and malignant) diseases and/or protein deficiency. Table 26-2 shows the normal blood serum ranges for these proteins.

The balance between total albumin and total globulin (known in medicine as the A-G ratio) is evaluated in relation to the total protein level. A reversed A-G ratio (decreased albumin and elevated globulins) with low total protein shows chronic liver disease; reversed A-G ratio with normal total protein shows myeloproliferative disease (e.g., leukemia and Hodgkin's disease) or certain chronic infectious diseases (e.g., tuberculosis (TB) and chronic hepatitis).

BLOOD UREA NITROGEN LABORATORY TEST

The blood urea nitrogen (BUN) laboratory test measures the blood's nitrogen fraction of urea, the chief product of protein metabolism. Formed in the liver from ammonia and excreted by the kidneys, urea constitutes 40% to 50% of the blood's nonprotein nitrogen. The BUN level reflects protein intake and kidney excretory capacity, but it is a less reliable indicator of uremia (urine in the blood) than the serum creatinine level (see "Serum Creatinine Laboratory Test," below).

With normal values ranging from 8 to 20 mg/dL, the BUN test helps to evaluate kidney function, aids in the diagnosis of kidney illness and assesses the body's hydration. An elevated BUN happens in reduced renal blood flow from dehydration, renal disease, urinary tract obstruction and increased protein catabolism, as in burns. Depressed BUN levels occur in severe liver damage, malnutrition and overhydration.

Note: Due to initial decreased dietary protein intake, a person following the Gerson Therapy will likely show a slightly reduced level of BUN.

SERUM CREATININE LABORATORY TEST

Providing a more sensitive measure of kidney damage than the BUN, the serum creatinine laboratory test is a quantitative analysis of the nonprotein end product of metabolism, creatinine. Kidney impairment is virtually the only cause of creatinine elevation in the blood; therefore, creatinine levels are directly related to the glomerular filtration rate. They assess renal glomerular function and screen for kidney damage.

Creatinine concentration in males normally ranges from 0.8 to 1.2 mg/dL; in females from 0.6 to 0.9 mg/dL. Elevation of serum creatinine means that serious renal disease is present with 50% damaged nephrons, as in gigantism and acromegaly. Interfering factors are too much absorption of ascorbic acid, barbiturates, diuretics and sulfobromophthalein. Also, athletes may have above-average creatinine levels, even with normal kidney function.

SERUM URIC ACID LABORATORY TEST

Used mainly to detect gout, the serum uric acid laboratory test measures levels of uric acid, a metabolite of purine in the blood. Glomerular filtration and tubular secretion gets rid of uric acid, but it is less soluble at a pH of 7.4 or lower, which occurs in certain diseases, such as gout, excessive cellular generation and destruction as in leukemia and kidney dysfunction.

Uric acid concentrations in men range from 4.3 to 8 mg/dL; in women, they range from 2.3 to 6 mg/dL. Although elevated levels of serum uric acid don't correlate with severity of disease, they do rise in congestive heart failure; glycogen storage disease; acute infectious diseases, such as infectious mononucleosis; hemolytic anemia; sickle cell anemia; hemoglobinopathies; polycythemia; leukemia; lymphoma; metastatic malignancy; and psoriasis. Depressed uric acid levels indicate defective acute hepatic atrophy or tubular absorption, as in Wilson's disease and Fanconi's syndrome.

Drug factors interfering in the serum uric acid laboratory test include loop diuretics, ethambutol, vincristine, pyrazinamide, thiazides, and low doses of salicylates, which elevate blood levels. Also starvation, a high-purine diet, stress and alcohol abuse raise uric acid. When uric acid is measured by the colorimetric method, false elevations come from acetaminophen, ascorbic acid, levodopa and phenacetin. Decreased uric acid is caused by high doses of aspirin, Coumadin®, clofibrate, cinchophen, adrenocorticotropic hormone and phenothiazines.

GLUCOSE, FASTING BLOOD
SUGAR LABORATORY TEST

Following a 12- to 14-hour fast, the glucose, fasting blood sugar (FBS) laboratory test measures glucose metabolism as required in diabetes mellitus. In the fasting state, blood glucose levels decrease, stimulating release of the hormone glucagon. Glucagon then raises plasma glucose by accelerating glycogenolysis, stimulating glyconeogenesis and inhibiting glycogen synthesis. Normally, secretion of insulin checks this rise in glucose levels. In diabetes, absence or deficiency of insulin allows persistently high glucose levels.

Normal ranges for fasting blood glucose on the FBS laboratory test after an eight- to 12-hour fast are:

- Fasting serum, 70 to 100 mg/dL
- Fasting whole blood, 60 to 100 mg/dL
- Nonfasting whole blood, 85 to 125 mg/dL in persons over age 50, and 70 to 115 mg/dL in persons under age 50

These laboratory readings help to screen for diabetes mellitus and other disorders of glucose metabolism. They also monitor drug or dietary therapy for diabetics, insulin requirements for uncontrolled diabetics and known or suspected hypoglycemics.

Fasting blood glucose levels of 140 to 150 mg/dL or higher obtained on two or more occasions are diagnostic of diabetes mellitus. Nonfasting levels that exceed 200 mg/dL also show diabetes. The elevated blood glucose may come from pancreatitis, hyperthyroidism, pheochromocytoma, chronic hepatic disease, brain trauma, chronic illness, chronic malnutrition, eclampsia, anoxia and convulsive disorders.

Depressed blood glucose occurs from hyperinsulinism, insulinoma, von Gierke's disease, functional or reactive hypoglycemia, hypothyroidism, adrenal insufficiency, congenital adrenal hyperplasia, hypopituitarism, islet cell carcinoma of the pancreas, hepatic necrosis and glycogen storage disease.

SERUM IRON AND TOTAL IRON-BINDING CAPACITY LABORATORY TEST

Two separate blood tests conducted with buffering and coloring reagents measure:

- The amount of iron bound to the glycoprotein transferrin; and
- The plasma's total iron-binding capacity (TIBC) if all the transferrin were saturated with iron.

The percentage of saturation is obtained by dividing the serum iron result by the TIBC, which reveals the actual amount of saturated transferrin. Normal transferrin is 30% saturated. Thus, the two tests:

- Estimate total iron storage;
- Diagnose hemochromatosis;
- Distinguish between iron deficiency anemia and chronic disease anemia; and
- Evaluate a person's nutritional status.

Normal serum iron and TIBC values are shown in Table 26-3.

In iron deficiency, serum iron falls and TIBC increases to decrease the saturation. With chronic inflammation, as in rheumatoid arthritis, serum iron is low in the presence of adequate body stores, but TIBC remains unchanged or drops to preserve normal saturation. Iron overload does not alter serum levels until relatively late in the pathology, but serum iron increases and TIBC remains the same to increase the saturation.

Table 26-3
Normal Serum Iron and
Total Iron-Binding Capacity

	Serum Iron	TIBC (mcg/dL)	Saturation (mcg/dL)
Men	70 to 150	300 to 400	20 to 50
Women	80 to 150	350 to 450	20 to 50

ERYTHROCYTE (RED BLOOD CELL) COUNT

Traditionally counted by hand with a hemacytometer, red blood cells (RBCs) are now commonly counted with electronic devices, which provide faster, more accurate results. This erythrocyte count does not provide qualitative information about the RBC's hemoglobin content, but it does tell mean corpuscular volume (MCV) and mean corpuscular hemoglobin (MCH). Thus, the erythrocyte blood count offers indices for RBC size and hemoglobin content, and supports other hematologic tests in diagnosing anemia and polycythemia.

Depending on age, sex, sample and geographic location, normal RBC values in adult males range from 4.5 to 6.2 million/microliter (µL) (4.5 to 6.2 x 10^{12}/L) of venous blood; in adult females from 4.2 to 5.4 million/µL (4.2 to 5.4 x 10^{12}/L) of venous blood; in children from 4.6 to 4.8 million/µL of venous blood; and in full-term infants from 4.4 to 5.8 million/µL (4.4 to 5.8 x 10^{12}/L). An elevated RBC count indicates polycythemia or dehydration; a depressed count shows anemia, fluid overload or recent hemorrhage. With total bed rest, RBC counts drop considerably from decreased oxygen requirements.

TOTAL HEMOGLOBIN LABORATORY TEST

The total hemoglobin (Hgb) concentration in a deciliter (100 ml) of whole blood is measured by the total Hgb laboratory test. The Hgb-RBC ratio (or MCH) and free plasma Hgb affect the RBC count. This test, a usual part of the complete blood count, measures the severity of anemia or polycythemia, monitors therapy response, and supplies figures for calculating MCH and mean corpuscular Hgb concentration.

Based on venous blood samples, normal values for different patients are illustrated in Table 26-4.

Table 26-4
Normal Hemoglobin Values

Age	Hemoglobin Level (g/dL)
Less than 7 days	17-22
1 week	15-20
1 month	11-15
Children	11-13
Adult males	14-18
Elderly males	12.4-14.9
Adult females	12-16
Elderly females	11.7-13.8

HEMATOCRIT LABORATORY TEST

The volume of RBCs packed in a whole blood sample is measured by the hematocrit (Hct) laboratory test. Number and size of the RBCs determine the Hct concentration, and such a read-out aids in the diagnosis of abnormal states of hydration, polycythemia, anemia, fluid imbalance, blood loss, blood replacement and red cell indices. According to a patient's sex, age, laboratory competence and type of blood sample, the test routinely screens one's blood in a complete blood count.

Hct reference values range from 40% to 54% (0.4 to 0.54) for men and from 37% to 47% (0.37 to 0.47) for women. Low Hct indicates anemia or hemodilution; high Hct shows polycythemia or hemoconcentration caused by blood loss. If a hematoma develops at the venipuncture site, ease discomfort by applying ice, followed later by warm soaks.

ERYTHROCYTE INDICES LABORATORY TEST

MCV, MCH and mean corpuscular hemoglobin concentration (MCHC) are the three measurements provided by the erythrocyte indi-

289

ces laboratory test. The MCV expresses the average size of erythrocytes and indicates whether they are undersized (microcytic), oversized (macrocytic) or normal (normocytic). MCH gives the weight of Hgb in an average red cell. MCHC defines the concentration of Hgb in 100 mL of packed red cells.

The normal RBC indices are:

- MCV: 84 to 99 cubic microliters/red cell (femtoliters (fl)/red cell)
- MCH: 26 to 32 picograms (pg)/red cell
- MCHC: 30% to 36% (300 to 360 g/L)

These indices aid in diagnosing and classifying anemia. Low MCV and MCHC show microcytic hypochromic anemias caused by iron deficiency anemia, pyridoxine-responsive anemia or thalassemia. High MCV indicates macrocytic anemia caused by megaloblastic anemias coming from folic acid or vitamin B_{12} deficiency, inherited disorders of DNA (deoxyribonucleic acid) synthesis or reticulocytosis.

ERYTHROCYTE SEDIMENTATION RATE

Measuring the time required for erythrocytes in a whole blood sample to settle to the bottom of a vertical tube, the erythrocyte sedimentation rate (ESR) is a sensitive but nonspecific test that indicates the presence of disease when other chemical or physical signs are normal. It rises in widespread inflammatory disorders caused by infection, autoimmune disease or malignancy.

Thus, the ESR monitors inflammatory or malignant illness and detects occult disease, such as TB, tissue necrosis or connective tissue disorders. The normal ESR ranges from 0 to 20 mm/hour. It rises in pregnancy, acute or chronic inflammation, TB, paraproteinemias, rheumatic fever, rheumatoid arthritis and some cancers. ESR also rises in anemia. ESR drops in polycythemia, sickle cell anemia, hyperviscosity and low plasma protein.

Note: ESR is frequently raised during and after reactions and fevers induced by the Gerson Therapy.

PLATELET COUNT

Platelets, or thrombocytes, are tiny formed elements in the blood which create the hemostatic plug in vascular injury. They promote coagulation by supplying phospholipids to the intrinsic thromboplastin pathway. The platelet count is vital for monitoring chemotherapy, radiation therapy, or severe thrombocytosis and thrombocytopenia. A platelet count that falls below 50,000 brings on spontaneous bleeding; below 5,000, fatal central nervous system bleeding or massive gastrointestinal hemorrhage is possible.

The platelet count evaluates platelet production, assesses effects of cytotoxic therapy, aids the diagnosing of thrombocytopenia and thrombocytosis, and confirms visual estimate of platelet number and morphology from a stained blood film. Normal platelet counts range from 130,000 to 370,000/μL (1.3 to 3.7 x 10^{11}/L).

A decreased count comes from aplastic or hypoplastic bone marrow; infiltrative bone marrow diseases like carcinoma, leukemia or disseminated infection; megakaryocytic hypoplasia; ineffective thrombopoiesis caused by folic acid or vitamin B_1 deficiency; pooling of platelets in an enlarged spleen; increased platelet destruction from drug use or immune disorders; disseminated intravascular coagulation; Bernard-Soulier syndrome; or mechanical injury to platelets.

Medications decreasing the count include acetazolamid, acetohexamide, antimony, antineoplastics, brompheniramine maleate, carbamazepine, chloramphenicol, ethacrynic acid, furosemide, gold salts, hydroxychloroquine, indomethacin, isoniazid, mephenytoin, mefenamic acid, methazolamide, methimazole, methyidopa, oral diaoxide, oxyphenbetazone, penicillamine, penicillin, phenylbutazone, phenytoin, pyrimethamine, quinidine sulfate, quinine, salicylates, streptomycin, sulfonamides, thiazide, thiazide-like diuretics and tricyclic antidepressants. Heparin causes transient reversible thrombocytopenia.

An increased platelet count results from such diseases as hemorrhage; infectious disorders; malignancies; iron deficiency anemia; myelofibrosis; primary thrombocytosis; polycythemia vera; myelogenous leukemia; recent surgery, pregnancy or splenectomy; and inflammatory disorders, such as collagen vascular disease.

LEUKOCYTE (WHITE BLOOD CELL) COUNT

Reporting on the number of white blood cells (WBCs) found in a microliter (cubic millimeter) of whole blood by use of a hemacytometer or Coulter counter, the leukocyte count varies with strenuous exercise, stress or digestion. It is used to detect infection or inflammation, the need for further tests such as the WBC differential or bone marrow biopsy and the response to chemotherapy or radiation therapy.

The WBC count ranges from 4.1 to 10.9 x 10^{11}. An elevated count signals infection, such as an abscess, meningitis, appendicitis or tonsillitis, and it may indicate leukemia, tissue necrosis from burns, MI or gangrene. A low count shows bone marrow depression from viral infections or from toxic reactions, such as those following treatment with antineoplastics, mercury or other heavy metal toxicity; benzene or arsenic exposure; and invasion by the organisms of influenza, typhoid fever, measles, infectious hepatitis, mononucleosis and rubella.

WHITE BLOOD CELL DIFFERENTIAL TEST

The WBC differential test determines the relative number of each type of WBC, calculated by multiplying the percentage value of each WBC type to give an absolute number of each kind of the 100 or more WBCs (e.g., granulocytes, agranulocytes, juvenile neutrophils, segmented neutrophils, basophils, eosinophils, large lymphocytes, small lymphocytes, phagocytes and histiocytes).

The WBC differential evaluates the body's capacity to resist and overcome infection, various types of leukemia, the stage and severity of infection, allergic reactions, severity of allergic reactions and parasitic infections. There is a long list of reference values in the WBC differential test, divided into adult and child (see Table 26-5 for some

Table 26-5
White Blood Cell Differentials

For Adults	Relative Value (%)	Absolute Value (mcL)
Neutrophils	47.6-76.8	1950-8,400
Lymphocytes	16.2-43	660-4,600
Monocytes	0.6-9.6	24-960
Eosinophils	0.3-7	12-760
Basophils	0.3-2	12-200

examples). To make an accurate diagnosis, the test examiner must consider both relative and absolute values of the differential counts.[1]

ROUTINE URINALYSIS

Elements of routine urinalysis include the measurement evaluations of physical characteristics, specific gravity and pH, protein, glucose and ketone bodies, plus examination of urine sediment, casts and blood cell crystals. The analysis of urine is an exceedingly important test that tells a lot about a person's internal workings. Routine urine test results have a great number of implications for how the physiology is functioning or how it is responding to the diet, nonpathologic conditions, specimen collection time and other factors.

For the vast number of variables and illnesses which are evaluated by urinalysis, please see Appendix I of the *Gerson Therapy Handbook: Companion Workbook to A Cancer Therapy: Results of Fifty Cases.*[2]

REFERENCES

1. For the vast number of variables and illnesses which are diagnosed by them, please see Appendix I of the *Gerson Therapy Handbook: Companion Workbook* to M. Gerson, *A Cancer Therapy: Results of Fifty Cases and The Cure of Advanced Cancer by Diet Therapy: A Summary of Thirty Years of*

Clinical Experimentation, 6th ed. (San Diego, CA: Gerson Institute, 1999). To acquire a copy of this handbook/workbook, contact the Gerson Institute in San Diego, California.

2. Ibid.

CHAPTER 27

Case Histories of Recovered Patients

The following well-documented stories of recovered Gerson patients are just a very small sample of the considerable collection of such records in our archive. All of them refer to patients thoroughly diagnosed by biopsy, done mostly in U.S. hospitals; almost all of them were in a so-called terminal condition with widespread cancers that have never been cured by orthodox means.

We chose them in an attempt to include as many kinds of malignant disease as possible, since we know from long experience that individuals who are thinking of pursuing the Gerson Therapy always want to know first whether anyone suffering from "their" cancer has ever recovered. This selection aims to answer their questions.

The Gerson protocol is often attacked on the grounds that it has never been subjected to a so-called proper test (i.e., a randomized, double-blind, placebo-controlled clinical trial). This kind of test, however, has taken over fairly recently from another, centuries-old way of judging medical treatments, which was based on clinical results. In other words, as Dr. Gerson often stated, "It's the result at the sickbed that counts," a self-evident view that would be hard to dispute.

The currently favored randomized, double-blind, placebo-controlled clinical trial, however, is not concerned with individual patients. It requires a large group of individuals and is called double-blind because neither the doctor nor the patients know who is receiving the new drug under testing and who is not; this is meant to exclude psychological or other external influences that might interfere with the working of the drug.

Clearly, this method is suitable for testing a single drug but useless for any therapy that involves a total change of lifestyle, such as the Gerson treatment. Just consider for a moment the impossibility of administering coffee enemas or serving fresh juices 13 times a day without patients realizing that something radical is going on. Besides, the mainstays of conventional oncology, namely radiation treatment and chemotherapy, have never been subjected to randomized, double-blind clinical trials. Only various kinds of chemotherapy have been tested against each other—never chemo versus nonchemo treatment. Yet, all the time, books and academic studies have been published by physicians and other scientists attesting to the failure of chemotherapy. One of the latest books is *The War on Cancer: an Anatomy of Failure* by Guy B. Faguet, MD.[1]

In view of this, critics of the Gerson Therapy should perhaps demand the application of randomized double-blind clinical trials of chemotherapy before attacking a method with which they are totally unfamiliar.

HIGHLY AGGRESSIVE LYMPHOMA

S. M. was 47 years old in 1990 when she developed several swollen lymph nodes and, after having them biopsied, was diagnosed with non-Hodgkins lymphoma. Two years later, in the summer of 1992, she arrived at the Gerson hospital with extensive edema (fluid accumulation) in her legs, hips, buttocks and around a large, melon-sized tumor in her abdomen. She embarked on the Gerson Therapy as the only treatment for her condition and was not "tapped" to remove the fluid from her body. In the first five days on the full Gerson program, with many trips to the bathroom, S. M. lost 28 pounds.

In February 1993, when the patient was reexamined by her doctor in Wenatchee, Washington, the MD's report read: "The generalized lymphadenopathy [disease of the lymph nodes] has resolved [medical term for 'gone']. I can no longer feel the abdominal mass. Marked carotenemia [harmless orange discoloration of the skin often present in Gerson patients] is noticed. Spleen is not palpable [cannot be felt]. ... She remains adamant, however, that she wants no conventional medical treatment. Dr. Bulger, Hematology/Oncology, Wenatchee Valley Clinic, Wenatchee, Washington."[2] Understandable, since she no longer had any swollen lymph nodes! S. M. continued in good health, testified about her recovery at a convention in Seattle in 1998 and was active in her husband's business at last report in 2002.

At age 32, W. S. was a struggling young artist with a wife and three small children. When he noted a mass in his abdomen, he was sent to surgery in May 1951 in Cincinnati, Ohio. The doctor reported "a cluster of lymph glands, the largest measuring 5 cm (2 inches)."[3] He removed as many as he could; afterwards, W. S. was given radiotherapy. A mere four months later, in September, a new mass appeared and the patient received more radiotherapy, which reduced the swollen glands. However, a few months later, the trouble recurred and W. S. tried other treatments since his doctors told him that he had only two months to live.

When W. S. found out about the Gerson Therapy, he traveled to New York to see Dr. Gerson (who reported on the case in his book, *A Cancer Therapy—Results of Fifty Cases*, as Case #18).[4] After about eight months on the Gerson program, W. S.'s condition improved dramatically, he recovered his energy and was able to continue working as a church artist. He did construction and decoration work, designed stained glass windows and mounted an art exhibition in San Diego. In 1983, W. S. wrote: "I am looking back on 33 years, eight children, 12 grandchildren and a wonderful productive life." In 2006, aged 88, he appeared in *Dying to Have Known*, Stephen Kroschel's Gerson documentary film, still functioning well and working in his artist's studio with several of his children.

ENDOMETRIOSIS TURNING INTO CERVICAL CANCER

The endometrium is the mucous membrane lining the uterus. During the fertile years of a woman, this lining is shed every month if the

297

secreted ovum is not fertilized and implanted in the tissue. When the organism or the hormone system is malfunctioning, the endometrium can spread to various sites throughout the pelvic area, including the abdominal wall. As the condition worsens and the menstrual cycle does not get regulated, endometrial tissue may spread throughout the body, becoming a malignancy "resembling metastatic pelvic carcinoma."[5]

The case of S.T. illustrates this progression perfectly. This patient had gynecological problems at the very start of her menstrual periods. Thirty-five years later, she was diagnosed with endometriosis and had a number of D and Cs (dilatation and curettage, or scraping of the uterus) to remove endometrial plaque. In the end, she had a partial hysterectomy yet her problems continued. Finally, in 1979, a Pap smear showed cancer of the cervix, with atypical (irregular, not conforming to the normal) cells in her blood. She also noticed lumps in her breast but these were not further investigated. A hysterectomy was arranged for her, but she declined the operation.

She began to investigate alternative treatments, changed her diet and fasted. Then she remembered a lecture she had heard many years before by Charlotte Gerson and decided to go on the Gerson Therapy. Having done so, she was surprised to experience severe healing reactions with nausea and vomiting, but then recalled being told that she had a great deal of scar tissue in her abdominal area, probably caused by earlier ulcers. S.T. stayed on the therapy for two years and declares, "Never once did a bite of food enter my mouth that I should not have eaten." She remains well (last report was in November 2006) and is busy taking care of her aged parents and in-laws, who are in their 90s, and occasionally her grandchildren.

BREAST CANCER

In 1988, K.B., aged 70, noticed redness and swelling in the nipple area of her breast. Her doctor in Modesto, California, took a biopsy that proved she had a malignant tumor; he also confirmed that he "hadn't got it all" and urged her to have a mastectomy. She refused. A second opinion by a physician at Stanford confirmed the original diagnosis and K.B. was advised to undergo surgery, followed by chemotherapy and/or radiation. Again she refused.

Rejecting any conventional treatment, K.B. embarked on the Gerson Therapy at home, at first eating only raw foods and having six enemas a day for eight months. Then she added some organic, vegetarian cooked foods. After one and one-half years, the cancer was gone but she still had some scar tissue which she chose to have removed. A biopsy showed that the tissue was clear of any malignancy. The Tumor Board noted in her medical records that the patient was "Cured by Diet."[6] K.B., now in her late 80s, shows up every year at a Los Angeles Health Convention! She still drinks juices but eats "a little meat." This case is all the more remarkable because the patient pursued the Gerson Therapy on her own, at home, without staying at the Gerson hospital or having a Gerson doctor to consult.

BREAST CANCER WITH LIVER METASTASES

E.B., aged 43, reported to her doctor with a lump in her breast in January 2002, was biopsied and told that she had breast cancer. She took no action. In January 2004, she reported to Loma Linda University Medical Center and was diagnosed as suffering from Stage 4 breast cancer with liver metastases. According to the medical report, her liver was "covered with tumors and was shutting down; her skin and the whites of her eyes were yellow."[7]

E.B. was offered chemotherapy and, not knowing otherwise, she accepted one treatment. Her oncologist stated that, in view of her advanced condition, he was not sure she could survive for two months, but he hoped that chemotherapy would give her a year of life. That was when the patient began to look for other options and found out about the Gerson Therapy. From her research she knew that, with conventional medical treatment, cases of breast cancer with liver metastases had less than a 1% two-year survival rate, so her only hope was to try an alternative protocol.

After completing two years on the Gerson Therapy, E.B. was well enough to go skiing in Tulluride, Colorado, one of the steepest mountains in the U.S. Now, after three years, judging by her PET/CT (positron emission tomography/computed tomography) scan of August 2006, she has a fully functioning liver and no malignancy or metastases anywhere in her body. E.B. enjoys skiing in winter and water skiing in the summer, rock climbing, playing golf and riding her motorcycle. She also travels frequently.

BREAST CANCER RECURRENCE
AFTER CHEMO AND RADIATION

A.F. discovered a lump in her breast in September 1985. She had a biopsy and a lumpectomy, followed by radiation and chemotherapy at the Virginia Mason Hospital in Seattle, Washington. By 1989, the cancer had spread to her throat. She had more surgery, followed again by radiation. Five months later, more recurrences occurred "all over" and more radiation was offered. Due to the extreme suffering caused by the earlier radiation, she refused the treatment and went instead to the Gerson hospital in Mexico. Before long, she was getting better and, after about a year, she was told that she didn't have cancer anymore.

Seven years later, the radiation damage causing A.F. severe dryness in her throat cleared at last and her health was truly excellent. When she returned to her original doctor and told him that she was on the Gerson Therapy, he simply walked out of the office. A.F. continues in good health.

MELANOMA

M.H., aged 40, was diagnosed with melanoma in her vaginal wall. This was confirmed by biopsy and subsequent surgery, followed by 25 radiation treatments and a four-month course of interferon. During this treatment, the cancer spread to her liver. The oncologists treating her thought that, with chemotherapy, the patient might live up to nine months. Although M.H. was extremely weak and in serious pain, she refused that option and, in November 1996, embarked on the Gerson treatment in spite of her oncologist's warning against it. In September 1997, a scan showed that M.H. was clear of melanoma. Ten years later, she remains fit and well.

W.E., born in 1943, is a registered nurse. In 1996, she discovered a large mole growing on her arm. The surgeon who removed it remarked that he had had to go very deep in order to obtain clear margins. The diagnosis was Stage 4 melanoma. The patient's condition deteriorated and some months later, in 1997, at the University of California at Los Angeles, spots were found on her hip as well as a large tumor in her liver; both were biopsied and confirmed to be melanoma. Her doctor advised her to get her affairs in order since she didn't have long to live. W.E. started the Gerson treatment in July 1997, made a full recovery and remains alive and well (last report was in 2006).

RECURRENT MELANOMA

N.P. had a 5 mm mole on his back, which began to bleed in October 1990. He consulted skin cancer specialist, Dr. Richard Ferderspiel, who was sure that the lesion was not melanoma. However, the biopsy proved him wrong, and on October 30, at the Berrien General Hospital in Michigan, a large area of skin was removed from the patient's back.

Six months later, in April 1991, an enlarged lymph node was discovered in N.P.'s right axilla. It was biopsied and found to be metastasized melanoma. The oncologist at the Borgess Medical Center of Kalamazoo, Michigan, told N.P., "I've treated several cases like yours and lost them all."[8] He then proposed an experimental treatment that might possibly extend the patient's life from the six-month prognosis to nine months. N.P. refused.

At that stage, he received a letter from the widow of an acquaintance, a man of his own age, who had received all available conventional treatments for metastatic melanoma and died five months later. This persuaded N.P. to go to the Gerson clinic in Mexico, where he arrived with his wife in May 1991. At the time, another tumor appeared, but vanished in six weeks. At the end of the therapy, N.P., aged 67, was in perfect health and regularly competed in the Senior Olympic Games in Michigan and Florida, winning Silver twice and Gold once in the Racewalk.

In time, he eased off the Gerson type of food and abandoned the diet completely while traveling in South America. In 1994, another lymph node had to be removed from the original site; it proved to be melanoma. N.P. immediately resumed the strict intensive Gerson Therapy and again made a full recovery. At present, he remains well and active.

COLORECTAL CANCER WITH LIVER METASTASES

C.T. was 58 years old when he noticed signs of rectal bleeding. The treatment he was given for suspected hemorrhoids proved useless, so he was sent to Shand Hospital in Gainesville, Florida, for thorough tests and diagnosis. The resulting surgery report showed that C.T. was suffering from a colon malignancy with metastases throughout his body. The hospital doctors told the patient that, because of his widely spread cancer, chemotherapy would be of no use, and gave him a prognosis of three to six months of life. C.T. embarked on the Gerson Therapy, using no other treatment and, over a period of two years, achieved a complete recovery. Twenty-five years later, aged 81, he remains well and active.

In 1992, Y.H., a Japanese professor of medicine, found himself unable to have a bowel movement. Surgery, combined with a liver biopsy, disclosed colon malignancy, which had already spread to the liver. Professor Y.H. agreed to four mild chemotherapy treatments, but these resulted in the growth of the liver metastases. The patient abandoned the chemotherapy and embarked on the Gerson Therapy, following the directions in Dr. Gerson's book. Fourteen years later, he is fully recovered, with a clean liver, and has successfully treated many cancer patients with the same method. He described his experience in his book (only available in Japanese) and has trained a few of his colleagues in the Gerson Therapy.

At present, he is following up some 500 cancer cases, which have shown positive responses to the Gerson protocol he now uses.

PANCREATIC CANCER

L. K. went to see his doctor, as he was feeling poorly, and was prescribed a medicine to reduce his stomach acid. Unfortunately, this remedy caused him severe pain and other problems. In November 1994, he was given a CT scan, which showed "an abnormal irregular mass at the head of the pancreas, contiguous [adjacent] with the superior mesenteric artery and superior vein." L. K.'s doctor stated, "You have pancreatic cancer and surgery is impossible, while neither radiation nor chemotherapy would work for you." [9]

After talking to recovered Gerson patients, and without any treatment on offer, the patient decided to go to Mexico and start the Gerson treatment. After 20 months of strictly adhering to the protocol, a second CT scan showed no sign of disease and everything came up as normal. L. K. points out that the regular severe migraine headaches that had plagued him for many years disappeared almost at once after he started the therapy. After more than 10 years, he remains fit, well and active.

Having lost some 25 pounds, in January 1986, P. A. was sent to a hospital in Victoria, British Columbia, Canada, for a CAT scan, whose results were verified by a needle biopsy. The diagnosis was pancreatic cancer. The specialist told her to get her affairs in order because her cancer was inoperable and added that the malignancy had spread to her liver, gallbladder and spleen. By then, the patient had lost 45 pounds and was vomiting blood. With no other option, she decided to try the Gerson Therapy, having heard about a local man who claimed to have recovered on it from pancreatic cancer.

In March 1986, she arrived at the Gerson clinic in Mexico and started the intensive therapy. By December of that year, a mere 11 months later, according to her doctor the patient had the cancer licked. In February 1990, her family doctor stated that "As of the present time, she has no evidence of recurrence and what evidence of malignancy was present in

1985 has now gone."[10] P. A. continues in good health and leads an active life, 20 years after being diagnosed with an apparently incurable and life-threatening disease.

PROSTATE CANCER

P. S. was 69 years old in 1991 when he was diagnosed with prostate cancer. He had several needle biopsies, three of which showed the presence of malignant cells, while three others were negative. His PSA (prostate-specific antigen) stood at 6—not very elevated, but above normal.

P. S. started the Gerson Therapy at the Gerson clinic in Mexico in 1991 and—as we often note—at first his PSA rose, reaching 14 at the end of three months. The patient was somewhat alarmed by this increase, but he persevered with the treatment. Indeed, after 18 months, his PSA went down to 0.3. Now in his 80s, P. S. is perfectly well, as shown by his regular annual check-ups. His prostate is normal and his present PSA stands at 2.1 (latest report was October 2006).

PROSTATE AND BONE CANCER,
AND A CASE OF LUNG CANCER

E. T., of Cairo, Illinois, presents the most remarkable case history. E. T. had dropped out of school after the sixth grade and had received no further education. He had spent all his life working in a junkyard, sorting various metals. In 1966, aged 69, he was advised by his doctors to put his affairs in order as he was dying of prostate cancer with extensive spreading into his bones and a large mass in his groin. He had been treated with hormones, but his doctors realized that those treatments were no longer effective and there was nothing more they could do.

When his doctors gave him what amounted to a death sentence, he remembered reading something about the Gerson Therapy. He contacted Dr. Gerson's eldest daughter, asking for help. She pointed him to her father's book, *A Cancer Therapy—Results of Fifty Cases,*[11] but after a short while he called her back and stated that he couldn't understand the book. So she told him simply to follow the chart on page 235.

E. T. obeyed her instructions but, having lost his wife years before, he found that pursuing the therapy at home was "the hardest thing he ever did." One day, leaning over the arm of a chair, he broke one of his ribs, weakened by metastases. He was in severe pain and felt tempted just to stay in bed. However, he forced himself to get up and prepare the food and juices since he knew that, without helping himself, he would die. In a short time, he was free from pain. After a month, his doctor could no longer feel the large mass that he had found in the patient's groin. E. T. soon felt well and had much greater energy.

One day he received a call from a friend in Kentucky, the chiropractor Dr. G. D., who told him that he was dying of lung cancer that had spread through both of his lungs. Could E. T. come and help him? E. T. traveled to G. D.'s home and set up the Gerson Therapy for him. Amazingly, both these terminal patients recovered! Fifteen years later, in 1981, both were alive and well. E. T. was 84 years old. Dr. G. D. was a good deal younger and lived for many more years. Eventually, we heard from his son that he had passed away.

ASTROCYTOMA

In 1987, just weeks before her 10th birthday, N. K., living in North Liberty, Indiana, began to suffer from headaches followed by vomiting. A CAT scan showed a brain tumor and the patient was taken to Riley Children's Hospital in Indianapolis for brain surgery. The surgeon removed what he could but found that some of the tumor was too close to a major blood vessel and could only be cauterized.

Subsequently, N. K. had annual check-ups. When she turned 13, an MRI (magnetic resonance imaging) showed a recurrence. The doctor said that, at this early stage, he could not operate, but N. K.'s mother felt unable to just sit by and wait for her daughter's brain tumor to grow. She found out about the Gerson treatment and, in 1990, the patient and her mother came to the Mexican hospital. Due to the demanding routine of the Gerson Therapy with the need for hourly juices, N. K. could not go to school, so her mother home-schooled her. Also, doing her enemas, the patient did a great deal of reading. First she read the classics, then she studied mathematics and finally philosophy. By the time she took her Scholastic Aptitude Test, she was not only free from her tumor but also scored extremely high on her test.

When her surgeon examined her new x-rays, he could not understand how it was possible for N. K. to have no more malignancy since he knew that he had left some tumor tissue in place at the time of her operation. Her fine motor skills were also perfectly restored, so much so that she was even able to play the violin. At the last report, N. K. continues fit and well; at 26, she is married and has a family. She graduated from college magna cum laude.

NICOTINE ADDICTION

A. C. started to smoke cigarettes at the age of 17. She looked barely 15 and hoped that smoking would make her look more grown-up. At first, she hated the smell and taste of cigarettes but quickly got hooked on them, and was still smoking 35 years later when she went down with malignant melanoma.

When she discovered the Gerson Therapy and decided to go to the Gerson clinic in Mexico, her main worry was the need to manage without smoking once she got there. It had been made clear to her that if she tried to smoke just one cigarette, she would be sent home at once. Having tried, and failed, to stop smoking more times than she cared to remember, A. C. felt very anxious indeed.

As soon as she arrived at the hospital, she found herself embroiled in the full intensive program: constant juicing, enema training, meals, instructions and meetings with other patients, which took up every waking minute. With all of his activity, it took A. C. almost two whole days to realize that she had neither smoked nor missed her lifetime habit. The real shock came a few hours later when, in the garden of the hospital, she met a visitor who was smoking. To her amazement, A. C. found the smoke highly offensive and quickly walked past the smoker. She suffered no serious withdrawal symptoms, but it took several weeks for the extremely unpleasant accumulated residue of her smoking years to evaporate through her skin and hair. She never looked back and—incidentally—also recovered from her melanoma.

ESOPHAGEAL CANCER

It is important to remember that, beside the most common malignancies—namely, cancer of the breast, prostate and colon, which respond so well to the Gerson Therapy—the same treatment is just as effective in healing rare cancers. To illustrate this, we present the case history of K. G.

Born in 1953, this man was a taxidermist living in Arizona. He was health-conscious and adopted a careful lifestyle: he didn't smoke or use drugs and only occasionally drank a glass of wine—but, as he put it, his diet consisted of "purely junk and convenience foods"! If he ate a whole wheat bread sandwich, he felt he was on a "health kick"; he didn't touch salads, which he dismissed as rabbit food. His annual intake of fruit consisted of perhaps four apples and two to four oranges. To make things worse, he didn't realize the devastating effects of the materials he used daily in his taxidermist business, such as formaldehyde, lacquer thinner, fiberglass and urethane foam and paints.

Slowly over the years, he became aware of some irritation in his throat. In due course, swallowing became difficult and his breathing was heavy. Aged 37, he consulted a doctor and the tests resulted in a diagnosis of esophageal cancer. K. G. was reluctant to consider the proposed treatment, especially in view of the extremely low rate of recoveries, and searched for an alternative, which turned out to be the Gerson Therapy.

He embarked on it and now admits that it had been a real struggle to overcome his aversion to the coffee enemas, but "once I experienced one, I could feel a difference, and realized their importance." The patient experienced very long healing reactions and was aware of the tumor "rotting in my throat with a terrible smell."[12] After some two and one-half months, K. G. reports, he felt the remaining tumor falling down his throat into his stomach. This made him terribly sick for a few days, but finally he expelled all the toxins and made a full recovery. He resumed his professional work, but has become extremely careful in the handling of the chemicals involved, and remains well some 15 years after his recovery.

A WHOLE FAMILY RECOVERS: BREAST AND PROSTATE CANCER AND PLEURISY

This report illustrates the effectiveness of the Gerson treatment in healing the different diseases suffered by the members of one family.

First we saw the mother, S. H., whose mammogram at the age of 53 showed some suspicious details. The surgeon removed two lumps from her breast; they were found to be malignant. He suggested that S. H. should have a mastectomy, possibly followed by radiation, but admitted that the latter would leave her lungs permanently burned and would also soften and damage her bones. The patient opted for a radical mastectomy, but the day before the surgery she decided to go to Mexico for the Gerson treatment. She started the therapy in February 1995, had no other treatment of any kind, recovered fully and remains well.

S. H.'s daughter T. had suffered from pleurisy since the age of three. Her condition worsened and, by the age of 37, as the mother of two children, she was seriously ill: she could hardly breathe and was unable to sit, lie down or sleep, even in a hospital bed. At the time, her mother, S. H., was in the 14th month of her Gerson Therapy. She traveled from California to her daughter's home in Wyoming, with one suitcase full of organic fruit and vegetables and another one containing her clothes.

S. H. reports that, after her first glass of carrot juice, her daughter T. started to feel better. She kept improving rapidly and, after three weeks, was walking, sleeping and recovering, until eventually she completely cleared the long-standing pleurisy for the first time in her life. She is now fully well and training to become a massage therapist.

Some years after the recovery of mother and daughter, S. H.'s husband C. was found to have a PSA of around 14 to 16 (the normal level is 1 or below). In July 2003, a biopsy proved that C. had prostate cancer. This was remarkable since, for years, he had been eating the same diet that had cured his wife, S. However, C. had heard a lot of commercial hype about soy products and their high protein content and, thinking he needed more protein, added a number of soy products to his food intake. He also took a fairly large amount of "aminos," which are high in sodium as well as being derived from soy. When C. stopped the soy and the aminos and went on the full Gerson Therapy, he, too, recovered, and has remained well and active for over four years.

EWING'S SARCOMA

In June 1993, T. I., an eight-year-old boy, was brought to the Gerson clinic in Mexico from Hungary. In March 1992, he had been diagnosed with Ewing's sarcoma, an endothelial myeloma forming tumors on the long bones, for which medical texts give a very poor prognosis. In Hungary, he had been treated with chemotherapy, but the cancer had spread from his pelvis into the soft tissues of his abdomen. He arrived at the hospital looking pale and thin and had lost his hair. Despite the unfamiliar surroundings and his inability to understand English, the boy showed remarkable discipline and consumed the unaccustomed saltless vegetarian food and the raw juices without any fuss.

After returning to Hungary, his mother reported that, in three months on the therapy, the boy's tumor had disappeared. Two years later, she sent us some photographs of T. I., showing a strong, well-developed, healthy-looking 10-year-old child.

His dramatic recovery was underscored by another fact. Prior to his journey to Mexico, being treated in Hungary with chemotherapy, he was one of a group of seven children, all suffering from Ewing's sarcoma and all receiving the same chemotherapy treatment at the same hospital. While T. I. had survived and was fit and well, the six other children from his group were all dead. The last news of the young patient was received in March 2006, when his mother reported that he was then 20 years old and enjoyed continued good health.

REFERENCES

1. Guy B. Faguet, MD, *The War on Cancer: An Anatomy of Failure* (New York: Springer, 2006).
2. Charlotte Gerson, *Healing Lymphoma the Gerson Way* (Carmel: Cancer Research Wellness Institute, 2002), p. 18.
3. Ibid., p. 8.
4. M. Gerson, *A Cancer Therapy: Results of Fifty Cases and The Cure of Advanced Cancer by Diet Therapy: A Summary of Thirty Years of Clinical Experimentation*, 6th ed. (San Diego, CA: Gerson Institute, 1999), Case #18, p. 313.
5. *Taber's Cyclopedic Medical Dictionary* (Philadelphia: F. A. Davis Company, 1993).
6. Personal communication to Charlotte Gerson.
7. Letter to Charlotte Gerson from patient.
8. Note 6, supra.
9. Ibid.
10. Ibid.
11. Note 4 (Gerson), supra.
12. *Gerson Healing Newsletter* 13 (2) (March/April 1998): 5-6.

Chapter 28

Recipes

L ast, but far from least, this chapter contains a treasury of recipes that add variety, pleasure and super-healthy nutrition to Gerson-style meals. However, there are some important points to remember:

- Study and learn by heart the basic rules for food preparation described in Chapter 12, "Preparing Food and Juices—The Basic Rules," p. 153.
- If you are a Gerson patient, newly embarked on the full intensive therapy, you need to limit your food intake to the basic recipes contained in that chapter for the first three months and eat no dairy produce for the first six to 10 weeks.
- After three months, you may introduce some variety by using different salads, dressings and vegetable courses.
- The "Special Soup or Hippocrates Soup" (see p. 313) and the baked potato are essential parts of the healing diet and must not be omitted.

If you are not ill but wish to improve your health and well-being by switching to the Gerson lifestyle, you may of course enjoy the recipes freely. Please use the slow, low heat, waterless or minimum-water cooking method, described in Chapter 12, in order to preserve precious nutrients.

SPECIAL NOTES

Bread

You will find no recipes for bread or other flour-based baked goods in this chapter. The only acceptable bread—unsalted, organic 100% rye bread—is available at good health food stores, so there is no point in baking bread at home. Patients are allowed two small slices of bread a day, but only after eating the complete Gerson meals consisting of salad, soup and potato with vegetables and fruit. Bread must not take the place of any of these items.

Yogurt

Yogurt, when permitted, must be certified organic and fat free (or extremely low fat). A few recipes refer to "thick yogurt." To make this, hang some regular yogurt, placed in several layers of cheesecloth, over the sink or in a cheesecloth-lined strainer over a bowl, and allow it to drain overnight

Sweeteners

The only permitted sweeteners are:
- Organic raw brown sugar, which is available in various shades ranging from light beige to dark brown
- Organic clear honey
- Organic maple syrup
- Unsulphured molasses
- Sucanat (also known as Rapadura)

In the recipes, these ingredients are referred to as "honey" and "sugar."

Washing Fruits and Vegetables

All fruits and vegetables must be washed before use. If the water supply in your area is not fluoridated, purified or distilled water (produced by reverse osmosis) may be used, both for washing produce and for cooking. If the water supply contains fluoride, only distilled water is permissible for cooking and as a final rinse for fruits and vegetables. (For distillers, see Chapter 9, "The Gerson Household," p. 133; for fluoride, see Chapter 5, "Breakdown of the Body's Defenses," p. 29.)

Baking

When baking, the oven should always be preheated.

Cooking Time/Serving Size

When a specific cooking time or a number of people served is omitted, it is because it depends on the size of the ingredient. For example, if a large potato is used, it takes much more time to bake or cook than a small one. Also, one or two large potatoes serve more people than the same number of small ones.

Special Soup or Hippocrates Soup

"Special Soup" or "Hippocrates Soup" are interchangeable terms for the same staple item of the Gerson diet. In some recipes, it is referred to as "soup stock." For a detailed description, see Chapter 12, "Preparing Food and Juices—The Basic Rules," p. 153.

Bon appetit!

RECIPES

Dips

Carrot and Dill Dip

Preparation time: 15 minutes
Cooking time: 30 minutes
Serves 4-8

1 lb. carrots, scrubbed, unpeeled
4 tbsp. thick yogurt
2 tbsp. dill weed (or 2 tsp. dried dill), finely chopped
1 tsp. flaxseed oil
juice of 1 small lemon

Simmer carrots until just tender. Drain and leave until cooled. Put through the food mill. Mix in thick yogurt, dill, flaxseed oil and lemon juice. Mix well. Chill in the refrigerator. Serve as part of a large salad or as a dip with carrot, zucchini and bell pepper sticks. Also delicious on bread.

Orange (or Red) Pepper Dip

Preparation time: 15 minutes
Serves 6

2 orange (or red) bell peppers
10 oz. yogurt
1/2 tsp. organic tomato purée

Seed and dice one of the peppers very finely and mix with the yogurt and tomato purée. Slice the remaining pepper lengthwise in half and remove the seeds. Place the yogurt mixture into each pepper half. Place on a serving dish with thin strips of carrot, zucchini and celery.

Appetizers

Celery Root Rémoulade Appetizer

Preparation Time: 10 minutes
Serves 2-4

celery root, grated
radicchio lettuce
2 or 3 varieties of loose leaf lettuce (butter or red leaf lettuce)
green onions (or chives), chopped
parsley (or tarragon)

Dressing:
vinegar
water
honey
yogurt

Combine the dressing ingredients. Grate the celery root and add the dressing. Place lettuce leaves on a plate and top with celery root. Sprinkle with chopped green onions (or chives) and parsley (or tarragon).

Eggplant Appetizer

Preparation time: 15 minutes
Cooking time: 50 minutes
Serves 2

1 eggplant
1 small onion, chopped
1/2 tbsp. organic tomato purée
parsley (or cilantro), chopped
lemon wedge
yogurt

Prick the skin of the eggplant all over. Place directly onto the oven rack (or use a small baking dish) and bake at 375° F (190° C) for about 40 minutes near the top of the oven, turning once after 20 minutes. Remove from oven and cool. When cool, peel away the stalk and skin, and chop the flesh until you have a rough purée. Heat a little water in a small pan and sauté the chopped onion over low heat for about 10 minutes or until soft. Stir in the tomato purée and the eggplant purée. Cook for another 2 minutes over high heat to remove excess moisture. Remove from heat and cool completely. Chop some parsley (or cilantro) and mix in with the purée. Lay on a bed of lettuce. Garnish with a wedge of lemon and a little yogurt.

Grapefruit Appetizer

Preparation time: 15 minutes
Serves 1 or 2

1 pink grapefruit
celery, chopped
1 red bell pepper, seeded
radicchio (or red leaf lettuce leaves)
grated horseradish (or chopped mint leaves)

Cut the grapefruit in half. Juice one-half and cut out the segments of the other half. Chop some celery and seeded red pepper. Arrange a layer of radicchio (or red leaf lettuce leaves) on a plate. Mix grapefruit segments, celery and red pepper together and put on top of lettuce. Make a dressing with grapefruit juice flavored with a little grated horseradish (or chopped mint leaves).

Variation: Put grapefruit segments on top of endive and watercress. Make a dressing with yogurt and a little grapefruit juice. Mix well and serve immediately.

How to segment a grapefruit: Cut a horizontal slice off the top and bottom. Sit the grapefruit flat and, using a sharp knife, remove the peel and outer white membrane by cutting downwards in sections. Using a container to catch any juice, cut between the membranes and the flesh of each segment to the core, taking care to point the knife blade away from you. Work around the grapefruit, easing out each segment as you go.

Jerusalem Artichoke Paté

Preparation time: 20 minutes
Cooking time: 40 minutes
Serves 2

1 lb. Jerusalem artichokes
1 tbsp. yogurt
1-2 tsp. lemon juice
parsley, chopped
flaxseed oil

Scrub the artichokes. Put in dish in oven to roast at 400° F (204° C) for 25 minutes. (It's a good idea to cook them with your baked potato.) Allow to cool and remove skin. Mash or purée (with electric blender or food mill) until it has a creamy consistency. Add the yogurt, lemon juice, chopped parsley and flaxseed oil, and beat together. Serve as an appetizer or a snack with toasted slices of bread and a smattering of various lettuce leaves and cherry tomatoes to decorate.

Melon and Mango Appetizer

Preparation time: 15 minutes
Serves 2-4

slices of honeydew and/or cantaloupe melon
slices of mango

Dressing:
1/2 tbsp. honey
1 tbsp. flaxseed oil
2 tbsp. lime (or lemon) juice
mint leaves

Cut the melon in half and remove the rind. Slice the melon and arrange in a fan shape on a shallow plate. Slice the mango lengthwise and peel, including the flesh left around the pit. Cut the mango flesh into slices and arrange between the melon slices on the plate. Pour the dressing over the melon.

Papaya and Lime Appetizer

Preparation time: 15 minutes
Serves 2

2 papayas
2 tbsp. honey
juice of 1 lime
1 lime for decoration, sliced

Peel the papaya and remove the seeds. Cut into slices (or cubes). Mix the honey with the lime juice and pour over papaya slices. Toss gently and refrigerate. Serve chilled, decorated with thin slices of lime.

Stuffed Zucchini Appetizer

Preparation time: 10 minutes
Cooking time: 5 minutes
Serves 2-4

8 medium zucchinis
1 large onion, chopped
1 green bell pepper, chopped
3 tomatoes, chopped
1 tsp. parsley, chopped
1 clove garlic, crushed
red leaf lettuce
4-6 tbsp. dressing

Dressing:
6 tbsp. apple cider vinegar (or lemon juice)

4 tbsp. water
herbs
flaxseed oil

Cook the zucchini whole (about 5 minutes on a very low heat) until half-cooked. Cut off both ends and cut each in half lengthwise. Scoop out the seeds and chop them. Sprinkle some dressing into the zucchini hollows and add a little chopped onion. Leave to marinate while preparing the stuffing. Take the remaining onion and chop the pepper and tomatoes, add the chopped parsley and crushed garlic, and mix with the chopped zucchini middles. Toss in the rest of the dressing and fill the hollows with the mixture. Arrange on a layer of red leaf lettuce to serve.

Yogurt and Apricot Sorbet Appetizer

Freezing time: 2-3 hours
Preparation time: 15 minutes
Cooking time: 40 minutes
Serves 2-4

8 oz. dried apricots
20 fl. oz. water
10 oz. yogurt
2 tbsp. honey

Place the apricots and a little water in a saucepan and bring to a boil. Cover and simmer for 30-40 minutes, or until soft. Add the rest of the water to bring the liquid content to 15 oz. Leave to cool. Place the apricots and liquid in a blender and blend until smooth. Add the yogurt and honey but do not blend these. Transfer the contents to a freeze-proof container and freeze until solid. Use an ice-cream scooper to serve one or two scoops into a bowl. Serve immediately.

Dressings

Baba Ghanoush (Eggplant and Lemon Dressing)

Preparation time: 10 minutes
Cooking time: 1 hour
Serves 3 or 4

1 large eggplant
1 or 2 cloves garlic
2 tbsp. lemon juice
1 tbsp. parsley, chopped

Bake the eggplant for 1 hour at 350-400° F (177-204° C). When cooled enough to peel, drain off excess juice, squeezing gently. Mash and blend with garlic until fairly smooth and add lemon juice and parsley. Mix well. Serve with lemon wedges. Good with crudités (raw veggies) and as a relish as well as a sauce.
    Variation: Mix with yogurt.

Basic Salad Dressing

Preparation time: 7 minutes
Serves 2

2 tbsp. lemon juice (or apple cider vinegar)
2 tbsp. water
pinch of sugar (optional)

Mix together and put into a container with any of the following:
tarragon, pushed in stalk first
shallots (or green onions), finely chopped
2 cloves garlic, peeled and crushed
fresh bay leaf
lemon grass (for a lemon flavor)

Dressing for Vegetables

Preparation time: 5 minutes
Serves 2

2 tbsp. lemon juice (or apple cider vinegar)
2 tbsp. water
pinch of sugar (optional)
yogurt

Mix lemon juice (or apple cider vinegar), water and sugar (if used). Mix in yogurt and beat well.

Flaxseed Oil and Lemon Juice Dressing

Preparation time: 5 minutes
Serves 2

1 tbsp. flaxseed oil
1/2 tbsp. lemon juice
(Use a ratio of 2/3 oil to 1/3 lemon juice)
garlic
fresh herbs
a little orange juice

Combine all the ingredients in a pitcher and stir vigorously. Pour over the salad and serve immediately.

Garlic and Green Onion Dressing

Preparation time: 5 minutes
Serves 1

1 tbsp. flaxseed oil
1/2 tbsp. lemon juice (or apple cider vinegar)
1 clove garlic, crushed
1 green onion, chopped
fresh parsley

chives
dill
fennel
a little mint

Mix flaxseed oil with lemon juice (or apple cider vinegar). Crush the garlic and add. Chop the green onion, parsley and chives and add, together with the dill, fennel and mint. Either pour over the salad and serve immediately, or put into a pitcher and allow guests to serve themselves.

Variation: If you have no fresh herbs, use a generous pinch of suitable dried herbs.

Basic Dressing

Preparation time: 5 minutes
Serves 6

2-1/3 cup apple cider vinegar
1 tsp. sugar
2/3 cup water

Mix ingredients together.

Variation: Add some or all of the following herbs (optional), letting them infuse: tarragon (pushed in stalk first); shallots or spring onions, finely chopped; 2 cloves of garlic, peeled and crushed with the back of a knife; and 1 fresh bay leaf.

Orange Vinaigrette

Preparation time: 6 minutes
Serves 1

1 clove garlic, chopped
2 tbsp. fresh parsley, chopped
2 tbsp. apple cider vinegar
1 tsp. sugar

4 tbsp. orange juice
1 tbsp. flaxseed oil

Chop the garlic and parsley, and add to vinegar, sugar, orange juice and flaxseed oil.

Yogurt, Garlic and Honey Dressing

Preparation time: 6 minutes
Serves 2

6 oz. yogurt
1 clove garlic, crushed
1 tsp. honey
watercress

Mix the ingredients, toss lightly and serve immediately. Garnish with watercress.

Yogurt, Herb and Vinegar Dressing

Preparation time: 4 minutes

apple cider vinegar
a little water
honey
yogurt
parsley
tarragon

Mix all together.

Yogurt, Onion and Apple Cider Vinegar Dressing

Preparation time: 4 minutes

yogurt
apple cider vinegar

chopped onion

Mix all together and serve with a green salad.

Salads

Apple and Carrot Salad

Preparation time: 15 minutes
Serves 2

1 small crisp red apple, grated
1 large carrot, grated
1 green onion, chopped
1 radish, sliced
apple juice
mint

Grate the apple and carrot into a dish and add a chopped green onion and a sliced radish. Pour over a little apple juice and sprinkle with mint. Serve on a bed of mixed colored salad leaves, such as radicchio, watercress or parsley.

Beet and Watercress Salad

Preparation time: 5 minutes

cooked beet, chopped
flaxseed oil
watercress

Chop cooked beet and toss in a little flaxseed oil. Serve with watercress.

Beet Salad Yolande

Preparation time: 20 minutes

cooked beets, diced

carrots, diced
celery, diced
apples, diced
parsley

Dressing:
yogurt
lemon juice
flaxseed oil

Dice the beets, carrots, celery and apples and put into a bowl. Make the dressing and mix in with the vegetables. Sprinkle with parsley.

Beet Thermidor

Preparation time: 6 minutes

cooked beets

Dressing:
yogurt
lemon juice
grated horseradish

Dice cooked beets, put into a bowl and add the dressing.

Carrot Salad

Preparation time: 15 minutes
Serves 2-4

8 oz. carrots, grated
1 medium crisp eating apple, quartered, cored and grated
5 oz. yogurt
juice of 1 large orange

Grate the carrots into a bowl. Cut the apple into quarters, remove core, then grate into the bowl and mix with the carrot. Mix the yogurt with the orange juice and stir into the salad.

Variation: Presoaked raisins (soak overnight in cold water, or pour boiling water over them and leave for a couple of hours until plump) or sultanas can also be added.

Carrot and Orange Salad with Fresh Dates

Preparation time: 15 minutes
Serves 2

1 large carrot, cut into strips
1 orange, segmented
a few fresh dates, chopped
toasted oats

Dressing:
lemon (or lime) juice
flaxseed oil

Cut the carrot into thin strips. Segment the orange and mix with the carrot. Chop the dates and add. Add dressing and garnish with toasted oats.

Carrot and Raisin Salad

*Preparation time: 10 minutes**
** Does not include presoaking*
Serves 2

3 large carrots, grated
2 oz. raisins, presoaked
lettuce
2 tsp. parsley, chopped

Dressing:
1 clove garlic, crushed
flaxseed oil
apple cider vinegar

1/2 tsp. honey
2 tsp. lemon juice

Mix grated raw carrots with presoaked raisins (soak the raisins over-night in cold water, or pour boiling water over them and leave for a couple of hours until plump). Add dressing and serve on lettuce garnished with chopped parsley.

Carrot, Apple and Onion Salad

Preparation time: 15 minutes
Serves 2

12 oz. carrots, shredded
8 oz. apples, shredded
1 medium onion, shredded
10 oz. yogurt
juice of 1/2 lemon

Shred the carrots, apples and onion. Combine with the yogurt and lemon juice. Serve with a mixed green salad.

Celery Salad

Preparation time: 10 minutes
Serves 2

2 stalks celery, chopped
2 crisp small eating apples, chopped
1/4 medium red bell pepper, finely sliced
mixed lettuce leaves

Dressing:
apple cider vinegar
flaxseed oil
1 tsp. honey

Chop the celery and apples and put into a large bowl. Add the finely sliced red bell pepper. Add the dressing. Line a salad plate with mixed lettuce leaves and pile the dressed salad on top.

Cherry Tomato and Watercress Relish

Preparation time: 15 minutes
Serves 2-4

cherry tomatoes (red and yellow), halved
watercress
fresh chives (or green onions), finely chopped
herbs, finely chopped

Halve the tomatoes and place in a bowl. Steam the watercress over boiling water for 10 seconds, rinse well in cold water and shake dry. Trim off any woody stems and cut or tear the remaining stems and leaves into small pieces. Add to the tomatoes. Add the finely chopped chives (or green onions) and herbs and toss together.

Chicory and Orange Salad

Preparation time: 15 minutes
Serves 2-4

1 lb. chicory heads, trimmed and sliced
2 large oranges, peeled and sliced
1 medium green onion, trimmed and chopped
juice of 1/2 lemon
1 tbsp. flaxseed oil
1 tsp. honey

Trim the chicory and slice into rounds about 1/2-inch thick. Push the rounds apart to make rings. Peel the oranges, removing the white pith, and slice into rounds. Place the chicory in a bowl and lay the oranges in overlapping rings around the top, leaving the center empty. Trim and chop the green onion and sprinkle into the center. Mix the lemon juice, flaxseed oil and honey, and pour over the salad. Leave for a few minutes before serving to allow the flavors to "marry."

Coleslaw

Preparation time: 15 minutes*
* Does not include presoaking

raisins, presoaked
white cabbage, thinly shredded
apple, thinly shredded
celery, finely chopped
onion, finely chopped

Dressing:
yogurt
lemon juice
flaxseed oil

Presoak the raisins (soak the raisins overnight in cold water, or pour boiling water over them and leave for a couple of hours until plump). Thinly shred the white cabbage and apple. Finely chop the celery and onion. Put all into a bowl and add the raisins. Toss in dressing.

Colorful Mixed Salad

Preparation time: 15 minutes
Serves 2

zucchini, grated
beet, grated
apple, grated
lettuce
tomato
orange

Dressing:
equal amounts of apple cider vinegar and water
honey (or maple syrup)
garlic
lemon (or orange) juice

Grate the zucchini, beet and apple. Add the dressing and mix them together or pile them in separate mounds onto a bed of lettuce. Decorate with slices of tomatoes and orange.

Colorful Three-Cabbage Salad

Preparation time: 15 minutes*
* Does not include presoaking
Serves 2

2 oz. raisins, presoaked
4 oz. each white, red and green cabbage, finely shredded
4 oz. carrot, grated
1 medium onion, finely sliced
1 small crisp eating apple, chopped
watercress

Dressing:
5 fl. oz. yogurt
a little flaxseed oil
1 clove garlic, crushed

Presoak the raisins (soak the raisins overnight in cold water, or pour boiling water over them and leave for a couple of hours until plump). Finely shred the cabbage. Grate the carrot. Put both in a bowl with the raisins, finely sliced onion and chopped apple. Mix well. Mix the dressing ingredients and pour over the salad just before serving, tossing lightly. Garnish with watercress.

Colorful Winter Salad

Preparation time: 20 minutes
Serves 4-6

3 tart eating apples, cored and roughly chopped
lemon juice
1/4 medium-sized red cabbage, cored and finely shredded
1 medium carrot, peeled and grated
1/2 medium red bell pepper, seeded and chopped
2 sticks celery, sliced
1/2 red onion, peeled and chopped
watercress

Core and roughly chop the apples and mix with lemon juice in a small bowl. Core and finely shred the red cabbage. Peel and grate the carrot. (This is the only time to peel the carrots. If they are grated with their skins on, they tend to turn brown.) Seed and chop the red pepper. Slice the celery. Peel and chop the red onion. Put all the above ingredients into a large bowl. Garnish with watercress.

Variations: Serve with cottage cheese (unsalted and uncreamed or fat-free) and your favorite dressing.

Crunchy Salad

Preparation time: 15 minutes*
* Does not include presoaking
Serves 4-6

2 oz. dried apricots, presoaked and chopped
3 oz. raisins, presoaked
1 lb. white cabbage, finely shredded
1 green bell pepper, chopped
1 red bell pepper (or 1/2 bunch of radishes), chopped
watercress

Dressing:
6 fl. oz. yogurt
1 clove garlic, crushed
1 tsp. honey

Presoak the apricots and raisins (soak overnight in cold water, or pour boiling water over them and leave for a couple of hours until plump). Finely shred the white cabbage. Chop the pepper (or radishes). Place into a bowl together with the raisins and chopped apricots. Mix well. Mix the dressing and pour over the salad. Toss lightly, garnish with watercress and serve.

Endive and Orange Salad

Preparation time: 15 minutes
Serves 2

1 small head of endive, chopped
1 red bell pepper, seeded and cut into strips
2 oranges, peeled
2 tomatoes
1 tbsp. herbs, chopped

Dressing:
juice of 2 oranges
5 oz. yogurt
1 tsp. honey

Chop the endive and put into a bowl. Seed the pepper, cut into thin strips and add to the bowl. Peel the oranges, removing the pith with the peel. Cut out segments between the membranes and add to the bowl with the tomatoes. Make the dressing and toss into the salad. Sprinkle with chopped herbs.

Fruity Winter Salad

Preparation time: 15 minutes*

* Does not include presoaking
Serves 2-4

2 oz. raisins, presoaked
2 oz. dried figs, presoaked
2 oz. dried apricots, presoaked
1/2 white cabbage, finely shredded
2 carrots, coarsely grated
2 red eating apples, coarsely grated
8 tbsp. yogurt
1 lemon
parsley, chopped

Presoak the raisins, figs and apricots (soak overnight in cold water, or pour boiling water over them and leave for a couple of hours until plump). Finely shred the cabbage. Coarsely grate the carrots and apples. (Sprinkle the apples with lemon juice to stop them from turning brown.) Put the above ingredients into a bowl. Combine the yogurt, lemon juice and chopped parsley in a jug and spoon over the salad. Toss together until well mixed.

Gerson Coleslaw

Preparation time: 15 minutes
Serves 2-4

onion, sliced or chopped
white cabbage, grated or sliced
carrot, grated

Dressing:
2 tbsp. lemon juice
2 tbsp. water
sugar (optional)
yogurt
cottage cheese (unsalted and uncreamed or fat-free)

Slice or chop the onion. Grate or slice the white cabbage. Grate the carrot. Mix all together. For the dressing, mix lemon juice with water (and sugar, if used). Mix yogurt with cottage cheese and beat well to get rid of any lumps. Then add the lemon juice and water mixture. Mix well and pour over salad.

Grated Zucchini Salad with Lime

Preparation time: 15 minutes
Serves 2-4

1 lb. zucchini, finely grated
juice of 1 lime (or lemon)
1 red bell pepper, grated
1 clove garlic, crushed
lettuce

Grate the zucchini finely. Mix with the lime (or lemon) juice and grated pepper. Add crushed garlic. Allow the flavors to blend a little before serving on a bed of lettuce.

Hungarian Tomato Salad

Preparation time: 15 minutes

whole tomatoes, skinned
lettuce
chopped chives

Dressing:
yogurt
lemon juice
flaxseed oil
grated horseradish

Skin the tomatoes by dipping them in boiling water for a minute. Make the dressing. Place the whole, skinned tomatoes on the lettuce leaves and cover with the dressing. Garnish with chopped chives.

Jumbo Salad

Preparation time: 20 minutes*
*Does not include presoaking
Serves 4-6

variety of shredded lettuce leaves
and salad greens, bite-sized and shredded

Any, or all, of the following:
tomato, chopped
green (or red) bell pepper, chopped
green onions, finely sliced
carrot, finely grated
beet, finely grated
radish, finely sliced
fennel, finely sliced
grape halves
lemon juice
flaxseed oil
dried dill weed
raisins, presoaked

Gradually build up the salad, beginning with the bite-sized shredded lettuce leaves and salad greens. Add any, or all, of the ingredients listed above. Presoak the raisins (soak overnight in cold water, or pour boiling water over them and leave for a couple of hours until plump). Sprinkle on top of the salad. Grate the carrot and/or beet and place to one side of the salad. (If you put it all on top, it tends to "smother" the salad.) Pour on the lemon juice and flaxseed oil. Sprinkle with dill. Serve with rice, oven-cooked and sliced potatoes or boiled small new potatoes.

Minted Apple and Celery Salad

Preparation time: 15 minutes*
* Does not include presoaking
Serves 2

1 red eating apple, cut, cored and chopped
apple cider vinegar
1 stalk of celery, chopped
raisins, presoaked
mint leaves
lettuce

Cut and core the apple and chop into bite-sized chunks. Mix with a little apple cider vinegar (diluted with water, if desired). Chop the celery and add, with the presoaked raisins (soak overnight in cold water, or pour boiling water over them and leave for a couple of hours until plump), to the apple and apple cider vinegar. Take the mint leaves and tear into small pieces. Add to the dish and serve on a bed of lettuce. (Leave for a little while before serving so the flavors have time to mix.)

Variation: Yogurt can be mixed with the apple cider vinegar for the dressing.

Orange, Chicory and Watercress Salad

Preparation time: 15 minutes
Serves 2-4

1 orange, peeled and segmented
2 heads of chicory
1 bunch of watercress

Dressing:
1 tbsp. flaxseed oil
1/2 tbsp. apple cider vinegar (or lemon juice)
1 clove garlic, crushed
1 green onion

parsley
chives
dill
fennel
mint

Peel the orange and split into segments. Separate the chicory leaves and arrange like the spokes of a wheel around a large dish. Put the watercress and orange in the middle. Combine all the dressing ingredients in a jug and stir vigorously. (If you have no fresh herbs, use a generous pinch of dried herbs.) Pour over the salad and serve immediately.

Radish, Apple and Celery Salad

Preparation time: 15 minutes*
* Does not include presoaking
Serves 2

radishes, chopped
green apples, chopped
celery, chopped
raisins, presoaked
lettuce

Dressing:
1 tbsp. apple cider vinegar
1 tbsp. water
1 tsp. sugar (or honey)
1 or 2 cloves garlic, crushed
dill, chopped
yogurt

Chop the radishes, green apples and celery into small chunks. Presoak the raisins (soak overnight in cold water, or pour boiling water over them and leave for a couple of hours until plump) and add. For the dressing, mix together the apple cider vinegar, water, sugar (or honey), garlic and dill. Add enough yogurt to make a creamy dressing. Pour over the salad and serve on a bed of lettuce (include radicchio or red leaf, if available).

Variations: Use other herbs instead of dill, omit the yogurt or add some flaxseed oil.

Raw Turnip, Watercress and Orange Salad

Preparation time: 15 minutes
Serves 2

1 turnip, peeled and cut
1 orange, segmented
watercress

Dressing:
orange juice
flaxseed oil

Peel and cut the turnip into matchstick-size pieces. Segment the orange and add to the turnip pieces. Add the watercress and toss in the dressing.

Rice Salad

Preparation time: 15 minutes
Serves 2

green bell pepper, chopped
red bell pepper, chopped
tomato, chopped
1 cup cooked brown rice

Dressing:
1 tbsp. flaxseed oil
1 tbsp. apple cider vinegar
1 clove garlic
sugar

Chop the peppers and tomato. Prepare the dressing, mix well and add the chopped peppers and tomato. Spoon onto the rice. Serve with a mixed green salad.

Romaine Lettuce with Yogurt Dressing

Preparation time: 10 minutes

Romaine lettuce
chives, chopped

Dressing:
yogurt
sugar
lemon juice
crushed garlic

Coarsely shred the lettuce. Pour on the dressing and sprinkle with chopped chives.

Salad Kebabs

Preparation time: 15 minutes

tomatoes, thinly sliced
zucchinis, thinly sliced
whole radishes, thinly sliced
lettuce hearts, thinly sliced
carrots, thinly sliced

Dressing:
lemon juice
yogurt
flaxseed oil
herbs (mint, dill or parsley)

Thread on wooden skewers thinly sliced pieces of tomato, zucchini, whole radishes, lettuce hearts and raw carrot. Dip into the salad dressing before serving.

Salad Lorette

Preparation time: 10 minutes

cooked beets, thinly sliced
celery stalks, thinly sliced
lettuce

Dressing:
flaxseed oil
lemon juice

Thinly slice the beets and celery and mix with lettuce. Add dressing.

Spanish Salad

Preparation time: 15 minutes
Serves 2

onions, thinly sliced
1 clove garlic
red bell peppers, seeded and sliced
tomatoes, sliced
parsley, chopped

Dressing:
flaxseed oil
1 tbsp. apple cider vinegar
1 tbsp. water
sugar (optional)

Thinly slice the onions and put into a bowl which has been rubbed over with a cut clove of garlic. Seed and slice the red peppers and lay them on top of the onion. Add a layer of sliced tomatoes. Crush the garlic and sprinkle on top. Pour over the dressing and sprinkle with chopped parsley.

Tomato and Zucchini Salad

Preparation time: 15 minutes
Serves 2

tomato, chopped
zucchini, chopped
green onion, sliced
beet
lettuce

Dressing:
flaxseed oil
yogurt
lemon juice

Chop the tomato and zucchini into chunks. Slice the green onion and add. Finely grate the raw beet (or chop cooked beet into chunks) and mix into the salad. Lay on a bed of lettuce. Pour over dressing.

Tomato Salad

Preparation time: 15 minutes
Serves 2

tomatoes, sliced
onion, sliced
1 tbsp. apple cider vinegar
1 tbsp. water
sugar (optional)
parsley, chopped
chives

Slice the tomatoes and spread out over a flat dish. Slice the onion and arrange the onion rings over the tomatoes. Mix the apple cider vinegar with water (and optional sugar, if used). Pour over the tomatoes and sprinkle with chopped parsley and chives.

Watercress, Endive and Grapefruit Salad

Preparation time: 10 minutes
Serves 2

watercress
endive (frisée or escarole, or both)
grapefruit
yogurt

Tear the watercress into smaller pieces, remove woody stems and put in a bowl with the endive leaves. Cut the grapefruit in half. Juice one half and segment the other half. Add the segments to salad leaves. Mix the grapefruit juice with yogurt and pour over the salad. Toss well and serve.

Zucchini Ribbon Salad

Preparation time: 10 minutes
Serves 2-4

3 large zucchinis, cut lengthwise
1 lb. tomatoes, quartered
6 green onions, thinly sliced

Dressing:
2 tbsp. apple cider vinegar
pinch of sugar
2 tbsp. flaxseed oil
freshly chopped cilantro

Using a vegetable peeler or cheese slicer, cut the zucchinis lengthwise into thin ribbons, running along the side so the ribbons include the green skin. Place into a bowl. Quarter the tomatoes and thinly slice the onions. Add to the bowl. Toss in the dressing just before serving.

Soups

Apple and Fennel Soup
Preparation time: 15 minutes
Cooking time: 30-45 minutes
Serves 4

1 lb. potatoes, peeled and diced
2 bulbs fennel, trimmed and chopped
2 leeks, sliced
2 Granny Smith apples, cored and chopped
1 tsp. sugar (optional)
1 tart eating apple

Peel and dice the potatoes, trim and chop the fennel, slice the leeks, and core and chop the apples into small pieces. Put these ingredients into a pot and cover with water. Bring to a boil, turn down the heat and simmer gently until potatoes and fennel are cooked. Purée (with electric blender or food mill). Add the chopped apples to the puréed soup. Serve immediately.
    Variation: Omit apples, if you wish.

Argyll Soup

Preparation time: 10 minutes
Cooking time: 45 minutes
Serves 4

2 large carrots, sliced
2 large onions, roughly chopped
4 sticks celery, sliced

1 lb. potatoes, peeled and chopped
2 cloves garlic, crushed
parsley

Slice the carrots, roughly chop the onions and slice the celery. Peel and chop the potatoes and crush the garlic. Put all into a large pot and cover with water. Bring to a boil. Turn down the heat and simmer gently for 45 minutes. Purée (with electric blender or food mill). Garnish with parsley and serve immediately.

Autumn Flame Soup

Preparation time: 15 minutes
Cooking time: 25 minutes
Serves 4

1 large onion, chopped
3 large cloves garlic, crushed
1 lb. squash (or pumpkin), peeled and chopped
4 large red bell peppers, seeded and chopped
1 lb. tomatoes, chopped
thyme
fresh green herbs (2 small bay leaves, fresh parsley or cilantro)

Chop the onion and crush the garlic. Peel and chop the squash into small chunks. Seed the peppers and chop into small pieces. Put it all into a pot and cover with water. Bring to a boil. Turn down the heat and add the chopped tomatoes, thyme and bay leaves. Simmer gently for no longer than 20 minutes. Purée (with electric blender or food mill). Serve immediately, garnished with fresh green herbs of your choice.

Beet Soup

Preparation time: 15 minutes
Cooking time: 1 hour
Serves 4

2 medium beets, unpeeled and chopped
1 large onion, peeled and chopped
1 medium carrot, unpeeled and chopped
2 large tomatoes, unpeeled and chopped
red cabbage leaves, chopped
1 bay leaf
water
1 tbsp. apple cider vinegar
juice of 1/2 lemon
herbs
yogurt
parsley

Chop beets, onion, carrot and tomatoes, without peeling (except for the onion!). Put into a large pot. Add chopped cabbage leaves and bay leaf. Cover with water and add apple cider vinegar, lemon juice and herbs. Bring to a boil, then lower heat and simmer gently for about 1 hour. When cooked, purée (with electric blender or food mill), serve with a swirl of yogurt and garnish with parsley.

Cabbage Soup

Preparation time: 10 minutes
Cooking time: 40 minutes
Serves 2-4

1 small green (or white) cabbage, coarsely chopped
2 leeks, coarsely chopped
2 potatoes, peeled and coarsely chopped
2 onions, coarsely chopped
2 sticks celery, coarsely chopped
1 clove garlic
yogurt
parsley, chopped

Coarsely chop the vegetables. Put in a pot and cover with water. Bring to a boil, lower the heat and simmer until vegetables are tender. Purée (with electric blender or food mill). Serve hot with swirls of yogurt and garnished with chopped parsley.

Broccoli Floret Soup

Preparation time: 15 minutes
Cooking time: 35 minutes
Serves 2-4

1 medium onion, peeled and chopped
6 oz. potato, peeled and chopped
1 lb. broccoli, trimmed and cut
bay leaf
yogurt

Peel and chop the onion and potato. Trim the broccoli and cut into florets. Keep a few florets to one side and put the rest into a pot with the chopped onion, potato and bay leaf, and cover with water. Bring to a boil and simmer for 20 minutes. Add the other florets and simmer for an additional 10 minutes. Remove the bay leaf. Take the whole florets from the soup and put onto a hot plate. Put the rest of the soup through the food mill. Add the other cooked florets. Reheat the soup gently. Serve immediately with a swirl of yogurt.

Carrot and Orange Soup

Preparation time: 10 minutes
Cooking time: 40 minutes
Serves 2-4

1 lb. carrots, chopped
8 oz. onions, chopped
8 oz. potatoes, peeled and chopped
juice of 1 orange

a pinch of thyme

Chop the vegetables and put them into a pot with the orange juice and the thyme, and cover with water. Bring to a boil, then simmer until vegetables are tender. Purée (with electric blender or food mill).

Cauliflower Soup

Preparation time: 10 minutes
Cooking time: 40 minutes
Serves 2-4

1 large cauliflower
1 onion, chopped
1 celery stick, sliced
10 oz. yogurt
parsley, chopped

Trim the cauliflower and break into small florets. Chop the onion and slice the celery. Put into a pot and cover with water. Bring to a boil, lower the heat and simmer gently for 30 minutes. Purée (with electric blender or food mill). Stir in the yogurt. Reheat gently before serving. Garnish with chopped parsley.

Celery, Carrot and Apple Soup

Preparation time: 10 minutes
Cooking time: 45 minutes
Serves 2-4

1 lb. celery, sliced
1 lb. carrots, diced
8 oz. sweet apples (Pink Lady or Gala), chopped
dill (or lemon grass)
celery leaves, chopped

Slice the celery, dice the carrots and chop the apples. Put into a large pot and cover with water. Bring to a boil, lower the heat, add the dill (or lemon grass) and simmer for 40 minutes. Purée (with electric blender or food mill). Serve immediately and garnish with chopped celery leaves.

Celery Root and Swiss Chard Soup

Preparation time: 10 minutes
Cooking time: 40 minutes
Serves 2-4

1 small celery root, scrubbed and chopped
1 medium leek, scrubbed and chopped
2 oz. Swiss chard, torn
apple cider vinegar (or lemon juice)
parsley

Scrub and chop the celery root and leek and tear the Swiss chard into small pieces. Put into a pot with apple cider vinegar (or lemon juice) and cover with water. Bring to a boil, turn down the heat and simmer until the vegetables are soft. Purée (with electric blender or food mill). Serve hot or cold and garnish with parsley.

Corn Chowder

Preparation time: 10 minutes
Cooking time: 45 minutes
Serves 2-4

3 sticks celery, diced
1 large potato, peeled and diced
1 large onion, diced
1 large green bell pepper, seeded and diced
1 bay leaf (or a pinch of ground bay leaf)
4 ears of corn, sliced off the cob
parsley, chopped

Dice the celery, potato and onion. Remove the seeds from the pepper and dice the flesh. Put into a pot with the bay leaf and cover with water. Simmer gently until the vegetables are almost cooked. Slice the corn from the cobs and add to the soup. Cook slowly until all the vegetables are soft but not broken (about 5 minutes.). Sprinkle with the chopped parsley and serve.

Potato, Cabbage and Dill Soup

Preparation time: 10 minutes
Cooking time: 40 minutes
Serves 2-4

1 medium potato, peeled and chopped
1 medium onion, chopped
1 medium leek, chopped
white cabbage, chopped
4 tsp. dried dill
chives, chopped

Chop the potato, onion and leek. Put into a pot with the chopped cabbage and cover with water. Bring to a boil, turn down the heat and add half the dill. Simmer gently until the potatoes are cooked. Purée (with electric blender or food mill). Add the rest of the dill and reheat gently. Garnish with chopped chives and serve immediately.

Potato Soup

Preparation time: 20 minutes
Cooking time: 1-1/2 to 2 hours
Serves 4-6

1 large onion, diced
1/2 small celery knob, diced
2 stalks celery, diced
2 large potatoes, diced

1 leek, diced
parsley
2 quarts water

Dice all vegetables. Place vegetables, parsley, and water in covered saucepan and bring to boil. Lower heat and cover. Simmer 1-1/2 to 2 hours. Mash through food mill.

Sweet and Sour Cabbage Soup

Preparation time: 10 minutes
Cooking time: 15 minutes
Serves 2-4

2 medium onions, sliced
1 medium white (or green) cabbage, cut into thin strips
2 cloves garlic, crushed
2 medium tomatoes, chopped
1 tbsp. sugar
juice of 1 large lemon
3 oz. raisins
1 qt. water

Slice the onion and sweat gently in a little water for a few minutes until it starts to soften. Cut the cabbage into thin strips and add to onion, mixing well. Add crushed garlic. Chop the tomatoes and add together with the sugar, lemon juice, raisins and water. Bring to a boil and simmer until the cabbage is al dente (about 10 minutes). Serve this hearty soup as a main dish with bread followed by fruit for dessert.

Tangy Tomato Soup

Preparation time: 10 minutes
Cooking time: 25 minutes
Serves 2-4

1 lb. tomatoes, chopped

1 carrot, chopped
1 stick celery, chopped
1 onion, chopped
1 red bell pepper, seeded and chopped
little orange juice
yogurt

Chop tomatoes, carrot, celery and onion. Seed pepper and chop. Put all into a large pot and cover with water. Bring to a boil, turn down the heat and simmer until vegetables are tender. Purée (with electric blender or food mill). Add the orange juice. Reheat gently. Add a swirl of yogurt before serving.

Tomato Soup with Potato and Onion

Preparation time: 20 minutes
Cooking time: 40 minutes
Serves 3-4

2 large tomatoes, diced
1 medium onion, diced
2 medium potatoes, diced
1 tsp. wine vinegar
small bay leaf

Dice all vegetables. Place all ingredients in covered saucepan, cover with water and cook over low flame for 35-40 minutes. Mash through food mill and serve hot.

Vegetables and Potatoes

Baked Pepper and Tomato Salad

Preparation time: 15 minutes
Cooking time: 30 minutes
Serves 2-4

3 red bell peppers
6 large tomatoes
1 medium red onion, finely sliced
3 cloves garlic, thinly sliced
juice of 1 large lemon
3 tbsp. fresh, chopped mint
flaxseed oil

Cook the peppers and tomatoes whole until somewhat cooked but still firm. Skin the peppers and tomatoes, chop roughly and place in a serving dish. Finely slice the onion and very thinly slice the garlic. Add to the mixture in the dish. Add the lemon and mint. Mix well. Sprinkle with a little flaxseed oil.

Baked Potato and Parsnip Rosti*

* Rosti means "broiled" or "roasted" (i.e., top-browned)
Preparation time: 15 minutes
Cooking time: 1-1/4 hour
Serves 2

8 oz. parsnips, cored, peeled and coarsely grated
8 oz. potatoes, peeled and coarsely grated
1 onion, finely chopped
2 tbsp. fresh chives, finely chopped
herbs
3-1/2 oz. yogurt
a little grated horseradish (optional)

Core the parsnips. Peel and coarsely grate the potatoes and parsnips into a large bowl. Add finely chopped onion, chives, herbs and yogurt. Mix until well combined. Put the vegetable mixture into a shallow dish and cover. Bake for 1 hour at 375° F (190° C). Remove the lid and bake a little longer until it begins to brown and the top is crispy. Serve with a crisp salad or a vegetable (or both).

Baked Potatoes

Preparation time: 5 minutes

Baked potatoes should be thoroughly washed, not scraped or peeled. Bake in a low oven at 300° F (149° C) for 2 or 2-1/2 hours or, alternatively, bake for 50 minutes to 1 hour at 350° F (177° C).

Baked Potato with Beet and Onion

Preparation time: 15 minutes
Cooking time: 1 hour

1 baking potato
1 large onion, peeled
beet, diced and cooked
yogurt
dill
1 tsp. flaxseed oil (optional)

Scrub the potato and place whole into a casserole dish with a large, peeled onion. Add a little water and bake until both are cooked. Chop the cooked onion and put into a saucepan with the diced, cooked beet. Heat through. Split open the potato and fill with the onion and beet mixture. Mix together the yogurt, dill and flaxseed oil (if using the flaxseed oil, wait until the potato is no longer steaming) and drizzle over the top. Serve with a green salad.

Baked Potato with Onion

Preparation time: 15 minutes
Cooking time: 1-1/2 hours

1 baking potato
1 onion, sliced
cooked beet, diced
yogurt
dill

Bake the potato in its skin. Slice the onion and cook gently until beginning to soften. Dice the beet, add to the onion and warm through. When the potato is cooked, split it open and spoon in the beet mixture. Top with dollops of yogurt and sprinkle with dill. Serve with a green salad.

Baked Tomatoes

Preparation time: 10 minutes
Cooking time: 20 minutes
Serves 2

1 lb. tomatoes, sliced
1 clove garlic, crushed
1 medium onion, chopped
bread crumbs (or a handful of rolled oats)
dill
flaxseed oil

Slice the tomatoes and put into a baking dish. Crush the garlic, chop the onion and sprinkle over the tomatoes. Cover with bread crumbs (or rolled oats) and bake for about 20 minutes at 325° F (170° C). Just before serving, sprinkle with dill and flaxseed oil.

Beets

Bake at 300-350° F (149-177° C) or boil beets in their jackets.

Beets, Cooked and Creamed

Preparation time: 15 minutes
Cooking time: 60-75 minutes

3 beets, cooked and chopped
6 tbsp. yogurt
1 tbsp. fresh chives, snipped
2 tbsp. onion, finely chopped

parsley, finely chopped

Put cooked, chopped beets into a saucepan with the yogurt, chives and onion and heat gently. Put into serving dish and sprinkle with chopped parsley.

Beets with Horseradish

Preparation time: 10 minutes
Cooking time: 1 to 1-1/2 hours
Serves 2-4

6 beets
yogurt
2 tsp. horseradish
chives

Cook the beets until tender. Remove the skin and cut into quarters. Combine the yogurt and horseradish and pour over the beets. Garnish with chopped chives and serve immediately.

Bessarabian Nightmare

Preparation time: 15 minutes
Cooking time: 40 minutes
Serves 2

tomatoes, skinned and sliced
onions, sliced
red (or green) bell pepper, seeded and sliced
garlic, crushed
herbs
flaxseed oil

Skin the tomatoes. Slice the tomatoes, onions and peppers. Arrange in layers in an oven-proof dish. Sprinkle with crushed garlic and herbs.

Cook slowly, then chill and serve cold, adding a little flaxseed oil before serving. A strange name for a delicious dish!

Braised Cabbage

Preparation time: 15 minutes
Cooking time: 1 hour
Serves 2

1 lb. green cabbage
4 oz. carrots, diced
4 oz. onion, diced
2 sticks celery, diced
dill seeds

Cut the cabbage into quarters. Remove the stalk, the core and any discolored leaves. Cook the cabbage in a little water in a saucepan for 10 minutes. Dice the carrots, onion and celery and put into a large oven-proof dish with very little water. Place the cabbage on top. Scatter with dill seeds. Bake covered for about 1 hour at 350° F (180° C) or until the vegetables are tender.

Braised Fennel with Orange and Tomato Sauce

Preparation time: 10 minutes
Cooking time: 30 minutes
Serves 2

1 medium head of fennel
1-1/2 lb. tomatoes
1 tbsp. tomato purée
juice of 1/2 orange
herbs
green fennel tops

Cut the fennel into quarters and remove the core. Cook gently for 8-10 minutes. Meanwhile, cook the tomatoes to a pulp and add the tomato purée, orange juice and herbs. Add the fennel and cook covered for 12-15 minutes. Garnish with fennel tops and serve.

Broccoli

Bake in a covered casserole in low oven at 300° F (149° C) with onions or a small amount of soup stock for 1-2 hours. Serve with tomato sauce.

Broccoli and Herbs

Preparation time: 20 minutes
Cooking time: 25 minutes
Serves 2

2 bunches of broccoli
4-6 cloves garlic
1/2 onion sliced
1/4 tsp. dill
1/4 cup soup stock

Peel the broccoli stems. Put garlic and onion in one pot and cook until onion becomes translucent. Add cut broccoli crowns and stems, dill and soup stock. Cook on low heat until broccoli is tender.

Broccoli, Green Beans and Pears

Preparation time: 5 minutes
Cooking time: 20 minutes
Serves 2

broccoli
green beans
2 pears, peeled and chopped

Dressing:
lemon juice (or apple cider vinegar)
flaxseed oil

Gently cook the broccoli and green beans. Allow to cool. Peel and chop the pears and put in a dish together with the broccoli and beans. Gently toss in dressing and serve with a baked potato and a mixed green salad.

Butternut Squash (Mashed)

Preparation time: 10 minutes
Cooking time: 35 minutes
Serves 2

butternut squash, peeled and cored
1 small onion
yogurt

Peel and core chunks of butternut squash. Place in pan with one small onion. You will probably not need cooking water as the butternut squash is a "wet" vegetable. Simmer until done. Mash with enough yogurt to make smooth.

Cabbage and Tomato Hot Pot

Preparation time: 15 minutes
Cooking time: 35 minutes
Serves 2

1 small cabbage
1 onion, chopped
1 dessert apple, chopped
4 large tomatoes, skinned and chopped
yogurt
bread crumbs
parsley, chopped

Cook the cabbage gently in water until cooked but still crisp. Chop the onion, apple and skinned tomatoes and cook gently until they form a thick purée. Shred the cabbage and add to the purée. Turn into a casserole dish. Mix the yogurt with the bread crumbs and sprinkle over the top. Top-brown under the broiler to heat a little. Sprinkle with chopped parsley and serve immediately.

Carrot and Leek Bake

Preparation time: 10 minutes
Cooking time: 1-2 hours
Serves 2-4

1 lb. carrots, diced or sliced
4 or 5 small leeks, sliced
2 medium oranges
handful of raisins

Dice or slice the carrots and slice the leeks. Put into a baking dish with the raisins. Add the juice of two oranges. Bake in a medium oven at 325° F (170° C) for 1 to 2 hours until done. If you wish, you can thicken the orange juice with corn starch to make a sauce. (Organic corn starch may be used occasionally.) Serve with a baked potato.

Carrot and Tomato Casserole

Preparation time: 15 minutes
Cooking time: 1 hour
Serves 2

8 oz. tomatoes, sliced or chopped
1/2 tbsp. chopped fresh sage (or 1/2 tsp. dried sage)
2 medium onions, sliced
1 lb. carrots, sliced

Slice or chop the tomatoes and put a layer into the bottom of a casserole dish. Add some sage. Slice the onions and place a layer on top of the tomatoes. Add another sprinkling of sage. Slice the carrot and place on top, finishing with a layer of tomato mixed with the last of the sage. Place the casserole in the oven and bake for 1 hour at 350° F (180° C) until the carrots are tender. Serve with a mixed green salad and a baked potato.

Carrots and Honey

Preparation time: 10 minutes
Cooking time: 45 minutes
Serves 1-2

carrots, sliced
soup stock
1/2 tsp. honey

Cut off the ends of the carrots and slice. Do not peel or scrape. Stew in a small amount of soup stock for 45 minutes or until tender. During the last 5 to 10 minutes of stewing, add honey for slight flavoring.

Cauliflower

Preparation time: 10 minutes
Cooking time: 45 minutes

cauliflower
2-3 tomatoes, sliced and chunked

Break cauliflower into sections. Add tomatoes, sliced and cut into chunks. Stew together for approximately 45 minutes (or until tender) on low heat.

Cauliflower and Carrot Sauce

Preparation time: 20 minutes
Cooking time: 50 minutes

1 small cauliflower
3 carrots
flaxseed oil

Separate the cauliflower florets, place them in a baking dish with a little water and cook at 250° F (121° C) for 40 minutes or until soft. When ready, drain off the water. At the same time, simmer the carrots on low heat with enough water until they are soft. Blend carrots in blender with the flaxseed oil. Pour sauce over the cooked cauliflower and place in warm oven at 250-300° F (121-149° C) (turned off) for 5-10 minutes before serving.

Chard Rolls, Stuffed

Preparation time: 40 minutes
Cooking time: 30 minutes

1/2 onion, sliced
6 medium potatoes
4 carrots
3 large cloves garlic, minced
1 bunch of chard

Cook onions and potatoes in one pot. In another pot, cook carrots and garlic. When done, purée (with electric blender or food mill) each potful separately, then mix together. Put chard leaves in very hot water, being sure not to overcook. Spread each leaf and remove tough center stem. Place purée in center of each leaf and roll tightly. Display on tray and serve with tomato sauce made with tomatoes, onion, garlic and small potato, which have been cooked and puréed.

Cooked Sweet Potato and Beet Salad

Preparation time: 10 minutes
Cooking time: 30 minutes
Serves 2

1 large (or 2 small) sweet potatoes
a few cooked small beets, sliced
arugula (or lettuce) leaves

Dressing:
yogurt
lemon juice
flaxseed oil
dill weed, dried or fresh

Cook the sweet potatoes gently in their skins until done. Allow to cool. Cut into slices and place the sweet potato and beet slices overlapping on a plate of arugula (or lettuce) leaves. Drizzle on the dressing and serve immediately.

Corn

Preparation time: 5 minutes

Corn may be baked in the husk wrapped in foil. Bake in low oven at 300° F (149° C) for 1 hour. If husked, place in boiling water for approximately 7 minutes.

Corn on the Cob Packets

Preparation time: 5 minutes
Cooking time: 1 hour
Serves 1-2

1 or 2 corn cobs
flaxseed oil
parsley, chopped

Leave the corn in its outer leaves and wrap in baking foil. Bake at 350° F (180° C) for about 1 hour. When cooked, peel back the leaves and allow to cool. Pour on some flaxseed oil to which some chopped parsley has been added. Serve as an appetizer or a side dish.

Corn with Mixed Vegetables

Preparation time: 15 minutes

Cooking time: 1 hour
Serves 2

2 ears of corn
3 stalks of celery, sliced
2 carrots, sliced
2 zucchinis squash, sliced

Husk the corn and cut the kernels off. Slice the other vegetables into small pieces. Put the corn in a baking dish and add the vegetables. Bake at 200° F (93° C) for 1 hour.

Corn with Orange Juice

Preparation time: 10 minutes

2 ears of corn
1 glass of orange juice

Husk the corn, cut off the kernels and put it in a baking dish with a lid. Bake at 250° F (121° C) until soft (approximately 25-30 minutes). Pour the corn juice off and add the orange juice. Let set 5 to 10 minutes before serving.

Creamed Corn

Preparation time: 20 minutes
Cooking time: 1-1/2 hours
Serves 2-3

3 ears of corn
1 green bell pepper, sliced

Husk corn and cut off the kernels. Put kernels from 2 ears in a blender and blend. Add the kernels from the third ear to the blended corn. Place in a baking dish and put the sliced green pepper on top and bake in the oven at 200-250° F (93-121° C) for 1-1/2 hours.

Creamed Green Beans

Preparation time: 5 minutes
Cooking time: 15 minutes
Serves 2

10 oz. whole green beans
yogurt
2 oz. onion, finely chopped

Cook the beans gently. Just before the beans are ready, gently heat the yogurt with the chopped onion. Put the beans into a warm serving dish and pour on the yogurt dressing.

Creamy Cabbage

Preparation time: 10 minutes
Cooking time: 30 minutes
Serves 2

white cabbage, shredded
1 small onion, chopped
2 tbsp. thick yogurt
1 tsp. dried dill tops, chopped (or crushed dill seeds)

Shred the cabbage and chop the onion. Add a little water to cook. When cooked and tender, add the thick yogurt mixed with the dill tops (or seeds).

Eggplant, Baked

Preparation time: 15 minutes
Cooking time: 2 hours
Serves 2

soup stock
1 onion, chopped
1 eggplant, sliced

2 tomatoes, sliced and skinned

Put some soup stock in bottom of large covered baking dish. Add onion, eggplant and tomatoes in layers. Cover and bake in a low oven at 300° F (149° C) for 2 hours.

Eggplant Fan

Preparation time: 15 minutes
Cooking time: 45 minutes
Serves 2

1 large onion, sliced
1 large eggplant, sliced
1 large firm, ripe tomato, sliced
thyme and marjoram
1 small clove garlic, chopped

Slice the onion into rings and cook gently in a thick-bottomed saucepan while preparing the other ingredients. Cut eggplant into 4 or 5 length-wise slices, stopping 3/4 inch from either end. Slice the tomato into twice as many slices as there are cuts in the eggplant. Arrange the egg-plant on top of the onions in a fan shape, and fill the cuts with the tomato slices. Sprinkle with herbs and chopped garlic. Cover and cook gently, on top of the stove, or bake gently in a low oven at 300° F (149° C) until the eggplant is soft.

Eggplant Salad

Preparation time: 15 minutes
Cooking time: 1 hour
Serves 2
1 eggplant
1 small onion, chopped
parsley, chopped
2 tomatoes, sliced

1-1/2 tbsp. vinegar
a little flaxseed oil

Bake the eggplant for about 1 hour at 350° F (180° C). Chop the onion and parsley and slice the tomatoes. Combine with the cooked eggplant. Add the vinegar and flaxseed oil.

Eggplant, Stewed

Preparation time: 20 minutes
Cooking time: 30 minutes
Serves 2

1 eggplant, cut into cubes
2 onions, chopped
3 tomatoes, peeled and chopped

Combine all ingredients in a stew pot. Stew approximately 30 minutes (until tender). Do not add water.

Fancy Garlic Potatoes

Preparation time: 5 minutes
Cooking Time: 1-1/2 to 2 hours

potatoes, sliced
flaxseed oil
garlic, crushed

Cut the potatoes into slices, not quite through to the base. Put into a casserole dish with only enough water to cover the bottom. Cook in the top of the oven at 325° F (170° C) for 1-1/2 to 2 hours or at 350° F (180° C) for 1 hour. Mix together the flaxseed oil and crushed garlic. Put the potatoes onto a serving dish and, when slightly cooled, pour on the dressing. Serve immediately.

Fennel Treat

Preparation time: 15 minutes
Cooking time: 1-2 hours
Serves 2

1 fennel bulb
1 large tomato, cut into 1/4-inch slices
2-3 cloves garlic, peeled and sliced thinly

Cut off stalks and leaves from fennel. Slice bulb in half lengthwise to give two flat halves. Rinse under running water to remove sand and put them in a baking dish with cut side up. Cover halves with tomato slices and place garlic slices on top of tomatoes. Cover the dish and bake at 250° F (121° C) for 1 to 2 hours. Serve with a baked potato and a salad of grated carrots on a bed of pretty greens.

Festive Broccoli (or Festive Green Beans)

Preparation time: 25 minutes
Cooking time: 45 minutes
Serves 2-3

1 large head broccoli (or 3-1/2 cups sliced green beans)
1 small onion, diced
1 clove garlic, minced
1 medium sweet red (or yellow) bell pepper, cut in strips
2 tsp. lemon juice (optional)
1/4 tsp. dried (or 1 tsp. fresh) dill weed

Select dark green head of broccoli with no yellowing. Cut into spears, peeling tougher stalks at base. Place onion and garlic in pot. Cover and stew on low flame for 45 minutes or until tender. Add pepper strips for the last 20 to 25 minutes of cooking. Add lemon juice just before serving (lemon will discolor broccoli if added during cooking). Sprinkle vegetables with dill and serve.

French Bean (Green Bean) Salad

Preparation time: 5 minutes
Cooking time: 10 minutes
Serves 2

French beans (green beans)
small onion, chopped
flaxseed oil
apple cider vinegar (or lemon juice)
parsley
chives

Cook the beans gently until just tender. Drain and add the chopped onion. Put into a serving dish and toss in the flaxseed oil and apple cider vinegar (or lemon juice). Add herbs and serve.

Fruited Red Cabbage

Preparation time: 10 minutes*
* Does not include soaking
Cooking time: 15 minutes
Serves 2

4 oz. raisins, presoaked
4 oz. dried apricots, presoaked
1 small red cabbage, shredded
2 dessert apples, cored and chopped
apple cider vinegar
a little sugar

Presoak the raisins and apricots (soak overnight in cold water, or pour boiling water over them and leave for a couple of hours until plump). Shred the red cabbage and sweat in a little water until slightly softened. Add raisins, chopped apricots and cored, chopped dessert apples. Toss in apple cider vinegar, to which a little water and sugar have been added. Pile into a bowl and serve with a baked potato.

Gerson Gardener's Pie*

*A bit like Shepherd's Pie but with vegetables instead of meat
Preparation time: 30 minutes
Cooking time: 2-1/2 hours
Serves 2-3

Topping:
1 lb. potatoes, peeled and cut into chunks
12 oz. celery root (or sweet potato or onion), peeled and cut into chunks

Peel the potato and other vegetable and cut into small chunks. Add water but only about 1/2 to 2/3 the height of the vegetables. Bring to a boil and reduce to a simmer. Cook slowly until all the water is gone and the vegetables are soft, and mash. If there is a little water left in the pan, beat it into the mash mixture.

Filling:
1 small onion (or a few shallots)
2 cloves garlic, crushed
8 oz. carrots, sliced, or chipped or diced (but not diced too thickly)
8 oz. zucchini, cut into half slices, not too thin
8 oz. leeks, trimmed and sliced
2 tomatoes, skinned and chopped
1-2 tbsp. chopped parsley
herbs to taste
2 oz. bread crumbs

Prepare vegetables and put them into a saucepan in the order listed above. Cook the vegetables very gently. You may need to use a simmer plate. This could take 1 to 1-1/2 hours. Prepare topping and bread crumbs. When vegetables are cooked, stir in bread crumbs and pour the mixture into a pie plate. Top with mashed potatoes. Drag a fork over the top to decorate and bake for about 45 to 60 minutes at 350° F (180° C). Place pie plate on baking sheet in case of leakage. Serve with green vegetables and salad.

Variations: Change the contents of the pie by adding green beans, peas and/or corn when in season. Jerusalem artichokes would be also good. You could leave the leeks out of the pie and purée them (with electric blender or food mill) to add to the topping instead of the sweet potato, onion or celery root.

Gerson Roast Potatoes

Preparation time: 5 minutes
Cooking time: 1 hour

1 baking potato

Cut a baking potato in half (or, if very large, into quarters). Score across the cut surface with a knife. Put into a casserole dish with a little water to just cover the bottom. Put lid on and bake in a hot oven at 400-425° F (204-218° C) for 1 hour. Before serving, remove the lid and leave to slightly brown.

Glazed Beets

Preparation time: 25 minutes
Cooking time: 1-1/2 hours
Serves 6 to 8

9 large beets

Scrub beets and boil in 2 to 3 inches of water until tender for 1 to 1-1/2 hours. Add more water if needed. Peel in cold water. Slice or cut into bite-sized pieces.

Glaze:
2/3 cup fresh orange juice
1 tsp. cornstarch
1-1/2 tsp. apple cider vinegar
1 tsp. honey (or sugar)

Combine ingredients for glaze. Cook over low flame until thick. Add beets and mix well.

Variation: Use 1/2 cup apple juice and 3 tsp. lemon juice in place of orange Juice.

Glazed Carrots and Turnips with Garlic

Preparation time: 10 minutes
Cooking time: 30 minutes
Serves 2

8 oz. carrots
8 oz. turnips

Dressing:
1 tbsp. lemon juice
1 clove garlic, crushed
flaxseed oil

Gently cook the carrots and turnips. Cut into thin slices and put into a serving dish. Pour on the dressing and garnish with cilantro or dill.

Glazed Carrots with Herbs and Lemon

Preparation time: 5 minutes
Cooking time: 30 minutes
Serves 2

1 lb. carrots
1 tsp. sugar
a little water
1 tbsp. lemon juice
mint
rosemary
parsley
flaxseed oil

Gently cook the carrots whole. When beginning to soften, remove from pan and cut into 2-inch sticks. Return to the saucepan with the sugar and a little water. Heat until the sugar is dissolved, the water has been absorbed and the carrots are cooked. Add the lemon juice and herbs and heat for an additional 2 minutes. Place on a warm serving dish, add flax-seed oil and serve immediately.

Glazed Carrots with Orange

Preparation time: 5 minutes
Cooking time: 30 minutes
Serves 2

1 lb. carrots
1 tbsp. sugar
juice of 1/2 orange
flaxseed oil

Gently cook the carrots whole. When beginning to soften, remove from the pan and cut into 2-inch sticks. Return to the saucepan with the sugar and orange juice. Heat until the sugar has been dissolved and the orange juice absorbed. Turn onto platter, add flaxseed oil and serve.

Green Beans in Honey and Tomato Sauce

Preparation time: 15 minutes
Cooking time: 20 minutes
Serves 2

1 lb. fine green beans

Sauce:
1 medium onion, chopped
2 cloves garlic, crushed
1 lb. tomatoes, roughly chopped
1 tsp. honey
herbs

Cut ends off the beans, cook until just tender and drain. To make the sauce, chop the onion and crush the garlic. Cook them both in a little water until just tender. When the onion is soft, add the roughly chopped tomatoes and bring to a boil. Simmer gently until sauce becomes fairly thick. Stir in the honey and herbs. Add the beans and allow to cool. Serve at room temperature.

Green Chard Rolls

Preparation time: 45 minutes
Cooking time: 2 hours

4 leaves of green chard
2 carrots
1/4 head broccoli
1/4 head cauliflower
2 small zucchini squash
1 ear of corn (cut kernels off)
1/2 cup uncooked rice

Sauce:
1-1/2 tomatoes
2 cloves garlic

Put the chard leaves in hot water long enough to wilt them so they will bend. Cut the broccoli, cauliflower, squash and corn into small pieces and put them in a pan with a little water to simmer. When cooked, drain the water off. Make a sauce in the blender with the tomatoes and garlic, and pour this sauce on top of the vegetables and uncooked rice. Place some of the vegetables/rice mixture in the center of each leaf and roll them up. Put these in a baking dish with a lid and bake in the oven at 250° F (121° C) for 1 to 1-1/2 hours.

Green Peppers

Preparation time: 10 minutes

Cooking time: 30 minutes
Serves 2-3

2-4 green peppers, sliced
2-4 onions, sliced

Stew in tightly covered pot for approximately 30 minutes. Do not add water.

Grilled Eggplant

Preparation time: 10 minutes
Cooking time: 20 minutes
Serves 1

1 eggplant
garlic
parsley, chopped
lemon (or lime) juice

Slice the eggplant lengthwise. Heat a griddle pan (preferably a "ridged" pan). When the pan is hot, turn down the heat, place the slices of eggplant on the griddle and allow them to cook slowly. Turn over the slices and repeat. Before serving, squeeze garlic over the slices, sprinkle with chopped parsley and drizzle lemon (or lime) juice over them. This is a good main course for lunch served with new potatoes.

Variations: You can do the same thing with large slices of peppers, halves of onions or zucchini halved lengthwise.

Leek and Potato Bake

Preparation time: 15 minutes
Cooking time: 40 minutes
Serves 2

1 lb. potatoes
1 small leek, very thinly sliced

fine oats (put some regular rolled oats in the blender)

Parboil the potatoes in their skins until they are hot through and just beginning to soften. Very thinly slice the leek (using the white section only). Peel the potatoes and coarsely grate them. Mix in the leek. Put into a shallow baking dish (sprinkled at the bottom with fine oats to prevent sticking). Cook on the top shelf of the oven at 350° F (180° C) until beginning to show signs of browning. (Don't leave it for too long or it will dry out.) Serve with either cooked vegetables or a green salad and tomatoes.

Leeks (or Zucchini) à la Grecque

Preparation time: 10 minutes
Cooking time: 30 minutes
Serves 2

1 lb. leeks (or zucchini), sliced
3 tomatoes, chopped (optional)
juice of 1 lemon
bay leaf
thyme
coriander seeds

Slice the leeks (or zucchini) into 1-inch pieces. Cook gently with chopped tomatoes (if used), lemon juice, bay leaf, thyme and coriander seeds. Serve hot or cold.

Lima Beans and Zucchini

Preparation time: 15 minutes
Cooking time: 20 minutes
Serves 1-2

1 large onion
1 clove garlic
1/2 cup soup stock

1 cup fresh lima beans
3 cups zucchini
4 medium tomatoes
1/2 tsp. cornstarch
4 sprigs fresh parsley
dash of thyme (or sage, or a pinch of dried parsley)

Mix together all ingredients except herbs. Simmer about 15 minutes (until tender). Thicken with cornstarch mixed with a little water. Just before serving, add herbs.

Lyonnaise Potatoes

Preparation time: 5 minutes
Cooking Time: 1 to 1-1/2 hours
Serves 2

1 lb. potatoes, thickly sliced
1 large onion, thickly sliced
2 tbsp. of water
flaxseed oil
garlic, crushed

Thickly slice the potatoes and onion. Arrange the potato slices in an oven-proof dish with a slice of onion between each potato slice. Pour on the water. Bake in oven at 300-350° F (149-177° C) until well done and beginning to brown. Allow to cool slightly, then pour on the flaxseed oil and crushed garlic. Serve immediately.

Mashed Carrot and Potato Bake

Preparation time: 10 minutes
Cooking time: 1 hour

carrots
potatoes

Cook the carrots and potatoes gently until just tender. Mash them and pile into an oven-proof dish. Decorate with diagonal fork marks and put into a hot oven at 400-425° F (204-218° C) to brown.

Mashed Potatoes

Preparation time: 20 minutes
Cooking time: 40 minutes

potatoes, peeled and cubed
1 small onion
yogurt

Peel and cube potatoes. Place in pan with one small onion and enough water to bring to a boil. Simmer until done (when there is no water left). Mash with enough yogurt to make smooth.

Mashed Potatoes and Chard

Preparation time: 15 minutes
Cooking time: 25 minutes
Serves 4

1 bunch green (or red) chard
4-5 tbsp. water (or soup stock)
3 large (or 4 medium) potatoes, peeled and cubed
6-8 oz. yogurt

Shred the chard and put in pan. Add water (or soup stock) and start to boil. When boiling, turn down to simmer. Meanwhile, peel potatoes, cube and place on top of the chard. Let simmer until potatoes are soft and done. Remove any remaining water and add yogurt. Mash all together. Add a little more yogurt if the mixture is too dry.

Variation: The same recipe can be used with kale. When using kale, strip out central stems before shredding into pan.

Mashed Potatoes Gerson Style

Preparation time: 10 minutes
Cooking time: 35 minutes

potatoes, peeled and cut into pieces
onion, peeled and chopped small

Place potatoes and onions in a pot. Add just enough water to reach the vegetables half-way up. Cover, bring to boil and simmer until potatoes are cooked. (Most of the cooking water will probably be gone.) Mash potatoes and onions using some (or all) of the cooking water. If not enough moisture, add some soup stock.

Variations: Add any herb of your choice, finely chopped. Parsley is very good; mint and dill will also work.

Oven-Browned Potatoes

Preparation time: 5-10 minutes

potatoes

Cut the potatoes like French fries (or in small cubes, or in thin slices) and brown on an oven tray in the oven. They will brown at a surprisingly low heat (300° F or 149° C), if left in long enough. Depending on the variety of potato, they can brown very quickly and puff up at high heat (425° F or 218° C). They can also be browned under the broiler, but watch them to avoid burning. This is meant to be an occasional treat!

Parsley Potatoes

potatoes
parsley, chopped
flaxseed oil

Boil several potatoes in their skins until done. Remove the peel and roll in some chopped parsley after slightly brushing with flaxseed oil.

Parsnips and Sweet Potatoes

Preparation time: 10 minutes
Cooking time: 40 minutes
Serves 2-4

1 lb. parsnips, cut into wedges
1 lb. sweet potatoes, cut into wedges
sprig of fresh rosemary

Cut the parsnips and sweet potatoes into wedges, leaving the skins intact. Put into a baking dish with a little water to cover the bottom. Add a sprig of rosemary. Cover and bake in a medium oven at 325° F (170° C) until just cooked. Serve with a baked potato.

Patate alla Francesca

Preparation time: 5 minutes
Cooking time: 40 minutes

new potatoes
tomatoes, chopped or sliced
fresh rosemary sprigs
garlic

Bake new potatoes in a covered dish at 300-350° F (149-177° C) with chopped or sliced tomatoes, fresh rosemary sprigs and plenty of garlic. Serve with lemon wedges and a green salad.

Piemontese Peppers

Preparation time: 10 minutes
Cooking time: 1 hour
Serves 2

2 tomatoes, skinned
2 red bell peppers, halved and seeded
2 cloves garlic, sliced

herbs

Skin the tomatoes. Halve the peppers and remove the seeds (but not the stalks). Place the peppers skin-side down in a baking dish. Place slices of garlic inside each pepper half and top each with half a skinned tomato. Bake covered at 350° F (180° C) until tender and sweet (about 1 hour). Serve hot or cold, sprinkled with herbs.

Potato and Celery Root Lyonnaise

Preparation time: 15 minutes
Cooking Time: 1-1/2 to 2 hours
Serves 2

1 small to medium onion, thinly sliced
1 small to medium celery root, scrubbed (and, if necessary, peeled) and thinly sliced
1 medium potato, scrubbed and thinly sliced

Slice all the ingredients thinly. Arrange in layers (onion, celery root and, potato) in a small soufflé dish. Add a very little amount of water. Bake for 1-1/2 to 2 hours at 325° F (170° C). The top layer will get crisp while the lower layers should be soft. Serve with green vegetable of your choice and a salad.

Potato Cakes

Preparation time: 25 minutes
Cooking time: 30 minutes
Serves 2-4

1 lb. potatoes
1 large carrot, thinly cut
1 green bell pepper, chopped
1 stick of celery, chopped
fine oats (put some regular rolled oats in the blender)

Parboil the potatoes in their skins until they are hot through and just beginning to soften. Put through the food mill. (This will also get rid of the skin.) Cut carrot into thin matchsticks. Chop the green pepper and celery. Add these to the potato purée and form into small cakes. Coat with oats and bake in the oven at 325° F (170° C) on a baking sheet sprinkled with fine oats to prevent sticking.

Potatoes and Carrots, Westphalian Style

Preparation time: 10 minutes
Cooking time: 35 minutes
Serves 4

6-8 small (or 4-5 large carrots) carrots, sliced
3 medium (or 2 large) potatoes, peeled and sliced
1 large onion, chopped
3-4 tbsp. of soup stock

Slice carrots into pan. Peel and slice potatoes and chop onion. Add all together in pan with soup stock. Let simmer until done, adding a bit more soup stock, if necessary. When done, no liquid should remain in pan.

Potatoes Anna

Preparation time: 20 minutes
Cooking time: 1 to 1-1/2 hours
Serves 2

onion, cooked
1 lb. potatoes, very thinly sliced
garlic, crushed
yogurt
parsley, finely chopped

Sweat the onions in a covered saucepan over very low heat for approximately 1 hour. Using a 10-inch flan (or quiche) tin with at least 1-inch sides, place a layer of sweated onions on the bottom of the tin. Sprinkle with a little water to stop the onions from sticking. Very thinly slice the potatoes and layer them in the dish on top of the onions. Sprinkle with crushed garlic and some of the yogurt. Add an additional two layers, again sprinkling with garlic and yogurt. Press down each layer and make sure the potatoes overlap each other very slightly so there are no spaces. Cover the dish (e.g., by using a base from a larger, loose-bottomed cake tin). Bake at 350° F (180° C) for about 1 to 1 to 1-1/2 hours or until the potatoes feel soft when pierced with a knife. Check the potatoes while cooking; if they look too dry, add a little more yogurt. To serve, turn the potato cake out of its dish and sprinkle with finely chopped parsley.

Potato Puffs

Preparation time: 5 minutes
Cooking time: 45-50 minutes

baking potato

Take a baking potato and cut it into 1/2-inch slices. Place the slices on the oven rack and, without any addition, bake at high heat (425° F (218° C)) to puff. Turn over and lower heat to 325° F (163° C) with oven door cracked open. Bake for another 20 minutes. The slices puff up and become crisp and tasty, almost like fried potatoes. Done when shiny brown on both sides. This is marginal food, so eat it occasionally.

Potato Salad

Preparation time: 10 minutes
Cooking time: 20 minutes
Serves 2

1 lb. small new potatoes
large sprig of mint
1 tbsp. fresh parsley

Dressing:
4 oz. yogurt
a little flaxseed oil
2 cloves garlic, crushed

Scrub the potatoes and put in a saucepan with a little water. Gently simmer until cooked but still firm. While the potatoes are still hot, slice them and put into a warm dish. Pour over the dressing. Finish by sprinkling fresh chopped mint and parsley.

Quick Bake Potatoes

Preparation time: 5 minutes
Cooking time: 1 hour

potatoes
flaxseed oil

Cut potatoes in half lengthwise and score cut surfaces with diagonal lines crossing each other (like lattice work). They will cook in about half the time (about 50 minutes) in the oven at 300-350° F (149-177° C); when cool enough, the surfaces can be coated with flaxseed oil.

Quick Tomatoes and Zucchini

Preparation time: 5 minutes
Cooking time: 30 minutes
Serves 2

2 medium tomatoes, sliced
1 clove garlic, crushed
1/4 to 1/2 tsp. sugar (optional)
1 medium zucchini, sliced

Slice the tomatoes and place in the bottom of a saucepan, along with the crushed garlic and sugar (if using). Slice the zucchini and place on top.

Set on a gentle heat. When the tomatoes begin to cook, stir, cover and cook for about 20 minutes.

Ratatouille

Preparation time: 15 minutes
Cooking time: 1 hour
Serves 2-4

8 oz. onions, sliced
8 oz. green/red/yellow bell peppers, seeded and thinly sliced
8 oz. eggplant
4 tomatoes, chopped
1 clove garlic, finely chopped
2 tsp. apple cider vinegar
marjoram

Slice the onions and place in a baking dish. Seed and thinly slice the peppers. Add to the dish. Cut the eggplants in quarters lengthwise and then into 1/4-inch slices and add. Chop the tomatoes and finely chop the garlic clove. Add to the dish together with the apple cider vinegar and a sprinkling of marjoram. Cook very gently in the oven at 325° F (170° C) until well done. Can also be cooked on top of the stove.

Red Cabbage

Preparation time: 25 minutes
Cooking time: 1 hour
Serves 2-3

1/2 red cabbage, shredded
3 tsp. vinegar
3 large onions, chopped
2 bay leaves
a little soup stock
3 apples, peeled and grated

1 tsp. sugar

Combine cabbage, vinegar, onions, bay leaves and soup stock in a pan. Stew over low heat for approximately 1 hour. At the 1/2-hour mark, add apples and sugar.

Red Cabbage and Apple Casserole

Preparation time: 15 minutes
Cooking time: 1-1/2 hours
Serves 2

medium red cabbage, shredded
apples (cooking or green), sliced
juice of 1 orange
apple cider vinegar
maple syrup

Shred the red cabbage and slice the apple. Place layers of red cabbage and apple in a casserole dish. Pour over the orange juice, apple cider vinegar and maple syrup. Cover with a tight-fitting lid and bake at 350° F (180° C) for about 1-1/2 hours or until tender. Stir and serve. Almost better as a reheated leftover!

Red Kuri Squash with Vegetables

Preparation time: 15 minutes
Cooking time: 30 minutes
Serves 2-4

1 red kuri squash
1 tbsp. water
1 small sweet potato, cooked
1 small zucchini, cooked
1 red (or green) bell pepper, cooked
1 tomato, peeled
onion (or garlic) powder

fresh herbs

Cut the red kuri squash in half. This is easily done with a very sharp, pointed knife. Scoop out the seeds, leaving the rest of the red flesh intact. Stand upright in an oven-proof dish to which the water has been added. Cover and bake at 300-350° F (149-177° C) until cooked (about 30 minutes; test by inserting a knife into the flesh). If there is enough room, the other vegetables could be cooked in the same dish. Otherwise, bake them in a separate dish in the same way, or cook them gently on top of the stove in a saucepan. When cooked, pile the vegetables into the squash halves. Sprinkle with onion (or garlic) powder or fresh herbs. Serve with a colorful mixed salad.

Roasted Zucchini and Pepper Salad

Preparation time: 10 minutes
Cooking time: 30 minutes
Serves 2

1 lb. small zucchini
2 red bell peppers, seeded and quartered
thick yogurt
3 tbsp. mint, roughly chopped

Dressing:
2 tbsp. lemon juice
2 cloves garlic, crushed
flaxseed oil

Cut the ends off the zucchini and cut in half lengthwise. Seed the peppers and cut into quarters. Put the zucchini and peppers skin-side up on a baking tray. Bake in oven at 325° F (170° C) for about 1/2 hour. When cooked and tender, cool slightly and cut into 1-inch lengths. Put into a serving dish, pour on the dressing and add the chopped mint. Serve with a smattering of cottage cheese (unsalted and uncreamed or fat-free).

Rolled Chard Parcels

Preparation time: 10 minutes
Cooking time: 30 minutes

chard leaves
green onions
snow peas
asparagus
broccoli
julienne of carrots
red chard stems

Set aside the chard leaves. Gently cook the green onions, snow peas, asparagus, broccoli, carrots and red chard stems in very little water and then chop them. Blanch the chard leaves. Fill with the cooked vegetable medley and form into "packets." Cook briefly in the oven at 300-350° F (149-177° C) for a few minutes until heated through. Serve hot or cold.

Root Vegetable Rosti*

* Rosti means "broiled" or "roasted" (i.e., top-browned)
Preparation time: 10 minutes
Cooking time: 1 hour
Serves 2

1 small onion, thinly sliced
8 oz. potatoes
4 oz. carrots
4 oz. swede (rutabaga)
dill

Thinly slice the onion and cook by "sweating" in a little water. Meanwhile, gently cook the potatoes, carrots and swede (rutabaga). Drain thoroughly and, when cool enough to handle, coarsely grate into a bowl. Stir in the softened onion and dill. Put the mixture into an oven-proof

387

dish. Bake for about 1/2 hour in the top of the oven at 350° F (180° C) or until cooked and slightly browning. Serve immediately.

Sauté of Sweet Potatoes

Preparation time: 15 minutes
Cooking time: 20 minutes
Serves 2-4

4 medium sweet potatoes
juice of 1 orange
a little sugar
flaxseed oil

Cook the sweet potatoes in their skins until just cooked. Allow to cool slightly, then cut into cubes. Put orange juice and sugar into a saucepan with the sweet potatoes. Heat gently but don't let the mixture boil. Put into a serving dish and allow to cool a little. Add the flaxseed oil, toss and serve immediately with fresh parsley (or chives) and a green salad.

Scalloped Potatoes (Without Yogurt)

Preparation time: 15 minutes
Cooking time: 1-2 hours

1 onion
potatoes, sliced
tomato, sliced
marjoram and/or thyme

Place a whole chopped onion in the bottom of a glass baking dish. Slice potatoes and place one layer on top of the onion. Add a layer of sliced tomato on top, then another layer of sliced or chopped onion. Sprinkle with a dash of marjoram and/or thyme and bake in a low oven at 300° F (149° C) for 1 to 2 hours or until done.

Scalloped Potatoes (With Yogurt)

Preparation time: 15 minutes
Cooking time: 1 to 1-1/2 hours
Serves 2

1 lb. potatoes
1 small onion, finely chopped
1 clove garlic, finely chopped
yogurt

Cook the potatoes gently until just cooked but firm. Slice thinly. Finely chop the onion and garlic. Arrange the slices of potato, layered with onion and garlic, in a pie dish. Pour over the yogurt and bake at 350° F (180° C) for 1 to 1-1/2 hours or until well cooked and beginning to brown on top.

Spinach

Preparation time: 10 minutes
Cooking time: 20 minutes

spinach
onions, chopped

After cutting off roots, wash spinach 3 to 4 times. Put in large, tightly covered pot that has a layer of chopped onions on the bottom of the pan. Do not add water. Stew over a low flame until spinach wilts. Pour off excess juice. Serve chopped with slice of lemon.

Spinach (or Chard) with Tomato Sauce

Preparation time: 15 minutes
Cooking time: 15 minutes

spinach (or chard)
lemon grass
sprig of rosemary

allspice (optional)

Cook the spinach (or chard) with some lemon grass and a sprig of rosemary. Add a pinch of allspice, if desired. Thinly cut the ribs of the spinach (or chard) and cook the leaves. Serve with tomato sauce.

Stuffed Eggplant

Preparation time: 20 minutes
Cooking time: 1 hour
Serves 2

1 eggplant
4 oz. tomatoes
1 medium onion
1 clove garlic, crushed
1 tbsp. fresh chopped parsley

Place the whole eggplant in a large saucepan and cover with boiling water. Let stand for 10 minutes, then plunge into cold water. Meanwhile, in another saucepan, very gently cook the tomatoes for 5 minutes. Press through sieve to get rid of the skins and set aside the pulp. Cut the cooled eggplants in half lengthwise. Scoop out the pulp, leaving a 1/2-inch thick outer shell. Chop the eggplant pulp and set aside. Place the eggplant shells in a shallow baking dish with just a little water in the bottom to prevent sticking. Bake for 30 minutes at 350° F (180° C). Sauté onion and crushed garlic in a small amount of boiling water until tender. Stir in the parsley. Add the sieved tomato pulp and chopped eggplant pulp, and cook for 20 minutes on moderate heat until it thickens. Spoon this mixture into the cooked eggplant shells. Keep warm in the oven until serving, or leave to cool and serve cold.

Stuffed Mixed Vegetables

Preparation time: 25 minutes
Cooking time: 30 minutes

Serves 2-4

1 zucchini
1 eggplant
2 small onions, chopped
garlic, crushed
marjoram
1 green (or red) bell pepper
soup stock

Cut the zucchini and eggplant in half, scoop out the pulp of the eggplant (carefully leaving a shell) and cook with the onion, crushed garlic and marjoram. Cut the peppers in half and take out the seeds. Stuff the eggplant, zucchini and peppers with the mixture and put in a shallow baking dish on a layer of onion rings. Bake at 300-350° F (149-177° C) until the pepper is done. Add a little soup stock if the dish seems to be getting dry. Serve with tomato sauce.

Stuffed Pepper

Preparation time: 10 minutes
Cooking time: 50 minutes
Serves 1

red (or green) bell pepper, seeded
leftover mixed, chopped vegetables
tomatoes, sliced

Halve the pepper and seed it. Place it open-side up in an oven-proof dish. Stuff leftover mixed, chopped vegetables into pepper halves. Place slices of tomato over the top. Cook at 350° F (180° C) for 40 to 50 minutes or until the pepper is soft. Serve with broccoli or another very green vegetable.

Variation: For a change from baked potato, serve with "Potato Puffs" (see p. 382).

Stuffed Squash

Preparation time: 30 minutes*
* Does not include presoaking
Serves 4-6

3-4 acorn squash
1/2 cup onion, diced
1/2 cup celery, diced
1/2 cup carrot, diced
1-1/4 cup cooked brown rice
1/2 cup lentils sprouted
1/4 cup raisins (or chopped prunes), presoaked and drained
3 tsp. fresh parsley, minced
1/2 tsp. rubbed sage
1/2 tsp. thyme
1 large clove garlic, crushed

Slice squash lengthwise and remove seeds. Presoak rains (or chopped prunes) (soak overnight in cold water, or pour boiling water over them and leave for a couple of hours until plump) and add. Combine remaining ingredients and fill squash halves. Cover and bake at 300-325° F (149-163° C) for 1-1/2 hours or until squash is tender. Delicious with carrot sauce in "Cauliflower and Carrot Sauce" (see p. 360).

Variation: For a delicious mild flavor, try using 6-8 whole garlic cloves. Crushing the fresh garlic releases its strong aromatic oils, whereas using it uncut imparts a mild taste.

Sweet Potato and Apple Bake

Preparation time: 15 minutes
Cooking time: 1 hour
Serves 2

8 oz. sweet potatoes
2 eating apples, sliced
a little water

a little sugar
allspice (optional)

Cook the sweet potatoes gently in their skins until just cooked. Allow to cool. Slice and put into a baking dish alternating with layers of apple. Over each layer, sprinkle some water and a little sugar (and allspice, if using). Bake at 300-350° F (149-177° C) covered for 20 minutes, then remove cover and bake for an additional 10 minutes. Serve as a main dish with a salad (if omitting the allspice) or as a dessert (if using allspice).

Tangy Sweet and Sour Casserole

Preparation time: 20 minutes
Cooking Time: 1-1/2 to 2 hours
Serves 2

1 large (or 2 small) cooking apples, peeled and sliced
a few slices of leek, sliced
1 small onion, peeled and sliced
1 small sweet potato, sliced
1 small parsnip, cored and chopped
bay leaf
1 tomato, skinned and sliced
1 large clove garlic, crushed
thyme
1 small zucchini, sliced

Peel and slice the apple, and arrange half the slices in the bottom of a casserole dish. Slice the leek and arrange on top of the apple. Peel and slice the onion and add a layer. Slice the sweet potato, core and chop the parsnip and add a further layer, intermingling with the rest of the apple slices. Put a bay leaf in the middle of the casserole. Skin the tomato and slice, adding a further layer to the casserole. Crush the garlic and sprinkle over the tomato with the thyme and add a layer of sliced zucchini. Cover and bake in the oven at 350° F (180° C) for 1-1/2 to 2 hours.

Vegetable Casserole

Preparation time: 20 minutes
Cooking time: 1 hour

onions, sliced
tomatoes, sliced
leeks, sliced
potatoes
zucchinis
peppers
carrots

Using a heavy saucepan with a tight-fitting lid, slice a layer of either onions, tomatoes or leeks (or all three) and put layer in the bottom of the pan. Take an assortment of sliced, chopped or cubed vegetables and put in layers until about 3/4 full. Add a little water if needed. Cook gently for 45 minutes or until done.

Winter Vegetable Casserole

Preparation time: 20 minutes
Cooking time: 2 hours
Serves 2

sweet potato
parsnip
swede (rutabaga)
celery root
celery stalks
fennel root
tomatoes
Brussels sprouts
bay leaves
water (or soup stock)
fresh parsley, chopped

Chop, slice or dice any or all of the above ingredients (with the exception of the Brussels sprouts and parsley). Put into a large casserole dish with the bay leaves and very little water (or soup stock) to stop the vegetables from sticking. Cover and cook slowly at 325° F (170° C) for 1-1/2 hours. Trim and halve the Brussels sprouts, add to the casserole and continue to cook for another 1/2 hour. Sprinkle with fresh, chopped parsley just before serving.

Zucchini and Potato Bake

Preparation time: 20 minutes
Cooking time: 1-1/2 hours
Serves 2

1 lb. zucchini, finely sliced
1 lb. potatoes, finely sliced
2 medium onions, finely sliced
2 cloves garlic, crushed
10 oz. yogurt
fresh parsley, chopped

Finely slice the zucchini, potatoes and onions. Place alternate layers of zucchini, potatoes and onions in a casserole dish, adding a sprinkling of crushed garlic between the layers. Cook in the oven at 300-350° F (149-177° C) for about 1-1/2 hours. Meanwhile, crush the second garlic clove and add to the yogurt. When the dish is cooked, remove from the oven and spread the yogurt mixture on top. Sprinkle chopped fresh parsley over the top and serve immediately.

Zucchini with Garlic and Parsley

Preparation time: 15 minutes
Cooking time: 35 minutes
Serves 2

1 lb. zucchini

3 tbsp. parsley, finely chopped
2 cloves garlic, crushed
juice of 1 lemon
flaxseed oil

Chop both ends off the zucchinis and cook whole. While they are cooking, finely chop the parsley and crush the garlic. Mix with the lemon juice and flaxseed oil. Put into a serving bowl. When the zucchinis are cooked, halve lengthwise (if small) or slice thickly (if large). While still hot, add to the serving bowl and toss in the mixture. Serve immediately with oven-roasted bell peppers, a baked potato and a green salad.

Zucchini with Mint

Preparation time: 10 minutes
Cooking time: 30 minutes
Serves 2

4 small zucchinis
2 tbsp. apple cider vinegar
2 tbsp. water
2 tbsp. chopped mint

Cook the zucchinis gently until just cooked but firm. Cut both ends off, then cut diagonally into thin slices. Put into a small casserole dish. Mix the apple cider vinegar, water and chopped mint and pour over the sliced zucchini. Bake gently in the oven at 300° F (149° C) until warmed through. Cool and serve with a baked potato and a green salad.

Desserts

Applesauce, Cooked

Preparation time: 10 minutes
Cooking time: 15-20 minutes
Serves 2

3 medium apples, pared, cored and sliced
honey (or sugar), if needed

Put apple slices in saucepan half covered with cold water. Add honey (or sugar) to taste. Boil about 15 minutes or until soft. Put through food mill.

Applesauce, Fresh

Preparation time: 10 minutes

3 medium apples, pared, cored and sliced
honey (or sugar)

Add honey (or sugar) to taste. Run apples through the grinder portion of the juicer.

Apple Spice Cake

1/4 cup honey (or maple syrup)
1 cup fresh applesauce
1-1/2 cups oat flour
3/4 cup triticale flour
3/4 cup sugar
a pinch of allspice
a pinch of mace
1/4 tsp. coriander
2 cups raisins (or chopped dates)

Crumb topping:
2/3 cup rolled oats
1/3 cup maple syrup (or honey)
a pinch of allspice
a pinch of mace

Combine honey (or maple syrup), applesauce and flours. Sift together sugar, allspice, mace and coriander. Add raisins (or dates). Combine wet and dry ingredients. Pour into nonstick oblong bake pan. For crumb topping, buzz oats briefly in blender to make a finer flake. Mix spices with oats. Mix in enough maple syrup (or honey) to make a crumbly mixture. When the crumb topping is made, sprinkle on top. Bake at 325° F (163° C) for 40 minutes or until cake tests done. Serve with a spoonful of fresh applesauce or yogurt.

Apple-Sweet Potato Pudding

Preparation time: 20 minutes
Cooking time: 30 minutes
Serves 2-3

1 sweet potato, boiled, peeled and sliced
1 apple, raw, peeled and sliced
1 tsp. raisins
1/2 cup bread crumbs
1 tsp. sugar
1/2 cup orange juice
3 tsp. yogurt

Place sweet potato slices in baking dish with apple slices and raisins spread with bread crumbs, sugar and orange juice. Bake in oven at 350° F (177° C) for 30 minutes. Serve hot with yogurt.

Banana (Broiled)

Preparation time: 5 minutes
Cooking time: 10 minutes
Serves 1

1 banana
1 tsp. sugar
lemon juice

Cut banana in half lengthwise and add sugar and a few drops of lemon. Place in pan and broil under low flame in its skin for 10 minutes. Serve hot.

Cherries (Stewed)

Preparation time: 10 minutes
Cooking time: 12 minutes
Serves 2

1/2 lb. cherries, stemmed
1 tsp. potato starch
2 tsp. cold water
2 tsp. sugar (if needed)

Place cherries in saucepan with water to cover. Cook 10 minutes over low flame. Add potato starch dissolved in cold water. Add to boiling cherries. Cook 2 minutes longer. Chill and serve. (Cherries are particularly healthful and are best enjoyed raw.)

Currants

Preparation time: 5 minutes
Serves 1-2

1/4 lb. red currants
3 tsp. sugar
yogurt

Clean currants thoroughly before removing stems. Place in dish, add sugar and serve. Yogurt, sweetened with sugar, may be used for sauce.

Fruit Combination

Preparation time: 5 minutes
Cooking time: 13-15 minutes
Serves 3

3 cups fresh cherries and apricots, halved, sliced and pitted
2 cups water
1/2 cup sugar
2 tsp. cornstarch, dissolved in 1/3 cup cold water

Place fruit with water and sugar in saucepan. Boil gently and slowly for 10 minutes. Add cornstarch. Cook 3 minutes longer. Cool and serve.

Glazed Pear Halves

Preparation time: 15 minutes
Cooking time: 15 minutes
Serves 4

4-5 ripe pears, halved and cored
4 oz. water
4 tbsp. honey (or sucanat, an organic dried cane sugar)

Cut ripe pears into halves and core. Add water to honey (or sucanat) and mix well. Place pear halves in baking dish and pour sugar mixture over them. Bake in slow oven at 250° F (121° C) until done. Baste with juice if necessary.

Oatmeal Cake

Preparation time: 20 minutes
Cooking time: 45 minutes
Serves 6

4 cups oatmeal (dry oats)
2 carrots, grated or blended
honey and raisins (as desired)

Combine all the above ingredients in a baking dish. Put in the oven without a lid and bake for 45 minutes at 250° F (121° C). Serve with yogurt.

Peaches

Preparation time: 15 minutes
Cooking time: 10 minutes
Serves 1-2

1/2 lb. peaches, skinned
2 tsp. sugar

Place peaches in boiling water for 1/2 minute, drain and peel. Cut in halves. Remove pits and place in saucepan with boiling water to half cover fruit level. Cover. Simmer for 10 minutes. Cool. Add sugar and serve chilled.

Pears

Preparation time: 5 minutes
Cooking time: 20 minutes
Serves 1

1 large pear, peeled, cored and halved
1 tsp. sugar

Place pear halves in saucepan with water to half cover. Add sugar and cook for 20 minutes

Plums

Preparation time: 10 minutes
Cooking time: 15 minutes
Serves 1

1/2 lb. plums, halved and pitted (or leave whole)
2 tsp. sugar

Cut plums in half and remove pits (or plums can be cooked whole). Place in saucepan with water to cover. Cook 15 minutes. Remove, cool and add sugar. Serve chilled.

Prune and Banana Whip

Preparation time: 10 minutes*
*Does not include presoaking
Cooking time: 10 minutes
Serves 2

1 cup dried prunes, presoaked and cooked
2 small bananas, mashed
juice of 1/4 lemon
1 tsp. sugar

Presoak the prunes (soak overnight in cold water, or pour boiling water over them and leave for a couple of hours until plump) and cook for 10 minutes. Whip all ingredients together thoroughly and put in refrigerator for 1 hour. May be served in slices decorated with sweetened yogurt.

Prunes and Apricots (Dried)

Preparation time: 5 minutes*
* Does not include presoaking
Cooking time: 15 minutes
Serves 2

1/2 lb. prunes, presoaked
1/2 lb. apricots, presoaked
1/3 cup barley

Presoak the prunes and apricots (soak overnight in cold water, or pour boiling water over them and leave for a couple of hours until plump). Use same water and let boil for 10 minutes or until barley is done. Cool and serve.

Additional Reference Material

A Cancer Therapy: Results of Fifty Cases and The Cure of Advanced Cancer by Diet Therapy: A Summary of Thirty Years of Clinical Experimentation, Max Gerson, MD (San Diego: Gerson Institute, 2002). Dr. Gerson's seminal work on his cancer therapy, developed over 35 years of clinical experience.

Dr. Max Gerson: Healing the Hopeless, Howard Straus (Carmel, CA: Totality Books, 2002). The official biography of Dr. Max Gerson, chronicling his life and the intertwined development of his therapy, flight from the Nazi Holocaust, and struggle against American allopathic medicine.

Censured for Curing Cancer: The American Experience of Dr. Max Gerson, S. J. Haught (San Diego: Gerson Institute, 1991). An investigative reporter who set out to expose Dr. Gerson as a cancer quack, but discovered who the quacks really were.

The Cancer Industry: Unraveling the Politics, Ralph W. Moss (New York: Paragon House, 1989). An exposé of the money and power politics, which drives the industry that it treats and victimizes the cancer patient.

Questioning Chemotherapy, Ralph W. Moss (Brooklyn: Equinox Press, 2000). An analysis of the practice and results of chemotherapy, and the reasons behind its widespread use despite its dismal record.

Death by Modern Medicine, Carolyn Dean, MD (Belleville, Ontario: Matrix Vérité, 2005). Dr. Dean painstakingly gathered government statistics and medical journal data, and published information to show that the #1 killer in the United States is ... our medical system.

The China Study: Startling Implications for Diet, Weight Loss and Long-term Health, T. Colin Campbell and Thomas M. Campbell II (Dallas: BenBella Books, 2005). One of the world's leading nutritionist sets out his tightly reasoned, experimentally proven case for avoiding animal products, the #1 carcinogen in the world.

A Time to Heal, Beata Bishop (Lydney, Gloucestershire, UK: First Stone Publishing Company, 2005; available from the Gerson Institute, San Diego). Ms. Bishop chronicles her own victory over spreading melanoma using the Gerson Therapy over 25 years ago, in very human terms, with insight and dry humor.

Living Proof: A Medical Mutiny, Michael Gearin-Tosh (London: Simon & Schuster UK, Ltd., 2002). An Oxford Don, faced with certain death from multiple myeloma or its allopathic treatments, chooses instead to use the Gerson Therapy and Chinese meditation, and survives his prognosis by over 10 years. Witty, incisive, and readable.

Fats & Oils, Udo Erasmus (Vancouver, BC: Alive Books, January 1989). The definitive book on fats and oils, and their structures, sources, uses and effects on human health and physiology. Excellent reference.

Fluoride: the Aging Factor, John Yiamouyiannis (Delaware, OH: Health Action Press, 1993). A survey of the suppressed literature on fluoridation of water, vitamins, toothpaste, and dental treatments. Chilling and vital information to protect your health and that of your loved ones.

The Root Canal Cover-Up, George Meinig (Ojai, CA: Bion Publishing, 1994). Root canal specialist and cofounder of the American Association of Endontists (root canal specialists) writes about the powerful negative effects of root canals on human health. A must read.

What Really Causes Schizophrenia, Harold D. Foster (Victoria, BC: Trafford Publishing, 2003). Professor Foster presents a novel analysis of the sources and cure of schizophrenia, viewing it as a deficiency or nutritional problem rather than a mental defect.

What Really Causes AIDS, Harold D. Foster (Victoria, BC: Trafford Publishing, 2002). Professor Foster shows the true cause of AIDS as a deficiency of selenium and that it is curable with the proper diet plus selenium supplementation.

Healing booklets by Charlotte Gerson (Carmel, CA: Cancer Research Wellness Institute, 2002; also available from the Gerson Institute, San Diego), 30 pages each. This is a series of nine booklets, eight of which detail the reason why cancer occurs, how and why the Gerson Therapy heals, a short outline of the Gerson Therapy, and about a dozen stories of recovered patients. The ninth booklet covers "Auto-Immune Diseases."

- *Healing Breast Cancer the Gerson Way*
- *Healing Prostate and Testicular Cancer the Gerson Way*
- *Healing Ovarian and Female Organ Cancer the Gerson Way*
- *Healing Colon, Liver and Pancreas Cancer the Gerson Way*
- *Healing Lung Cancer & Respiratory Diseases the Gerson Way*
- *Healing Lymphoma the Gerson Way*
- *Healing Melanoma the Gerson Way*
- *Healing Brain and Kidney Cancer the Gerson Way*
- *Healing "Auto-immune" Diseases the Gerson Way*

Doctor Max, Giuliano Dego (Barrytown, NY: Station Hill Press, 1997; available from Gerson Institute, San Diego, California). This biographical novel is a broad fictional saga based on the life and times of medical giant Dr. Max Gerson, developer of the Gerson Therapy. One of Italy's leading poets, and winner of the Italian National Paperback Book Prize for this book, Dr. Dego spent decades researching this opus.

DVDs:

- *The Gerson Miracle,* Stephen Kroschel (Haines, AK: Kroschel Films, 2004). Winner of the 2004 Golden Palm for "Best Picture," Beverly Hills Film Festival, Beverly Hills, CA.

- *Dying to Have Known,* Stephen Kroschel (Haines, AK: Kroschel Films, 2006). Awarded Honorable Mention, Feature-length documentary category, 2006 New York International Independent Film and Video Festival, New York City, NY.

Author Index

407

Subject Index

411

Item	Qty.	Price	Extended
BOOKS			
Healing the Gerson Way	____	$29.95	____
Dr. Max Gerson: Healing the Hopeless	____	$19.95	____
A Time to Heal	____	$12.95	____
DVDs			
The Gerson Miracle	____	$24.95	____
Dying to Have Known	____	$24.95	____
BOOKLETS			
Healing Breast Cancer the Gerson Way	____	$3.95	____
Healing Prostate and Testicular Cancer the Gerson Way	____	$3.95	____
Healing Ovarian and Female Organ Cancer the Gerson Way	____	$3.95	____
Healing Colon, Liver and Pancreas Cancer the Gerson Way	____	$3.95	____
Healing Lung Cancer & Respiratory Diseases the Gerson Way	____	$3.95	____
Healing Lymphoma the Gerson Way	____	$3.95	____
Healing Melanoma the Gerson Way	____	$3.95	____
Healing Brain and Kidney Cancer the Gerson Way	____	$3.95	____
Healing "Auto-immune" Diseases the Gerson Way	____	$3.95	____
Subtotal			____
* Shipping/handling			____
Sales tax (California residents only)			____
Total			____

* *This is an estimated shipping/handling charge. Actual charge will be calculated by Totality Books. Federal Express charges extra for next-day deliveries for orders placed on Friday.*

Personal checks and major credit cards accepted.

Name _____

Address _____

City/State/Zip _____

Credit Card Number _____ Exp. Date_____

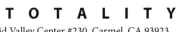

T O T A L I T Y B O O K S
316 Mid Valley Center #230, Carmel, CA 93923   (831) 625-3565   hdstraus@sbcglobal.net

Now also available from Totality Books   (use order form on overleaf)

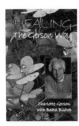
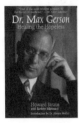

Healing the Gerson Way: Defeating Cancer and Other Chronic Diseases, by Charlotte Gerson with Beata Bishop. This book is the most up-to-date and fully documented and detailed "how to" book on the Gerson Therapy. Explanation of Gerson tests, variations for treating both cancer and nonmalignant diseases and health maintenance. Nearly 100 pages of recipes.

456 pages $29.95

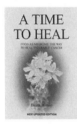

Dr. Max Gerson: Healing the Hopeless, by Howard Straus with Barbara Marinacci. Inspiring and uplifting biography of the originator of the Gerson Therapy, chronicling Dr. Gerson's life, development of his world-famous dietary therapy, flight from the Nazi Holocaust and successful search for a holistic and effective treatment for cancer in the United States.

412 pages $19.95

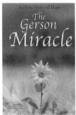

A Time to Heal, by Beata Bishop. British psychologist, BBC writer, novelist and lecturer Beata Bishop's account of her successful fight against stage IV spreading melanoma *over 25 years ago!* The co-author of *Healing the Gerson Way*, Ms. Bishop lectures widely in both Eastern and Western Europe on the Gerson Therapy, how she beat the odds and how you can, too.

320 pages $12.95

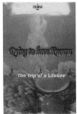

The Gerson Miracle (DVD), a stunningly beautiful and moving documentary. Master cinematographer Stephen Kroschel (*I Spy, Seven Years in Tibet*) explains visually how the Gerson Therapy heals, interviews recovered cancer patients on their experiences and shows the deep interrelationship between the health of the planet and our own. Winner, "Best Picture," 2004 Beverly Hills Film Festival.

91 minutes $24.95

Dying to Have Known (DVD), Cinematographer Stephen Kroschel's second Gerson Therapy documentary with interviews from patients and advocates—including two Japanese medical school professors, one of them a 16-year survivor of colon/liver cancer on the Gerson Therapy—as well as from detractors. This DVD is international in scope, sweeping in cinematographic splendor, moving and inspiring.

80 minutes $24.95

T O T A L I T Y   B O O K S
316 Mid Valley Center #230, Carmel, CA 93923   (831) 625-3565   hdstraus@sbcglobal.net

Item	Qty.	Price	Extended
BOOKS			
Healing the Gerson Way	___	$29.95	___
Dr. Max Gerson: Healing the Hopeless	___	$19.95	___
A Time to Heal	___	$12.95	___
DVDs			
The Gerson Miracle	___	$24.95	___
Dying to Have Known	___	$24.95	___
BOOKLETS			
Healing Breast Cancer the Gerson Way	___	$3.95	___
Healing Prostate and Testicular Cancer the Gerson Way	___	$3.95	___
Healing Ovarian and Female Organ Cancer the Gerson Way	___	$3.95	___
Healing Colon, Liver and Pancreas Cancer the Gerson Way	___	$3.95	___
Healing Lung Cancer & Respiratory Diseases the Gerson Way	___	$3.95	___
Healing Lymphoma the Gerson Way	___	$3.95	___
Healing Melanoma the Gerson Way	___	$3.95	___
Healing Brain and Kidney Cancer the Gerson Way	___	$3.95	___
Healing "Auto-immune" Diseases the Gerson Way	___	$3.95	___
Subtotal			___
* Shipping/handling			___
Sales tax (California residents only)			___
Total			___

* *This is an estimated shipping/handling charge. Actual charge will be calculated by Totality Books. Federal Express charges extra for next-day deliveries for orders placed on Friday.*

Personal checks and major credit cards accepted.

Name _____

Address _____

City/State/Zip _____

Credit Card Number _____ Exp. Date_____

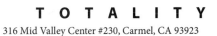

T O T A L I T Y B O O K S
316 Mid Valley Center #230, Carmel, CA 93923   (831) 625-3565   hdstraus@sbcglobal.net

Now also available from Totality Books (use order form on overleaf)

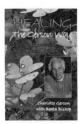

Healing the Gerson Way: Defeating Cancer and Other Chronic Diseases, by Charlotte Gerson with Beata Bishop. This book is the most up-to-date and fully documented and detailed "how to" book on the Gerson Therapy. Explanation of Gerson tests, variations for treating both cancer and nonmalignant diseases and health maintenance. Nearly 100 pages of recipes.

456 pages $29.95

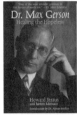

Dr. Max Gerson: Healing the Hopeless, by Howard Straus with Barbara Marinacci. Inspiring and uplifting biography of the originator of the Gerson Therapy, chronicling Dr. Gerson's life, development of his world-famous dietary therapy, flight from the Nazi Holocaust and successful search for a holistic and effective treatment for cancer in the United States.

412 pages $19.95

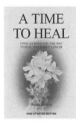

A Time to Heal, by Beata Bishop. British psychologist, BBC writer, novelist and lecturer Beata Bishop's account of her successful fight against stage IV spreading melanoma *over 25 years ago!* The co-author of *Healing the Gerson Way,* Ms. Bishop lectures widely in both Eastern and Western Europe on the Gerson Therapy, how she beat the odds and how you can, too.

320 pages $12.95

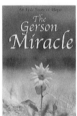

The Gerson Miracle (DVD), a stunningly beautiful and moving documentary. Master cinematographer Stephen Kroschel (*I Spy, Seven Years in Tibet*) explains visually how the Gerson Therapy heals, interviews recovered cancer patients on their experiences and shows the deep interrelationship between the health of the planet and our own. Winner, "Best Picture," 2004 Beverly Hills Film Festival.

91 minutes $24.95

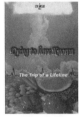

Dying to Have Known (DVD), Cinematographer Stephen Kroschel's second Gerson Therapy documentary with interviews from patients and advocates—including two Japanese medical school professors, one of them a 16-year survivor of colon/liver cancer on the Gerson Therapy—as well as from detractors. This DVD is international in scope, sweeping in cinematographic splendor, moving and inspiring.

80 minutes $24.95

T O T A L I T Y **B O O K S**

316 Mid Valley Center #230, Carmel, CA 93923   (831) 625-3565 hdstraus@sbcglobal.net